New Strategies in Preventing Inflammatory and/or Oxidative Stress-Induced Damages in Ischemia-Reperfusion Injury, 2nd Edition

New Strategies in Preventing Inflammatory and/or Oxidative Stress-Induced Damages in Ischemia-Reperfusion Injury, 2nd Edition

Guest Editors

Borja Herrero de la Parte
Ignacio García-Alonso
Ana Alonso-Varona

MDPI

Basel • Beijing • Wuhan • Barcelona • Belgrade • Novi Sad • Cluj • Manchester

Guest Editors
Borja Herrero de la Parte
Department of Surgery, Radiology and Physical Medicine
University of the Basque Country (UPV/EHU)
Leioa
Spain

Ignacio García-Alonso
Department of Surgery, Radiology and Physical Medicine
University of the Basque Country (UPV/EHU)
Leioa
Spain

Ana Alonso-Varona
Department of Cell Biology and Histology
University of the Basque Country (UPV/EHU)
Leioa
Spain

Editorial Office
MDPI AG
Grosspeteranlage 5
4052 Basel, Switzerland

This is a reprint of the Special Issue, published open access by the journal *Antioxidants* (ISSN 2076-3921), freely accessible at: https://www.mdpi.com/journal/antioxidants/special_issues/61WG1KX18K.

For citation purposes, cite each article independently as indicated on the article page online and as indicated below:

Lastname, A.A.; Lastname, B.B. Article Title. *Journal Name* **Year**, *Volume Number*, Page Range.

ISBN 978-3-7258-5849-1 (Hbk)
ISBN 978-3-7258-5850-7 (PDF)
https://doi.org/10.3390/books978-3-7258-5850-7

Contents

About the Editors

Borja Herrero de la Parte

Borja Herrero de la Parte is a faculty member at the Department of Surgery of the University of the Basque Country (UPV/EHU) and serves as the academic secretary of the department. His research focuses on surgical pathophysiology, particularly ischemia–reperfusion injury, neonatal brain damage, and liver regeneration. He has also led experimental studies in the field of bariatric and metabolic surgery. His work often integrates surgical models with pharmacological and radiological approaches, aiming to better understand the underlying mechanisms of tissue damage and recovery. In recent years, he has coordinated several interdisciplinary projects involving both preclinical and translational perspectives. He is also active in surgical education and has co-edited textbooks and other teaching resources for undergraduate medical students. His academic activity combines laboratory research, teaching, and editorial work, with a strong emphasis on collaboration across specialties.

Ignacio García-Alonso

Ignacio García-Alonso is a Professor of Surgery at the University of the Basque Country (UPV/EHU) and Head of the Department of Surgery at the same institution. His main research interests include liver regeneration, ischemia–reperfusion injury, and experimental models of surgical disease. Over the years, he has directed multiple funded projects and led collaborations between surgical and biomedical research teams. His work combines a solid clinical background with long-standing experience in experimental surgery and translational research. In addition to his scientific contributions, he has played a leading role in curriculum development and academic governance within the medical school. He is also a co-author and editor of several surgical textbooks aimed at medical students and residents.

Ana Alonso-Varona

Ana Alonso-Varona is a Full Professor of Histology at the Faculty of Medicine and Nursing of the University of the Basque Country (UPV/EHU). Her research focuses on cell and molecular biology applied to ischemia–reperfusion injury, cancer biology, and the development of nanostructured systems for drug delivery. She has extensive experience in in vitro and in vivo models of oxidative stress and has participated in numerous multidisciplinary projects involving collaboration with surgeons, pharmacologists, and materials scientists. Her work combines fundamental research with a strong translational orientation. She is also actively involved in academic teaching and has contributed to the training of undergraduate and postgraduate students in biomedical sciences.

antioxidants

MDPI

Editorial

New Strategies in Preventing Inflammatory and/or Oxidative Stress-Induced Damages in Ischemia–Reperfusion Injury (2nd Edition)

Borja Herrero de la Parte [1,*], Ignacio García-Alonso [1] and Ana Alonso-Varona [2]

1 Department of Surgery, Radiology and Physical Medicine, Faculty of Medicine and Nursing, University of the Basque Country (UPV/EHU), 48940 Leioa, Spain
2 Department of Cell Biology and Histology, Faculty of Medicine and Nursing, University of the Basque Country (UPV/EHU), 48940 Leioa, Spain
* Correspondence: borja.herrero@ehu.eus

Ischemia–reperfusion injury remains one of the most fascinating and challenging paradoxes in modern biomedicine. The restoration of blood flow, which is essential for preserving tissue viability, triggers a cascade of biochemical events that often exacerbate the initial damage. The overproduction of reactive oxygen species, mitochondrial dysfunction, the activation of inflammatory pathways, and endothelial dysfunction form a complex network that compromises organ function. Despite decades of research, effective prevention of this syndrome remains a challenge in many clinical settings, from transplantation and cardiovascular surgery to neurovascular events and intestinal ischemia.

The first edition of this Special Issue of *Antioxidants* served to highlight the central role of oxidative stress and antioxidant therapies in ischemia–reperfusion injury, as well as to bring together promising experimental strategies aimed at mitigating its effects. In this second edition, the focus broadens to a more integrative view, in which redox, immunological, and metabolic mechanisms are conceived as an interdependent and dynamic system. This perspective allows us to explore new therapeutic approaches capable of acting synergistically on the different levels of the lesion cascade.

The articles collected in this edition offer an updated and diverse view of the problem. Among the experimental works, the study by Sánchez-Bonet (contribution 1) and colleagues stands out, demonstrating the protective potential of a *Fucus vesiculosus* extract against intestinal ischemia, restoring the activity of antioxidant enzymes and reducing mucosal inflammation. In the cerebral sphere, Romaus-Sanjurjo et al. (contribution 2) show how the administration of low doses of TWEAK can mobilize endothelial progenitors and promote vascular repair after intracerebral hemorrhage, while Sigdel et al. (contribution 3) describe the beneficial effect of extracellular vesicles released after physical exercise on cerebral endothelial cells exposed to hypoxia and angiotensin II, opening up the door to non-pharmacological interventions based on "cell preparation".

At the heart of this research, two complementary approaches highlight the relevance of molecular and epigenetic modulation of oxidative stress. Cucinotta et al. (contribution 4) document the cardioprotective effect of the prolyl endopeptidase inhibitor KYP-2047, which attenuates inflammatory infiltration and apoptosis after myocardial reperfusion. Park et al. (contribution 5) demonstrated that the inhibition of microRNA-25 restores Sestrin3 expression and reduces oxidative burden, consolidating the role of microRNAs as modulators of redox balance.

In the field of experimental nephrology, the work of Jang et al. (contribution 6) provides an innovative insight by demonstrating that intermittent fasting mitigates epithelial–mesenchymal transition and renal fibrosis after ischemia, pointing to the relevance of metabolism and caloric restriction as modulators of the progression from acute injury to chronic disease. Complementarily, Troise and his team review (contribution 7) the involvement of the complement system in renal graft dysfunction after transplantation and propose the targeted inhibition of its components as an effective tool to reduce reperfusion injury and improve early function of the transplanted organ.

The two review articles included in this Special Issue offer a conceptual framework that broadens our understanding of IRI. Dery et al. (contribution 8) analyze the feedback loops between oxidative stress and the immune response in the liver, highlighting the relevance of redox metabolites and endoplasmic reticulum stress as mediators of inflammatory activation, while Dhalla et al. (contribution 9) provide a comprehensive update on the mechanisms of myocardial reperfusion injury, from mitochondrial ROS generation to impaired calcium handling, and review the most promising antioxidant therapeutic approaches.

Finally, Berzenji et al. (contribution 10) provide a review focusing on pulmonary ischemia–reperfusion injury in the context of transplantation. This review summarizes the pathophysiology of primary graft dysfunction and the oxidative and inflammatory mechanisms involved. It also discusses advances in ex vivo lung preservation and perfusion techniques. This review emphasizes the importance of integrated protection strategies—pharmacological, mechanical, and physiological—to optimize lung viability and reduce postoperative complications.

Together, these works reflect the maturity of a field that has evolved from the simple neutralization of free radicals to a much more sophisticated understanding of the interconnected processes that underlie reperfusion injury. Recent research clearly indicates that oxidative, inflammatory, and metabolic mechanisms do not act in isolation but rather as part of a complex regulatory network. Hence, emerging strategies tend to combine approaches: mitochondria-targeted antioxidants, complement modulators, microRNA inhibitors, or redox-sensitive controlled-release systems. Therapeutic nanotechnology and gene therapies appear to be promising tools for achieving precise, localized, and safe intervention.

At the same time, the studies included in this edition remind us of the importance of biological and behavioral factors that had traditionally been overlooked in antioxidant therapy. The influence of physical exercise, diet, and intermittent fasting on the cellular response to ischemic stress shows that the concept of "physiological conditioning" can be as relevant as pharmacology. This holistic view, in which the body prepares itself to resist oxidative stress, opens up a line of research that transcends the classic boundaries between prevention and treatment.

The future of ischemia–reperfusion research lies in integrating these approaches and transferring them to the clinical setting with rigorous and translational criteria. It will be essential to define robust biomarkers that allow for the optimal therapeutic window to be identified, rational combinations of treatments to be selected, and their long-term functional impact to be evaluated. IRI is not a single, uniform process: its manifestation varies according to the organ, time, and metabolic context. Consequently, therapeutic strategies must be equally specific and dynamic.

The second edition of this Special Issue of *Antioxidants* reflects the vitality of a field undergoing continuous transformation. The papers collected here not only expand our knowledge of the mechanisms of damage and defense but also point to a paradigm shift in the approach to ischemia–reperfusion: from isolated antioxidant therapy to the integrated modulation of redox, immune, and metabolic responses. We trust that this collection will inspire new lines of research, foster interdisciplinary collaboration, and contribute to bringing the advances currently being developed in the laboratory closer to clinical practice.

Author Contributions: Writing—original draft preparation, B.H.d.l.P.; writing—review and editing, B.H.d.l.P., I.G.-A. and A.A.-V. All authors have read and agreed to the published version of the manuscript.

Funding: This research received no external funding.

Conflicts of Interest: The authors declare no conflict of interest.

List of Contributions

1. Sánchez-Bonet, D.; Padrón-Sanz, C.; Lloris-Cejalvo, J.M.; Lloris-Carsí, J.M.; Cejalvo-Lapeña, D. Antioxidant Effect of a *Fucus vesiculosus* Extract on Intestinal Ischemia/Reperfusion Injury in Rats: A Biochemical and Histological Study. *Antioxidants* **2025**, *14*, 624. https://doi.org/10.3390/antiox14060624.
2. Romaus-Sanjurjo, D.; López-Arias, E.; Rodríguez, C.; Hervella, P.; Rodríguez-Arrizabalaga, M.; Debasa-Mouce, M.; Pías-Peleteiro, J.M.; Iglesias-Rey, R.; Aguiar, P.; Almeida, Á.; et al. Blood Progenitor Cell Mobilization Driven by TWEAK Promotes Neovascularization and Reduces Brain Damage in a Rat Model of Intracerebral Hemorrhage. *Antioxidants* **2025**, *14*, 601. https://doi.org/10.3390/antiox14050601.
3. Sigdel, S.; Chen, S.; Udoh, G.; Wang, J. Exercise-Intervened Circulating Extracellular Vesicles Alleviate Oxidative Stress in Cerebral Microvascular Endothelial Cells Under Hypertensive Plus Hypoxic Conditions. *Antioxidants* **2025**, *14*, 77. https://doi.org/10.3390/antiox14010077.
4. Cucinotta, L.; Palermo, N.; Ardizzone, A.; Capra, A.P.; Campolo, M.; Esposito, E.; Casili, G.; Lanza, M. The Inhibition of Prolyl Endopeptidase (PREP) by KYP-2047 Treatment to Reduce Myocardial Ischemia/Reperfusion Injury. *Antioxidants* **2025**, *14*, 442. https://doi.org/10.3390/antiox14040442.
5. Park, M.; Cho, S.; Jeong, D. Restoration of Sestrin 3 Expression Mitigates Cardiac Oxidative Damage in Ischemia–Reperfusion Injury Model. *Antioxidants* **2025**, *14*, 61. https://doi.org/10.3390/antiox14010061.
6. Jang, Y.; Kim, Y.S.; Kim, S.R.; Lee, D.W.; Lee, S.B.; Kim, I.Y. Intermittent Fasting Protects Against the Progression from Acute Kidney Injury to Chronic Kidney Disease. *Antioxidants* **2025**, *14*, 119. https://doi.org/10.3390/antiox14010119.
7. Troise, D.; Allegra, C.; Cirolla, L.A.; Mercuri, S.; Infante, B.; Castellano, G.; Stallone, G. Exploring Potential Complement Modulation Strategies for Ischemia–Reperfusion Injury in Kidney Transplantation. *Antioxidants* **2025**, *14*, 66. https://doi.org/10.3390/antiox14010066.
8. Dery, K.J.; Chiu, R.; Kasargod, A.; Kupiec-Weglinski, J.W. Feedback Loops Shape Oxidative and Immune Interactions in Hepatic Ischemia–Reperfusion Injury. *Antioxidants* **2025**, *14*, 944. https://doi.org/10.3390/antiox14080944.
9. Dhalla, N.S.; Ostadal, P.; Tappia, P.S. Involvement of Oxidative Stress and Antioxidants in Modification of Cardiac Dysfunction Due to Ischemia–Reperfusion Injury. *Antioxidants* **2025**, *14*, 340. https://doi.org/10.3390/antiox14030340.
10. Berzenji, L.; Hendriks, J.M.H.; Verleden, S.E.; Yogeswaran, S.K.; Wen, W.; Lauwers, P.; Verleden, G.; Paep, R.D.; Mertens, P.; Rodrigus, I.; et al. Lung Ischemia–Reperfusion Injury in Lung Transplant Surgery: Where do We Stand? *Antioxidants* **2025**, *14*, 1295.

antioxidants

MDPI

Article

Antioxidant Effect of a *Fucus vesiculosus* Extract on Intestinal Ischemia/Reperfusion Injury in Rats: A Biochemical and Histological Study

Desirée Sánchez-Bonet [1], Carolina Padrón-Sanz [2,*], José Miguel Lloris-Cejalvo [1], José Miguel Lloris-Carsí [3] and Dolores Cejalvo-Lapeña [2]

1 Escuela de Doctorado, Universidad Católica de Valencia "San Vicente Mártir", Plaza de San Agustín, 3, 46001 Valencia, Spain; desanbo@gmail.com (D.S.-B.); jmllorisc@gmail.com (J.M.L.-C.)

2 Centro de Investigación Traslacional San Alberto Magno, Universidad Católica de Valencia "San Vicente Mártir", C/Quevedo, 2, 46001 Valencia, Spain; dolores.cejalvo@ucv.es

3 Facultad de Medicina, Departamento de Cirugía, Universidad de Valencia, Avda. Blasco Ibáñez, 13, 46010 Valencia, Spain; jm_lloris@mac.com

* Correspondence: carolina.padron@ucv.es

Abstract: *Fucus vesiculosus* is a brown seaweed known for its strong antioxidant properties, mainly attributed to its high polyphenolic content. This study aimed to evaluate the antioxidant protective effect of an optimised *F. vesiculosus* extract in an experimental model of intestinal ischemia/reperfusion (I/R) injury, considering the intestine as particularly vulnerable to this pathology. Seventy-two male Wistar albino rats were randomly divided into twelve groups: Sham, I/R groups (3 and 24 h reperfusion), I/R plus vehicle groups (three application times, 3 h reperfusion), and I/R plus *F. vesiculosus* extract groups (three application times, 3 and 24 h reperfusion). Intestinal injury was assessed through biochemical markers (malondialdehyde [MDA], superoxide dismutase [SOD], catalase [CAT], glutathione peroxidase [GPx], and mieloperoxidase [MPO]), inflammatory cytokines (interleukin 1 β [IL-1β] and interleukin [IL-10]), and histological analysis. Results demonstrated that treatment with *F. vesiculosus* significantly reduced oxidative stress and inflammation caused by I/R injury ($p < 0.05$), restoring analysed parameters (MDA, SOD, CAT, IL-10) to levels comparable to the Sham group. Histological examination confirmed the preservation of intestinal mucosal integrity following *F. vesiculosus* administration. These findings suggest that the antioxidant extract from *F. vesiculosus* effectively protects against intestinal I/R injury, highlighting its potential for clinical use in preventing and managing this pathological condition, particularly in surgical contexts.

Keywords: *Fucus vesiculosus*; antioxidant; polyphenols; intestinal ischemia/reperfusion

1. Introduction

Molecular oxygen is essential for all aerobic organisms, but environmental conditions and pollutants can disrupt the functioning of electron transport chains and lead to the formation of oxygen free radicals (ROS) [1]. ROS are highly reactive molecules that can cause significant damage to cellular components including lipids, proteins and nucleic acids [2,3]. Under normal conditions, organisms are able to maintain stable ROS levels through endogenous antioxidant mechanisms [4]. These antioxidant systems are composed of enzymes such as superoxide dismutase (SOD), catalase (CAT) and glutathione peroxidase (GPx). However, when an imbalance occurs between ROS production and the organism's capacity to neutralise them, a biological phenomenon known as oxidative stress occurs [1,2,5,6].

There are several pathophysiological processes in which oxidative stress plays an important role, ischemia/reperfusion (I/R) being one of them [7,8]. During the ischemic phase, the lack of oxygen and nutrients causes a shift in cellular metabolism to anaerobic pathways. This shift results in a loss of cell function that can lead to cell death [7,9]. In the second phase (reperfusion), the restoration of blood flow could be seen as a recovery process, but paradoxically, the opposite effect occurs. The sudden increase in oxygen availability leads to an overproduction of free radicals, like superoxide (O_2^-) and hydrogen peroxide (H_2O_2), both presenting a high potential to damage cellular structures [8,10,11].

The small intestine is recognised as one of the most vulnerable organs to this type of injury, with one of the highest morbidity and mortality rates [12]. Intestinal I/R injury is associated with numerous acute pathological conditions, including small bowel transplantation, cardiopulmonary resuscitation, septic shock and mesenteric artery embolisation [13]. This phenomenon is usually caused by obstruction of arterial mesenteric vessels, although in rare cases, it can also involve venous vessels, as a result of thrombi or emboli [14]. Oxidative stress occurring during an intestinal I/R process can trigger the destruction of the intestinal mucosal barrier, increase vascular permeability, promote bacterial translocation, and trigger the release of inflammatory mediators. In addition, it can cause a cellular response involving apoptosis, autophagy and necroptosis [15,16].

Antioxidants are considered an essential resource to control the overproduction of ROS and prevent oxidative damage, as they are able to neutralise free radicals in the body's cells, producing a more stable and less harmful radical [17]. Currently, there is an increasing interest in obtaining new antioxidants from natural sources, as they are considered safer and more effective treatments to combat diseases associated with oxidative damage [18]. In this context, numerous studies have focused on marine-derived products, especially seaweeds, which have gained relevance due to their ability to synthesise a wide variety of secondary metabolites [17,19]. The production of this wide variety of bioactive compounds is attributed to the extreme environmental conditions to which these organisms have adapted, especially those algae that grow in intertidal zones, where they are exposed to fluctuating ocean levels that produce constant and alternating changes in high and low salinity, low or high temperature, high pressure, low nutrient availability and low or high exposure to sunlight [20,21]. These adverse conditions favour the formation of ROS and other oxidative agents [22,23]; however, the absence of oxidative damage to membrane lipids suggests that algal cells have developed a complex defence system based on potent antioxidant compounds [21,24].

Among the bioactive compounds found in marine algae, polyphenols have gained significant interest due to their high antioxidant potential [25]. The chemical configuration of these compounds enables them to scavenge free radicals through their hydroxyl groups [26], making their mechanism of action primarily centred on ROS scavenging, inhibition of lipid peroxidation, and activation of the endogenous antioxidant system [26–30].

Numerous studies have shown that brown algae (Phaeophyceae) present higher antioxidant potential compared to green (Chlorophyta) and red (Rhodophyta) algae [22,31–34]. In addition, a higher concentration of polyphenols has been observed in this group, highlighting florotannins, a type of polyphenol with potent antioxidant properties that are exclusively synthesised by brown algae [26,32,35–37]. Within the brown algae, the order Fucales stands out for its higher antioxidant potential [32,38]. In particular, *Fucus vesiculosus* has attracted considerable attention in recent years due to its remarkable bioactivity, outperforming other species in comparative studies [32,39,40], as well as for its richness in bioactive compounds, such as polyphenols [32].

Therefore, the aim of this study is to determine the efficacy of polyphenols extracted from the algae *Fucus vesiculosus* on intestinal ischemia/reperfusion injury using an animal experimental model.

2. Materials and Methods

2.1. Seaweed Pre-Treatment

Fucus vesiculosus seaweed was purchased by the pharmaceutical company FAGRON (Terrassa, Barcelona) already pre-treated: dehydrated and ground into a homogeneous powder in a hermetically sealed container with a capacity of 1 kg.

2.2. Seaweed Extracts Preparation

In an Erlenmeyer flask, 5 g of algae sample was mixed with 30 mL of 70% acetone. The mixture was then subjected to an extraction process using an orbital incubator (Sartorius Stedim Biotech GmbH, Göttingen, Germany) at a temperature of 25 °C for 60 min. After this time, the samples were centrifuged at 2000× *g* for 20 min (Thermo Scientific Heraeus, Waltham, USA), and the supernatants were filtered using 0.45 µm nylon filters. Before its administration to the rats, the extract was rotary evaporated (Büchi Labortechnik AG, Flawil, Switzerland) to remove all acetone, then resuspended in 10 mL of 10% ethanol (*v/v*). The smallest amount of alcohol possible was used, but enough to ensure resuspension of the entire dried extract.

2.3. Characterisation of Polyphenols and Determination of the Extract's Antioxidant Activity

The Folin–Ciocalteu method was used to determine the total polyphenol content in accordance with Julkunen-Tiito [41]. Antioxidant activity was measured using the 2,2-diphenyl-1-picrylhydrazyl free radical scavenging activity (DPPH-RSA) method described by Chu et al. [42] with some modifications. Chromatographic analyses for the description of the polyphenolic profile were performed using a method adapted from López et al. [43] with a reverse-phase high-performance liquid chromatography (RP-HPLC) equipment coupled to a diode array detector (DAD). The detailed procedural descriptions of these methodologies have been published in a previous study in which the extraction of the alga *F. vesiculosus* was optimised [44].

2.4. Animals

Male Wistar albino rats (n = 72) weighing between 200 and 300 g were used in the present study. The animals underwent a 7-day acclimatisation period in a controlled environment with temperatures ranging from 22 to 24 °C and humidity levels between 50 and 70%. They had unrestricted access to food and water. The care and treatment of the rats were conducted in compliance with the animal welfare guidelines outlined in the Guide for the Care and Use of Laboratory Animals, following European Union regulations. The animal experimentation procedure described in this study was approved by the Generalitat Valenciana (General Directorate of Agricultural Production and Livestock), in accordance with current animal welfare regulations (Royal Decree 53/2013).

2.5. Experimental Groups

The impact of *F. vesiculosus* extract on I/R injury was assessed in two phases. The first phase involved 60 min of ischemia followed by 3 h of reperfusion to evaluate the effect of the extract on early injury events, such as oxidative stress and inflammation. The second phase, with 60 min of ischemia followed by 24 h of reperfusion, allowed for the evaluation of injury progression, systemic inflammatory responses, and tissue repair processes. On the other hand, the antioxidant extract was administered at three different time points: t.1 (24 h before ischemia), to evaluate its potential protective or preventive effect; t.2 (at the onset of ischemia), to assess whether the extract can act on the damage initiated during the hypoxic phase; and t.3 (at the initiation of reperfusion), to evaluate its reparative capacity during the reperfusion phase.

The excipient group allowed us to verify that the substance used to resuspend the seaweed extract (10% ethanol) had no effect on the lesion produced by IR and to verify that the effects produced are only due to the seaweed extract. To reduce the number of animals used, the excipient and sham groups were not studied in the second phase once it was determined that their conditions did not influence the I/R injury.

This study involved twelve groups of animals (n = 6 animals per group), distributed as follows (Table 1):

Table 1. Experimental Groups.

	Groups	N	Treatment/Excipient	Ischemia	Reperfusion
Control	SHAM:	6	-	-	-
	I/R 3H	6	-	60 min	3 h
	I/R 24H	6	-	60 min	24 h
Excipient	Excip. t.1	6	0.5 mL of 10% ethanol	60 min	3 h
	Excip t.2	6	0.5 mL of 10% ethanol	60 min	3 h
	Excip t.3	6	0.5 mL of 10% ethanol	60 min	3 h
Algae Extract	Extract t.1	6	0.5 mL of extract (222 mg/kg)	60 min	3 h
	Extract t.2	6	0.5 mL of extract (222 mg/kg)	60 min	3 h
	Extract t.3	6	0.5 mL of extract (222 mg/kg)	60 min	3 h
	Extract t.1	6	0.5 mL of extract (222 mg/kg)	60 min	24 h
	Extract t.2	6	0.5 mL of extract (222 mg/kg)	60 min	24 h
	Extract t.3	6	0.5 mL of extract (222 mg/kg)	60 min	24 h

t.1: Treatment administered 24 h before surgery. t.2: Treatment administered at the initiation of ischemia. t.3: Treatment administered at the time of initiation of reperfusion.

2.6. Surgical Procedure

Following an overnight fast, animals were anesthetised with ketamine 80 mg/kg (Merial Laboratory, Barcelona, Spain) and xylazine 10 mg/kg (Calier Laboratory, Barcelona, Spain) via intraperitoneal injection. The rats were allowed to breathe on their own during the procedure. A heating lamp was employed to maintain their body temperature at approximately 37 °C. The abdominal area was shaved and disinfected with Betadine® prior to aseptic surgery. After performing a midline laparotomy, the superior mesenteric artery (SMA) was carefully exposed and occluded just below the aorta, resulting in collateral interruption, for 60 min using atraumatic microvascular clamps (Scanlan International, St. Paul, MN, USA). Following 60 min of ischemia, the clamp was taken out, and reperfusion was initiated.

For animals subjected to I/R for 24 h, the abdominal incisions were sealed using continuous 2/0 silk sutures (B. Braun Surgical SA, Rubí, Spain). All rats were anesthetised and euthanised 24 h after reperfusion. Tissue samples were taken at 3 h or 24 h of reperfusion to assess the intestinal damage caused by I/R. Segments of jejunum (2 cm from the third intestinal loop) were excised, frozen using liquid nitrogen, and stored at −80 °C for subsequent biochemical analysis of lipoperoxidation (measured by malondialdehyde

[MDA] levels), enzymatic activity of superoxide dismutase (SOD), catalase (CAT), glutathione peroxidase (GPx) and myeloperoxidase (MPO), as well as the quantification of inflammation markers (Il-1β and IL-10).

2.7. Intestinal Samples Pre-Treatment

The selected bowel segment was placed into a tube containing phosphate-buffered saline (PBS) as a washing buffer, along with protease inhibitors to prevent degradation of the target proteins. The next step involved mechanically homogenising the tissue sample for 1 min using an Ultraturrax™ (IKA T10 basic) at maximum speed. This procedure was performed at a low temperature to minimise protein degradation. To break down cell membranes, 20 μL of Triton X-100 (Sigma-Aldrich, St. Louis, MO, USA) was added. Lastly, the samples were centrifuged at 10,000× *g* for 10 min at 4 °C, and the supernatant was stored at −80 °C for future analysis.

2.8. Biochemical Analysis

2.8.1. Malondialdehyde (MDA) Activity Assay

The assay method used was based on the procedure carried out by Ozkan et al. [45]. Firstly, 50 μL of tissue sample, 150 μL of 60% perchloric acid (Fisher Scientific UK Ltd., Loughborough, UK) and 150 μL of thiobarbituric acid (Merck KGaA, Darmstadt, Germany) were mixed and incubated at 95 °C for 55 min with continuous agitation at 300 rpm. Afterwards, the mixture was cooled to −20 °C for 10 min. Then, 100 μL of 20% trichloroacetic acid (Merck KGaA, Darmstadt, Germany) and 250 μL of *n*-butanol (Acros Organics, Geel, Belgium) were added to the vials. The mixture was vortexed and centrifuged at 13,000× *g* for 6 min. Finally, the absorbance of the butanol layer was measured at 532 nm using a Nanodrop 2000c (Thermo Fisher Scientific, Waltham, MA, USA). MDA concentration was determined from a standard calibration curve generated using 1,1,3,3-tetraethoxypropane (TEP). The results were expressed in nmol per mg of protein.

2.8.2. Measurement of Superoxide Dismutase (SOD) Activity

SOD activity was assessed using a commercial kit (Superoxide Dismutase Assay Kit, Cayman Chemical Company, Ann Arbor, MI, USA), which utilises a tetrazolium salt to detect superoxide radicals generated by xanthine oxidase and hypoxanthine. In the assay, one unit of SOD is set as the amount of enzyme required to produce 50% of the superoxide radical dismutation, which is measured by the change in absorbance at a wavelength of 450 nm. Victor X5 Microplate Reader (PerkinElmer, Waltham, MA, USA) was used to determine absorbance values, and final results were expressed in U/mg.

2.8.3. Measurement of Catalase (CAT) Activity

CAT activity in the tissue was measured using a commercial assay kit (Catalase Assay Kit, Cayman Chemical Company, Ann Arbor, MI, USA). The method relies on the enzyme's reaction with methanol in the presence of an optimal concentration of H_2O_2. The resulting formaldehyde was quantified colourimetrically in the tissue homogenate at a wavelength of 540 nm with a Victor X5 Microplate Reader (PerkinElmer, Waltham, MA, USA). The results were given in nmol/min/mg.

2.8.4. Measurement of Glutathione Peroxidase (GPx) Activity

GPx activity was indirectly measured using a commercial assay kit (Glutathione peroxidase Assay Kit, Cayman Chemical Company, Ann Arbor, MI, USA), which involves a reaction coupled with glutathione reductase. The oxidised glutathione formed during the reduction of hydroperoxides by the enzyme is converted back to its reduced form by GPx and nicotinamide adenine dinucleotide phosphate (NADPH). The decrease in NADPH concentration is monitored by measuring lower absorbance at 340 nm with a Victor X5 Microplate Reader (PerkinElmer, Waltham, MA, USA). Final results were expressed in nmol/min/mg.

2.8.5. Mieloperoxidase (MPO) Activity Assay

For the analysis of MPO in intestinal tissue, a rat ELISA kit (Hycult Biotech, Uden, The Netherlands), based on a sandwich solid phase enzyme-linked immunosorbent assay, was used. The MPO level was determined by measuring the colour change at a wavelength of 450 nm using a Victor X5 Microplate Reader (PerkinElmer, Waltham, MA, USA). The results were expressed as ng/mg prot.

2.8.6. Determination of Interleukins Il-1β and Il-10

The commercial kits Quantikine® ELISA Rat IL-1β Immunoassay and Quantikine® ELISA Rat IL-10 Immunoassay (R&D Systems, Minneapolis, MN, USA) were used to determine intestinal tissue inflammation based on IL-1β and Il-10 levels. The assays are based on the quantification of Rat IL-1β and IL-10 in cell and tissue lysates using the sandwich-type quantitative enzyme-linked immunosorbent assay technique with the corresponding antibody in each kit. Absorbance readings of the samples were taken with a Victor X5 Microplate Reader (PerkinElmer, Waltham, MA, USA) set at 450 nm, and the concentrations were determined based on standard curves established with recombinant rat IL-1β and recombinant rat IL-10. Final results were given in pg/mL.

2.9. Histological Study

The jejunal tissue segments were fixed by immersion in a 10% formaldehyde solution via connection to a Minipuls® 3 peristaltic pump (Gilson, Middleton, WI, USA), and the specimens were embedded in paraffin using a Leica ASP3005 tissue processor (Leica Biosystems, Nussloch, Germany). The tissues were then sectioned into 5 μm slices (four slices per animal) with a Leica RM2235 rotary microtome (Leica Biosystems, Nussloch, Germany), mounted on glass microscope slides, and stained with haematoxylin and eosin. Each histological section was divided into four quadrants, and one microscopic field per quadrant was randomly selected for analysis. To minimise spatial clustering and ensure a more representative sampling, care was taken to select fields that were not in close proximity to one another. A total of sixteen fields were analysed per animal. The sections were examined under 100× magnification with a Leica microscope, and microphotographs were used to measure villus length from the basal membrane to the tip of the microvilli. Results were expressed in millimetres (mm). Intestinal lesions were evaluated and classified according to five levels of ischemia/reperfusion (I/R) injury, following the scoring system of Chiu et al. [46]: Grade 0, normal mucosa; Grade 1, development of subepithelial space at the villus tip, often accompanied by oedema and vascular congestion; Grade 2, detachment of the epithelial layer from the lamina propria with moderate extension of the subepithelial space, villus tip fragmentation, and haemorrhage; Grade 3, partial loss of villus tips, extensive epithelial detachment, and fragmentation with the loss of the upper third of the villi; Grade 4, dilated and exposed capillaries with lost villi, though crypts remain present; Grade 5, haemorrhage, ulceration, disintegration of the lamina propria, and complete mucosal necrosis.

2.10. Statistical Analysis

Statistical analyses were conducted using SPSS Statistics® 23.0 version. The Kruskal–Wallis test was used to assess the statistical significance of differences. For comparisons between two groups, the Mann-Whitney U test was applied. A significance level of $p < 0.05$ was considered. The Pearson chi-squared test was employed to analyse the severity of bowel tissue injury ($p < 0.05$). Data are presented as the mean ± standard deviation.

3. Results

3.1. Polyphenolic Content and Antioxidant Activity of F. vesiculosus Extract

In a previous study conducted by this research group, the optimisation of the extraction process of *Fucus vesiculosus* was carried out [44]. The results demonstrated that extraction times of 60 min and temperatures of 25 °C resulted in the *F. vesiculosus* extract with the highest antioxidant potential, obtaining a value of 89.74% with the 2,2-diphenyl-1-picrylhydrazyl free radical scavenging activity (DPPH-RSA) assay. The Folin–Ciocalteu method determined that this extract had a total phenolic content (TPC) of 13.61 mg phloroglucinol equivalents per 1 g of dry algae (PGE/g algae). In addition, the chromatographic characterisation of the extract by a reverse-phase high-performance liquid chromatography equipment coupled to a diode array detector (RP-HPLC-DAD) identified and quantified 10 polyphenols: floroglucinol (621.43 ± 7.28 μg/g), epicatechin (31.08 ± 1.47 μg/g), catechin (30.01 ± 1.95 μg/g), chlorogenic acid (20.27 ± 0.72 μg/g), rutin (17.10 ± 0.93 μg/g), gallic acid (15.26 ± 0.95 μg/g), vanillic acid (6.86 ± 0.07 μg/g), ferulic acid (6.07 ± 0.12 μg/g), caffeic acid (3.95 ± 0.14 μg/g) and coumaric acid (2.68 ± 0.07 μg/g). Among these, floroglucinol stood out due to its higher concentration compared to the others.

3.2. Effect of F. vesiculosus Treatment on Lipid Peroxidation: Determination of Malondialdehyde (MDA) Concentration in Intestinal Tissue

In Figure 1, an increase in lipid peroxidation damage was observed in the I/R group, in which MDA values increased, showing significant differences ($p < 0.01$) compared to the sham group. However, similar values to the sham control group were re-established in the groups treated with the algae extract. On the other hand, no significant differences were observed either in the different treatment times (t.1, t.2, t.3) or in the reperfusion times (3 and 24 h). The excipient-treated groups showed no significant differences compared to the I/R group.

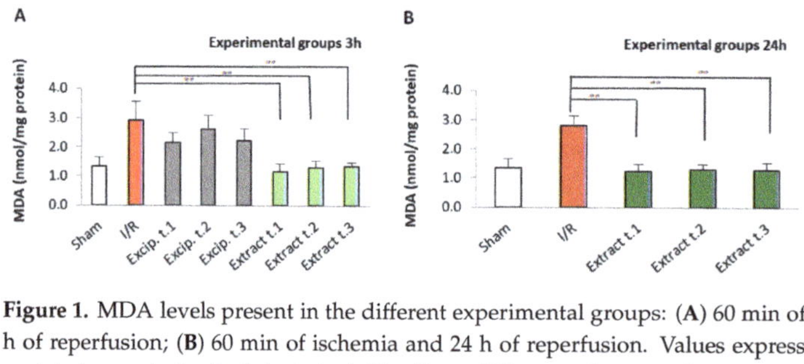

Figure 1. MDA levels present in the different experimental groups: (**A**) 60 min of ischemia and 3 h of reperfusion; (**B**) 60 min of ischemia and 24 h of reperfusion. Values expressed in nmol/mg protein (mean ± standard deviation). Significant differences between the treatment groups and the I/R group are indicated (** $p < 0.01$); Mann–Whitney U test, SPSS.

3.3. *Effect of F. vesiculosus Treatment on Superoxide Dismutase (SOD) Activity*

The results presented in Figure 2 illustrates the impact of *F. vesiculosus* extract on SOD activity. When compared to the sham group, the level of intestinal SOD in the I/R group was significantly higher ($p < 0.01$). However, the enzyme level in the algae extract-treated group was significantly lower than in the I/R group ($p < 0.01$). Additionally, no significant differences were observed between the different administration times for groups with reperfusion periods of 3 h (Extract t.1, Extract t.2, and Extract t.3), while Extract t.1 showed significant differences with respect to the Extract t.3 group ($p < 0.05$) for groups subjected to 24 h of reperfusion. Furthermore, Extract t.3 (3 h reperfusion) differed significantly from Extract t.3 (24 h reperfusion). Lastly, no differences were found between the excipient-treated groups and the I/R group.

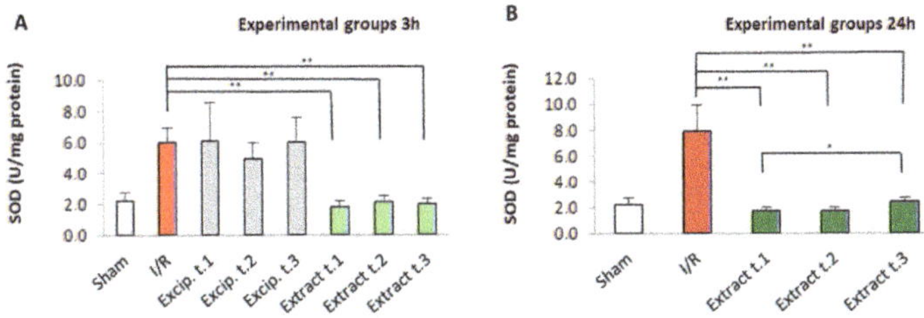

Figure 2. SOD levels present in the different experimental groups: (**A**) 60 min of ischemia and 3 h of reperfusion; (**B**) 60 min of ischemia and 24 h of reperfusion). Values expressed in U/mg protein (mean ± standard deviation. Significant differences between the treatment groups and the I/R group are indicated (* $p < 0.05$, ** $p < 0.01$); Mann–Whitney U test, SPSS.

3.4. *Effect of F. vesiculosus Treatment on Catalase (CAT) Activity*

The effects of *F. vesiculosus* extract on CAT activity are shown in Figure 3. The activity of the antioxidant enzyme was significantly lower in the I/R group compared to the sham group and algae extract-treated groups ($p < 0.01$). In addition, no significant differences between the sham group and the algae extract-treated groups were shown. On the other hand, the excipient-treated groups showed no significant differences from the I/R group. In terms of the comparison between the different extract application times (Extract t.1, Extract t.2, and Extract t.3), as well as reperfusion times (3 and 24 h), no significant differences were observed for any of the groups compared.

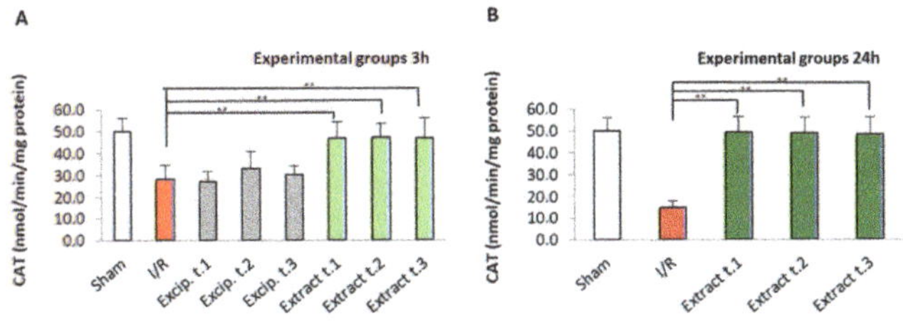

Figure 3. CAT levels present in the different experimental groups: (**A**) 60 min of ischemia and 3 h of reperfusion; (**B**) 60 min of ischemia and 24 h of reperfusion. Values expressed in nmol/min/mg protein (mean ± standard deviation). Significant differences between the treatment groups and the I/R group are indicated (** $p < 0.01$); Mann–Whitney U test, SPSS.

3.5. *Effect of F. vesiculosus Treatment on Glutathione Peroxidase (GPx) Activity*

GPx enzyme activity increased significantly in the untreated I/R groups, whereas the algae extract-treated groups exhibited a significant reduction in GPx values following the I/R process ($p < 0.01$). On the other hand, the excipient-treated groups showed no significant differences compared to the I/R group. No significant differences were observed in the treatment in terms of time of application (Extract t.1, Extract t.2, and Extract t.3) for any of the reperfusion periods (3 and 24 h). These results can be seen in Figure 4. However, differences were observed between Extract t.1 (3 h reperfusion)/Extract t.1 (24 h reperfusion) and Extract t.2 (3 h reperfusion)/Extract t.2 (24 h reperfusion).

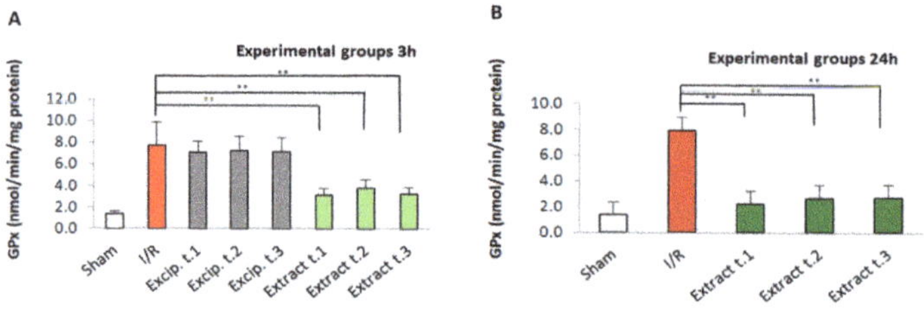

Figure 4. GPx levels present in the different experimental groups: (**A**) 60 min of ischemia and 3 h of reperfusion; (**B**) 60 min of ischemia and 24 h of reperfusion. Values expressed in nmol/min/mg protein (mean ± standard deviation. Significant differences between the treatment groups and the I/R group are indicated (** $p < 0.01$); Mann–Whitney U test, SPSS.

3.6. Effect of F. vesiculosus Treatment on Mieloperoxidase (MPO) Concentration

MPO values were significantly higher ($p < 0.01$) in the I/R group compared to the sham group, indicating oxidative damage. All groups treated with *F. vesiculosus* exhibited a significant reduction in MPO levels ($p = 0.009$). However, the excipient-treated groups did not show any significant decrease in MPO levels. Significant differences were also observed between the different application times of the seaweed extract. In this sense, *p*-values below 0.05 were obtained for the comparisons between Extract t.1/Extract t.2 and Extract t.1/Extract t.3 in rats reperfused for 3 h, as well as between the groups Extract t.1/Extract t.2, Extract t.1/Extract t.3 and Extract t.2/Extract t.3 in rats subjected to 24 h of reperfusion. These results are shown in Figure 5. The comparative analysis between the two reperfusion periods showed significant differences between Extract t.2 (3 h reperfusion)/Extract t.2 (24 h reperfusion).

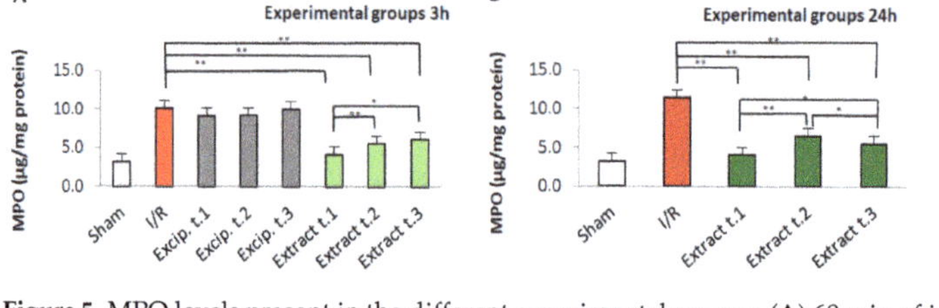

Figure 5. MPO levels present in the different experimental groups: (**A**) 60 min of ischemia and 3 h of reperfusion; (**B**) 60 min of ischemia and 24 h of reperfusion. Values expressed in µg/mg protein (mean ± standard deviation). Significant differences between the treatment groups and the I/R group are indicated (* $p < 0.05$, ** $p < 0.01$); Mann–Whitney U test, SPSS.

3.7. Effect of F. vesiculosus Treatment on Inflammation Markers: Interleukins Il-1β and IL-10

The levels of interleukins, both Il-1β and Il-10, were significantly higher in the untreated I/R group compared to the sham group ($p < 0.05$). In contrast, the groups treated with the seaweed extract showed a significant reduction in their interleukin levels. For IL-10, values comparable to those of the sham group were restored in all treated groups, regardless of application time and reperfusion period. In the case of IL-1β, sham values were restored in all three groups (Extract t.1, t.2 and t.3) reperfused for 24 h, whereas this restoration was not observed in these groups after 3 h of reperfusion. No significant differences were observed for either Il-1β or Il-10 between the different treatment application times. All these results are presented in Figures 6 and 7. However, when comparing the effect of the reperfusion period, differences in IL-1β levels were noted between the groups Extract t.3 (3 h reperfusion)/Extract t.3 (24 h reperfusion), while differences in IL-10 levels were observed in all three groups: Extract t.1 (3 h reperfusion)/Extract t.1 (24 h reperfusion), Extract t.2 (3 h reperfusion)/Extract t.2 (24 h reperfusion) and Extract t.3 (3 h reperfusion)/Extract t.3 (24 h reperfusion). The groups treated with the excipient showed no differences when compared to the I/R group.

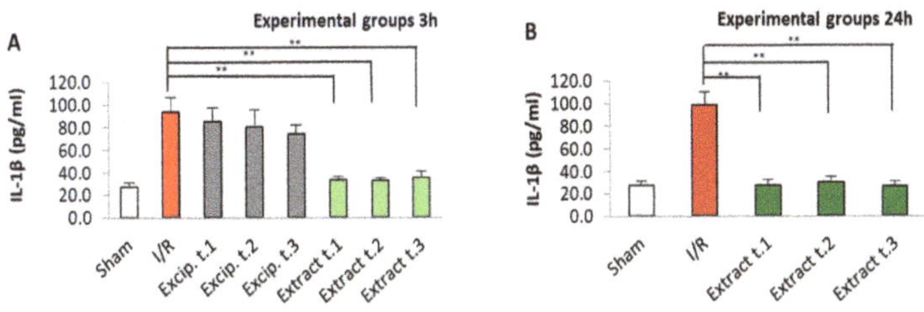

Figure 6. Il-1β levels present in the different experimental groups: (**A**) 60 min of ischemia and 3 h of reperfusion; (**B**) 60 min of ischemia and 24 h of reperfusion. Values expressed in μg/mg protein (mean ± standard deviation). Significant differences between the treatment groups and the I/R group are indicated (** $p < 0.01$); Mann–Whitney U test, SPSS.

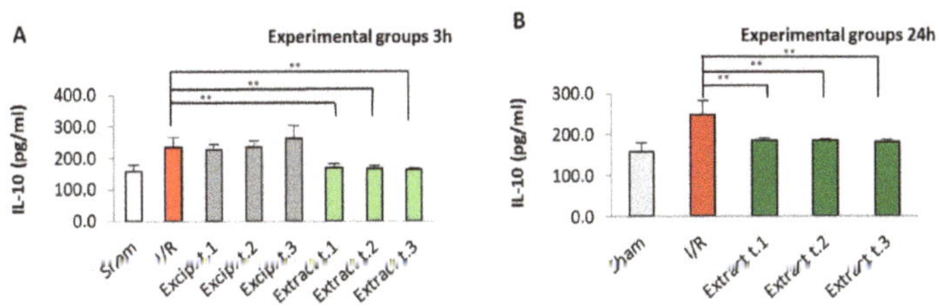

Figure 7. Il-10 levels present in the different experimental groups: (**A**) 60 min of ischemia and 3 h of reperfusion; (**B**) 60 min of ischemia and 24 h of reperfusion. Values expressed in μg/mg protein (mean ± standard deviation. Significant differences between the treatment groups and the I/R group are indicated (** $p < 0.01$); Mann–Whitney U test, SPSS.

The complete data for all biochemical parameters and their statistical analysis as well as the comparison between the two reperfusion times are provided in the Supplementary Materials (Tables S1 and S2).

3.8. Effects of F. vesiculosus Extract on Histological Alterations Induced by Intestinal I/R

Damage to the intestinal mucosa by I/R was assessed using the scoring scale outlined by Chiu et al. [46], with the results shown in Figures 8B and 9B. In the sham group, histopathological examination revealed a typical mucosal structure (G0), characterised by well-organised, tall, and evenly spaced villi with consistent thickness. The crypts appeared tightly packed and contained a thin layer of lamina propria. In contrast, the I/R group displayed significant mucosal damage, with notable villus loss, atrophy, and fragmentation. Most sections were classified under grade G3, with some showing G4 damage. On the other hand, in the treated groups after 3 h of reperfusion (Figure 8B), the intestinal mucosa showed more favourable outcomes when the extract was administered either 24 h prior to ischemia (Extract t.1) or at the onset of ischemia (Extract t.2), with significant differences ($p < 0.01$) compared to the I/R group. In contrast, in the treated groups subjected to 24 h of reperfusion (Figure 9B), greater mucosal recovery was observed when the extract was administered at the beginning of the reperfusion phase (Extract t.3). Comparative analysis between the two reperfusion periods revealed significant differences in all three groups: Extract t.1 (3 h reperfusion) vs. Extract t.1 (24 h reperfusion) ($p = 0.000$), Extract t.2 (3 h reperfusion) vs. Extract t.2 (24 h reperfusion) ($p = 0.001$), and Extract t.3 (3 h reperfusion) vs. Extract t.3 (24 h reperfusion) ($p = 0.001$). No differences were observed in the groups treated with the excipient compared to the I/R group.

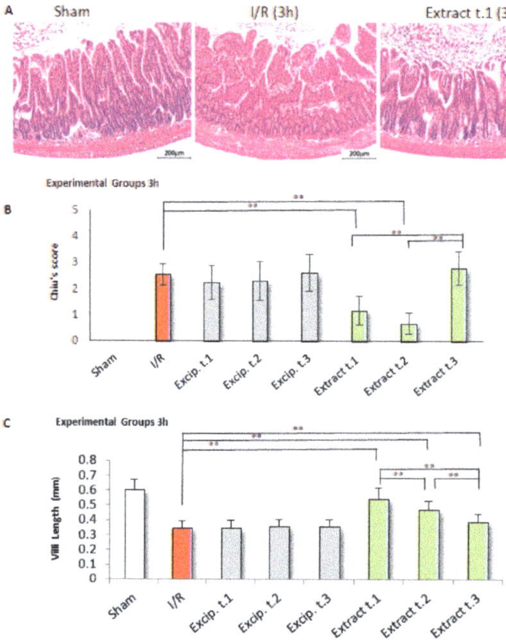

Figure 8. Histological results for the experimental groups after 3 h of reperfusion: (**A**) Tissue sections of small intestinal mucosa stained with H&E (100× magnification) revealed significant villus fragmentation and loss in the I/R group. In contrast, the villous structure was better preserved in the *F. vesiculosus* extract group. (**B**) Distribution of intestinal injury according to the Chiu scoring system (G0 = normal mucosa; G1 = development of subepithelial space at the villus tip, often accompanied by oedema and vascular congestion; G2 = detachment of the epithelial layer from the lamina propria with moderate extension of the subepithelial space, villus tip fragmentation, and haemorrhage; G3 = partial loss of villus tips, extensive epithelial detachment, and fragmentation with loss of the upper third of the villi; G4 = dilated and exposed capillaries with lost villi, though crypts remain present; G5 = haemorrhage, ulceration, disintegration of the lamina propria, and complete mucosal necrosis) indicated that the I/R group exhibited significant alterations, including fragmentation of the upper villus regions and loss of crypts (**C**) Furthermore, a marked reduction in villus length was noted in the I/R group compared to *F. vesiculosus* extracts with significant differences (** $p < 0.01$).

The villi in the groups treated with seaweed extract exhibited greater length and preservation compared to the untreated I/R group (Figures 8C and 9C). Regarding the timing of administration, in the treated groups after 3 h of reperfusion (Figure 8C) significant differences were observed ($p < 0.05$) between groups, with the Extract t.1 showing a greater villus height, while no significant differences were observed between the treated groups after 24 h of reperfusion (Figure 9C). Comparison of the reperfusion times showed significant differences ($p < 0.001$) between Extract t.2 (3 h reperfusion) vs. Extract t.2 (24 h reperfusion) and Extract t.3 (3 h reperfusion) vs. Extract t.3 (24 h reperfusion). The groups treated with the excipient showed no differences when compared to the I/R group.

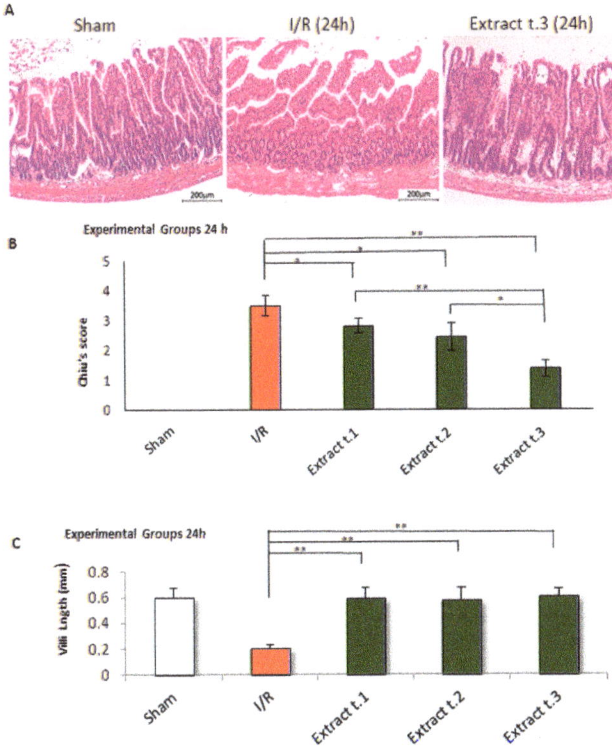

Figure 9. Histological results for the experimental groups after 24 h of reperfusion: (**A**) Tissue sections of small intestinal mucosa stained with H&E (100× magnification) revealed significant villus fragmentation and loss in the I/R group. In contrast, the villous structure was better preserved in the *F. vesiculosus* extract group. (**B**) Distribution of intestinal injury according to the Chiu scoring system (G0 = normal mucosa; G1 = development of subepithelial space at the villus tip, often accompanied by oedema and vascular congestion; G2 = detachment of the epithelial layer from the lamina propria with moderate extension of the subepithelial space, villus tip fragmentation, and haemorrhage; G3 = partial loss of villus tips, extensive epithelial detachment, and fragmentation with loss of the upper third of the villi; G4 = dilated and exposed capillaries with lost villi, though crypts remain present; G5 = haemorrhage, ulceration, disintegration of the lamina propria, and complete mucosal necrosis) indicated that the I/R group exhibited significant alterations, including fragmentation of the upper villus regions and loss of crypts (**C**) Furthermore, a marked reduction in villus length was noted in the I/R group compared to *F. vesiculosus* extracts with significant differences (* $p < 0.05$, ** $p < 0.01$).

4. Discussion

Intestinal ischemia/reperfusion (I/R) injury is associated with numerous acute pathological conditions and plays a crucial role in several clinical and surgical procedures [13,47]. This pathophysiological process leads to a significant release of reactive oxygen species

(ROS), which contribute to oxidative stress [2,6]. To combat ROS overproduction, organisms have developed a complex endogenous antioxidant defence system [1,48]. However, in the face of an overwhelming challenge, as may occur in the case of regional arterial occlusion, the provision of exogenous antioxidants helps ensure tissue survival [49].

Lipoperoxidation is a metabolic process where ROS cause the oxidative degradation of lipids, leading to the formation of malondialdehyde (MDA), a biomarker used to assess oxidative damage in tissues [50]. All intestinal samples treated with *F. vesiculosus* showed a significant decrease in MDA levels compared to the I/R group, suggesting that the antioxidants in the seaweed extract may inhibit ROS formation. Similar results have been reported in studies on other natural extracts, such as *Ganoderma lucidum* [51], *Phyllantus amarus* [12] and *Himathalia elongata* [52], where the extracts also reduced MDA levels, highlighting their potential to mitigate oxidative damage.

Antioxidant enzymes, including superoxide dismutase (SOD), catalase (CAT) and glutathione peroxidase (GPx), form the primary endogenous defence system against oxidative stress [53]. The main function of SOD is to convert the superoxide anion (O_2^-) into hydrogen peroxide (H_2O_2) and oxygen [54]. Then, CAT and GPx break down the H_2O_2 into water and oxygen [55]. An increase in SOD and GPx during mesenteric injury may indicate oxidative stress, with the cell possibly using this as an adaptive response to counter ROS production [56–59]. In this study, mesenteric obstruction significantly increased the levels of these enzymes compared to the sham group. However, the administration of the extract resulted in a reduction in enzyme activity, suggesting potential protective effects against tissue damage. These findings align with other studies, where increased SOD and GPx levels during I/R were associated with adaptive responses, and treatments with melatonin and thymoquinone [60], *Parquetina nigrescens* extract [59] and astaxanthin [61] reduced enzyme levels compared to the I/R group. On the other hand, CAT activity may decrease under oxidative stress, despite elevated ROS levels, possibly due to the presence of multiple isoenzymes with different functions. The assay used in our study measured total catalase activity without distinguishing between isoforms. But several studies have reported that CAT activity can be inversely correlated with oxidative damage [62–64]. In this context, the reduced CAT activity observed in the I/R group supports the presence of oxidative stress, whereas treatment with the algal extract significantly increased the enzyme levels. Previous studies evaluating the antioxidant potential of some polyphenols in experimental I/R models support our findings [65–68], showing a decrease in CAT activity in the I/R group, followed by a significant increase in enzyme activity after treatment with polyphenols. Moreover, since GPx and CAT use the same substrate, H_2O_2, the reduction in CAT activity could be leading to an increase in GPx activity as a compensatory mechanism, likewise the increased SOD levels could also be contributing to an accumulation of H_2O_2 [60].

Myeloperoxidase (MPO) is a lysosomal haemoprotein present in leukocytes and macrophages [69], and its activity is associated with inflammatory and oxidative stress processes [70]. MPO catalyses the conversion of chloride ions (Cl^-) and H_2O_2 into hypochlorous acid (HClO), a potent oxidant that generates ROS [71,72]. In this study, the results reveal that *F. vesiculosus* treatment significantly reduces the increased MPO levels during the intestinal I/R process, suggesting that the algae extract is able to attenuate the oxidant–antioxidant imbalance during I/R. Other studies have also demonstrated that polyphenols present in natural products, such as quercetin, rutin, resveratrol, and ferric acid, can inhibit MPO activity, offering potential for reducing I/R injury [70].

One of the main responses of tissues when subjected to I/R is the inflammatory response, as the release of pro- and anti-inflammatory cytokines is directly related to the formation of ROS [73]. Tissues subjected to I/R experienced an increase in interleukin-1β

(Il-1β) levels, which is justified by the increase in MPO, which promotes the infiltration of leukocytes and pro-inflammatory cytokines [12]. On the other hand, an increase in interleukin-10 (IL-10) expression was also observed. IL-10 is an anti-inflammatory cytokine that suppresses the expression of IL-1 β. However, several studies have found that both IL-1β and IL-10 increase after reperfusion in intestinal samples, rather than exhibiting an inverse relationship [74,75]. This could be interpreted as an adaptive mechanism by the organism to regulate the immune response in the damaged tissue [76]. Pretreatment with *F. vesiculosus* significantly attenuated the inflammatory response in the damaged tissues, reducing both IL-1β and IL-10 levels, suggesting that our treatment inhibits ROS production and attenuates the inflammatory response. These results are consistent with those of Ucar et al. [77], who also observed increases in both cytokines during intestinal I/R, and the administration of a treatment based on receptor blockade significantly decreased their expression.

Histopathological examination of jejunal tissue revealed that superior mesenteric artery occlusion for 60 min, followed by 3 and 24 h of reperfusion, caused severe damage to the intestinal mucosa. However, this damage was significantly reduced with treatment using *F. vesiculosus* extract. The injury grades, reflected in the Chiu score, were higher in the I/R group (grades 3–4) compared to the sham group (grade 0). In contrast, the treated samples showed a significant reduction in the score (grades 0–1–2). Additionally, the results demonstrated that the extract helped preserve the structure of the villi, with treated groups showing significant improvement in villus length compared to the I/R group.

The comparative study of treatment application times, in terms of degrees of injury, showed that in experimental groups subjected to 3 h of reperfusion, treatment at times t.1 and t.2 were most effective in reducing I/R injury. However, in groups subjected to 24 h of reperfusion, better results were observed when the extract was administered at the beginning of reperfusion (Extract t.3). Furthermore, t.1 and t.2 showed a greater reduction in damage with 3 h of reperfusion compared to the 24 h reperfusion period. However, t.3 showed better results after 24 h of reperfusion. These results suggest that when the treatment is administered before (t.1) or at the time of ischemia (t.2), it reduces oxidative injury, possibly due to its protective effect, as it proves effective even with just 3 h of reperfusion. On the other hand, when the extract is applied after ischemia (t.3), this protective effect is not observed, but a significant improvement in injury is noted after 24 h of reperfusion, suggesting it may act on ROS during this time interval. The comparative analysis of villus length also suggests that, for 3 h of reperfusion, Extract. t.1 yields better results, but Extract. t.3 works better with a long reperfusion period (24 h) than with a short one (3 h).

Overall, our results highlight not only the complexity of the mechanisms involved in intestinal ischemia/reperfusion injury but also the current limitations in understanding their temporal progression. The observed variability in the analysed parameters suggests that distinct pathological processes may be activated or suppressed at different time points during reperfusion. This highlights the need for future studies to more precisely define when and how oxidative, inflammatory and apoptotic mechanisms contribute to tissue damage in this model.

Finally, the groups that were treated with the excipient exhibited no significant differences when compared to the I/R group. This confirms that the observed effect is exclusively due to the extract, and the excipient shows no effect on the I/R injury.

5. Conclusions

In conclusion, our findings demonstrated that the *F. vesiculosus* extract holds significant potential in mitigating I/R injury in the intestines of rats. The extract effectively reduced lipid peroxidation, as evidenced by lower MDA levels, and helped preserve the antioxidant enzymatic balance by maintaining CAT, SOD, GPx and MPO activities. Furthermore, the treatment modulated the inflammatory response by reducing IL-1β and IL-10 cytokine levels towards normal levels. Histological analysis confirmed that the extract helped preserve intestinal mucosal architecture and reduce tissue damage. Nevertheless, the variability observed among the different extract administration times highlights the complexity of ischemia/reperfusion injury and underscores the need for further studies to better understand its temporal progression. Therefore, the use of *F. vesiculosus* extract appears promising and warrants further investigation as a potential treatment for preventing ischemic processes in mesenteric thromboembolism and during surgical procedures.

Supplementary Materials: The following supporting information can be downloaded at: https://www.mdpi.com/article/10.3390/antiox14060624/s1, Table S1: Analytical parameter results. Statistical comparison between treatments and I/R or Sham groups. Table S2: Analytical parameter results. Statistical comparison between treatments at different reperfusion times.

Author Contributions: Conceptualization, Methodology, Validation, Formal Analysis, Investigation, Data curation, Writing—original draft, Writing—review & editing, Visualization, D.S.-B.; Data curation, Software, Validation, J.M.L.-C. (José Miguel Lloris-Cejalvo); Conceptualization, Methodology, Investigation, Validation, Data curation, Writing—review & editing, Supervision, Visualization, C.P.-S.; Conceptualization, Resources, Project administration, Funding acquisition, J.M.L.-C. (José Miguel Lloris-Carsí); Conceptualization, Resources, Supervision, Project administration, Funding acquisition, D.C.-L. All authors have read and agreed to the published version of the manuscript.

Funding: The authors gratefully acknowledge the financial support provided by the Universidad Católica de Valencia for covering the publication costs of this article.

Institutional Review Board Statement: The animal study protocol was approved by the Institutional Review Board of GENERALITAT VALENCIANA (protocol code 2017VSC/PEA/00097 tipo2 and date of approval 21 May 2015).

Informed Consent Statement: Not applicable.

Data Availability Statement: It is not possible to publicly share the research data because the data are from the doctoral thesis of the researcher Desiree Sánchez-Bonet. However, after the defence of her work, access to the data can be requested by email to: desanbo@gmail.com.

Conflicts of Interest: The authors declare no conflicts of interest.

References

1. Aranda-Rivera, A.K.; Cruz-Gregorio, A.; Arancibia-Hernández, Y.L.; Hernández-Cruz, E.Y.; Pedraza-Chaverri, J. RONS and oxidative stress: An overview of basic concepts. *Oxygen* **2022**, *2*, 437–478. [CrossRef]
2. Kotha, R.R.; Tareq, F.S.; Yildiz, E.; Luthria, D.L. Oxidative stress and antioxidants—A critical review on in vitro antioxidant assays. *Antioxidants* **2022**, *11*, 2388. [CrossRef] [PubMed]
3. Namirah, I.; Wimbanu, K.S.; Rompies, A.M.E.; Prayogo, Y.S.; Arozal, W.; Fadilah; Hanafi, M.; Hardiany, N.S. The effect of ethanol-based coriander (*Coriandrum sativum* L.) seed extract on oxidative stress, antioxidant level and cellular senescence in the heart of obese rat. *J. Pharm. Pharmacogn. Res.* **2024**, *12*, 1111–1120. [CrossRef]
4. Di Meo, S.; Napolitano, G.; Venditti, P. Physiological and pathological role of ROS: Benefits and limitations of antioxidant treatment. *Int. J. Mol. Sci.* **2019**, *20*, 4810. [CrossRef]
5. Sies, H. Oxidative stress. *Acad. Press* **1985**, *86*, 715–748. [CrossRef]
6. Isgör, M.; Küçükgül, A.; Alasahan, S. Antioxidant and anti-inflammatory activities of Gallic acid in Japanese quails induced by oxidative stress. *Rev. Cient. Fac. Cienc. Vet.* **2023**, *33*, 1–6. [CrossRef]

7. Wu, L.; Xiong, X.; Wu, X.; Ye, Y.; Jian, Z.; Zhi, Z.; Gu, L. Targeting oxidative stress and inflammation to prevent ischemia-reperfusion injury. *Front. Mol. Neurosci.* **2020**, *13*, 28. [CrossRef]
8. Andrés, C.M.C.; Pérez de la Lastra, J.M.; Juan, C.A.; Plou, F.J.; Pérez-Lebeña, E. Chemistry of hydrogen peroxide formation and elimination in mammalian cells, and its role in various pathologies. *Stresses* **2022**, *2*, 256–274. [CrossRef]
9. Lin, L.; Wang, X.; Yu, Z. Ischemia-reperfusion injury in the brain: Mechanisms and potential therapeutic strategies. *Biochem. Pharmacol.* **2016**, *5*, 213. [CrossRef]
10. Wu, M.Y.; Yiang, G.T.; Liao, W.T.; Tsai, A.P.; Cheng, Y.L.; Cheng, P.W.; Li, C.-Y.; Li, C.J. Current mechanistic concepts in ischemia and reperfusion injury. *Cell Physiol. Biochem.* **2018**, *46*, 1650–1667. [CrossRef]
11. Nieuwenhuijs-Moeke, G.J.; Pischke, S.E.; Berger, S.P.; Sanders, J.S.F.; Pol, R.A.; Struys, M.M.R.F.; Ploeg, R.J.; Leuvenink, H.G.D. Ischemia and reperfusion injury in kidney transplantation: Relevant mechanisms in injury and repair. *J. Clin. Med.* **2020**, *9*, 253. [CrossRef] [PubMed]
12. Afolabi, A.O.; Akhigbe, T.M.; Odetayo, A.F.; Anyogu, D.C.; Hamed, M.A.; Akhigbe, R.E. Restoration of hepatic and intestinal integrity by *Phyllanthus amarus* is dependent on Bax/Caspase 3 modulation in intestinal ischemia/reperfusion-induced injury. *Molecules* **2022**, *27*, 5073. [CrossRef] [PubMed]
13. Wen, S.; Li, X.; Ling, Y.; Chen, S.; Deng, Q.; Yang, L.; Li, Y.; Shen, J.; Qiu, Y.; Zhan, Y.; et al. HMGB1-associated necroptosis and Kupffer cells M1 polarization underlies remote liver injury induced by intestinal ischemia/reperfusion in rats. *FASEB J.* **2020**, *34*, 4384–4402. [CrossRef] [PubMed]
14. Bertoni, S.; Ballabeni, V.; Barocelli, E.; Tognolini, M. Mesenteric ischemia-reperfusion: An overview of preclinical drug strategies. *Drug Discov. Today* **2018**, *23*, 1416–1425. [CrossRef]
15. Liu, C.; Ding, R.; Huang, W.; Miao, L.; Li, J.; Li, Y. Sevoflurane protects against intestinal ischemia-reperfusion injury by activating peroxisome proliferator-activated receptor gamma/nuclear factor-kappaB pathway in rats. *Pharmacology* **2020**, *105*, 231–242. [CrossRef]
16. Li, G.; Wang, S.; Fan, Z. Oxidative stress in intestinal ischemia-reperfusion. *Front. Med.* **2022**, *8*, 750731. [CrossRef]
17. Abo-Shady, A.M.; Gheda, S.F.; Ismail, G.A.; Cotas, J.; Pereira, L.; Abdel-Karim, O.H. Antioxidant and antidiabetic activity of algae. *Life* **2023**, *13*, 460. [CrossRef]
18. Anwar, H.; Hussain, G.; Mustafa, I. Antioxidants from natural sources. In *Antioxidants in Foods and its Applications*; InTech: London, UK, 2018. [CrossRef]
19. Veluchamy, C.; Palaniswamy, R. A review on marine algae and its applications. *Asian J. Pharm. Biol.* **2020**, *13*, 21–27. [CrossRef]
20. Wang, T.; Jonsdottir, R.; Liu, H.; Gu, L.; Kristinsson, H.G.; Raghavan, S.; Ólafsdóttir, G. Antioxidant capacities of phlorotannins extracted from the brown algae *Fucus vesiculosus*. *J. Agric. Food Chem.* **2012**, *60*, 5874–5883. [CrossRef]
21. Tziveleka, L.A.; Tammam, M.A.; Tzakou, O.; Roussis, V.; Ioannou, E. Metabolites with antioxidant activity from marine macroalgae. *Antioxidants* **2021**, *10*, 1431. [CrossRef]
22. Heffernan, N.; Smyth, T.J.; Soler-Villa, A.; Fitzgerald, R.J.; Brunton, N.P. Phenolic content and antioxidant activity of fractions obtained from selected Irish macroalgae species (*Laminaria digitata, Fucus serratus, Gracilaria gracilis* and *Codium fragile*). *J. Appl. Phycol.* **2015**, *27*, 519–530. [CrossRef]
23. Cikos, A.M.; Jokic, S.; Subaric, D.; Jerkovic, I. Overview on the application of modern methods for the extraction of bioactive compounds from marine macroalgae. *Mar. Drugs* **2018**, *16*, 348. [CrossRef]
24. Matsukawa, R.; Dubinsky, Z.; Kishimoto, E.; Masaki, K.; Masuda, Y.; Takeuchi, T. A comparison of screening methods for antioxidant activity in seaweeds. *J. Appl. Phycol.* **1997**, *9*, 29–35. [CrossRef]
25. Pereira, L.; Cotas, J. Therapeutic potential of polyphenols and other micronutrients of marine origin. *Mar. Drugs* **2023**, *21*, 323. [CrossRef]
26. Jimenez-Lopez, C.; Pereira, A.G.; Lourenço-Lopes, C.; Garcia-Oliveira, P.; Cassani, L.; Fraga-Corral, M.; Prieto, M.; Simal-Gandara, J. Main bioactive phenolic compounds in marine algae and their mechanisms of action supporting potential health benefits. *Food Chem.* **2021**, *341*, 128262. [CrossRef]
27. Ferreira, I.C.F.R.; Martins, N.; Barros, L. Phenolic compounds and its bioavailability: In vitro bioactive compounds or health promoters? *Adv. Food Nutr. Res.* **2017**, *82*, 1–44. [CrossRef] [PubMed]
28. Kumar, N.; Goel, N. Phenolic acids: Natural versatile molecules with promising therapeutic applications. *Biotechnol. Rep.* **2019**, *24*, e00370. [CrossRef]
29. Vuolo, M.M.; Lima, V.S.; Maróstica Junior, M.R. Phenolic Compounds: Structure, Classification, and Antioxidant Power. In *Bioactive Compounds: Health Benefits and Potential Applications*; Segura Campos, M.R., Ed.; Woodhead Publishing: Cambridge, UK, 2019; pp. 33–50. ISBN 978-0-12-814774-0. [CrossRef]

30. Rudrapal, M.; Khairnar, S.J.; Khan, J.; Bin Dukhyil, A.; Ansari, M.A.; Alomary, M.N.; Alshabrmi, F.M.; Palai, S.; Deb, P.K.; Devi, R. Dietary polyphenols and their role in oxidative stress-induced human diseases: Insights into protective effects, antioxidant potentials and mechanism(s) of action. *Front. Pharmacol.* **2022**, *13*, 283. [CrossRef]
31. Balboa, E.M.; Conde, E.; Moure, A.; Falqué, E.; Dominguez, H. In vitro antioxidant properties of crude extracts and compounds from brown algae: A review. *Food Chem.* **2013**, *138*, 1764–1785. [CrossRef]
32. Catarino, M.D.; Silva, A.M.S.; Cardoso, S.M. Fucaceae: A source of bioactive phlorotannins. *Int. J. Mol. Sci.* **2017**, *18*, 1327. [CrossRef]
33. Agregán, R.; Munekata, P.; Franco, D.; Carballo, J.; Barba, F.J.; Lorenzo, J.M. Antioxidant potential of extracts obtained from macro-algae (*Ascophyllum nodosum, Fucus vesiculosus* and *Bifurcaria bifurcata*) and micro-algae (*Chlorella vulgaris* and *Spirulina platensis*) assisted by ultrasound. *Medicines* **2018**, *5*, 33. [CrossRef]
34. El-Sheekh, M.M.; el-Shenody, R.A.E.K.; Bases, E.A.; el Shafay, S.M. Comparative assessment of antioxidant activity and biochemical composition of four seaweeds, Rocky Bay of Abu Qir in Alexandria, Egypt. *Food Sci. Technol.* **2020**, *41*, 29–40. [CrossRef]
35. Obluchinskaya, E.D.; Pozharitskaya, O.N.; Zakharov, D.V.; Flisyuk, E.V.; Terninko, I.I.; Generalova, Y.E.; Smekhova, I.E.; Shikov, A.N. The biochemical composition and antioxidant properties of Fucus vesiculosus from the Arctic region. *Mar. Drugs* **2022**, *20*, 193. [CrossRef] [PubMed]
36. Hermund, D.B.; Plaza, M.; Turner, C.; Jonsdottir, R.; Kristinsson, H.G.; Jacobsen, C.; Nielsen, K.F. Structure dependent antioxidant capacity of phlorotannins from Icelandic Fucus vesiculosus by UHPLC-DAD-ECD-QTOFMS. *Food Chem.* **2018**, *240*, 904–909. [CrossRef]
37. Mateos, R.; Pérez-Correa, J.R.; Domínguez, H. Bioactive properties of marine phenolics. *Mar. Drugs* **2020**, *18*, 501. [CrossRef]
38. Zubia, M.; Fabre, M.S.; Kerjean, V.; Lann, K.L.; Stiger-Pouvreau, V.; Fauchon, M.; Deslandes, E. Antioxidant and antitumoural activities of some Phaeophyta from Brittany coasts. *Food Chem.* **2009**, *116*, 693–701. [CrossRef]
39. O'Sullivan, A.M.; O'Callaghan, Y.C.; O'Grady, M.N.; Queguineur, B.; Hanniffy, D.; Troy, D.J.; Kerry, J.; O'brien, N. In vitro and cellular antioxidant activities of seaweed extracts prepared from five brown seaweeds harvested in spring from the west coast of Ireland. *Food Chem.* **2011**, *126*, 1064–1070. [CrossRef]
40. Monteiro, M.; Santos, R.A.; Iglesias, P.; Couto, A.; Serra, C.R.; Gouvinhas, I.; Barros, A.; Oliva-Teles, A.; Enes, P.; Díaz-Rosales, P. Effect of extraction method and solvent system on the phenolic content and antioxidant activity of selected macro and microalgae extracts. *J. Appl. Phycol.* **2020**, *32*, 349–362. [CrossRef]
41. Julkunen-Tiitto, R. Phenolic constituents on the leaves of northern willows: Methods for the analysis of certain phenolics. *J. Agric. Food Chem.* **1985**, *33*, 213–217. [CrossRef]
42. Chu, Y.-H.; Chang, C.; Hsu, H. Flavonoid content of several vegetables and their antioxidant activity. *J. Sci. Food Agric.* **2000**, *80*, 561–566. [CrossRef]
43. López, A.; Rico, M.; Rivero, A.; Suáez de Tangil, M. The effects of solvents on the phenolic contents and antioxidant activity of *Stypocaulon scoparium* algae extracts. *Food Chem.* **2011**, *125*, 1104–1109. [CrossRef]
44. Sánchez-Bonet, D.; García-Oms, S.; Belda-Antolí, M.; Padrón-Sanz, C.; Lloris-Carsi, J.M.; Cejalvo-Lapeña, D. RP-HPLC-DAD determination of the differences in the polyphenol content of *Fucus vesiculosus* extracts with similar antioxidant activity. *J. Chromatogr. B* **2021**, *1184*, 122978. [CrossRef] [PubMed]
45. Ozkan, O.V.; Yuzbasioglu, M.F.; Ciralik, H.; Kurutas, E.B.; Yonden, Z.; Aydin, M.; Bulbuloglu, E.; Semerci, E.; Goksu, M.; Atli, Y.; et al. Resveratrol, a natural antioxidant, attenuates intestinal ischemia/reperfusion injury in rats. *Tohoku J. Exp. Med.* **2009**, *218*, 251–258. [CrossRef]
46. Chiu, C.; McArdle, A.H.; Brown, R.; Scott, H.J.; Gurd, F.N. Intestinal mucosal lesion in low-flow states: I. A morphological, hemodynamic, and metabolic reappraisal. *Arch. Surg.* **1970**, *101*, 478–483. [CrossRef]
47. Wang, J.; Zhang, W.; Wu, G. Intestinal ischemic reperfusion injury: Recommended rats model and comprehensive review for protective strategies. *Biomed. Pharmacother.* **2021**, *138*, 111482. [CrossRef] [PubMed]
48. Jomova, K.; Raptova, R.; Alomar, S.Y.; Alwasel, S.H.; Nepovimova, E.; Kuca, K.; Valko, M. Reactive oxygen species, toxicity, oxidative stress, and antioxidants: Chronic diseases and aging. *Arch. Toxicol.* **2023**, *97*, 2499–2574. [CrossRef]
49. Pisoschi, A.M.; Pop, A.; Lordache, F.; Stanca, L.; Predoi, G.; Serban, A.I. Oxidative stress mitigation by antioxidants—An overview on their chemistry and influences on health status. *Eur. J. Med. Chem.* **2021**, *209*, 112891. [CrossRef]
50. Mas-Bargues, C.; Escrivá, C.; Dromat, M.; Borrás, C.; Viña, J. Lipid peroxidation as measured by chromatographic determination of malondialdehyde. Human plasma reference values in health and disease. *Arch. Biochem. Biophys.* **2021**, *709*, 108941. [CrossRef]
51. Gömeç, M.; Kulăh, B.; Ercan, U.; Sahin, S. The healing effects of *Gonoderma lucidum* on intestinal ischemia-reperfusion damage in rats. *J. Surg. Med.* **2022**, *6*, 476–482. [CrossRef]

52. Belda-Antolí, M.; Padrón-Sanz, C.; Cejalvo-Lapeña, D.; Prieto-Moure, B.; Lloris-Cejalvo, J.M.; Lloris-Carsí, J.M. Antioxidant potential of *Himanthalia elongata* for protection against ischemia-reperfusion injury in the small bowel. *Surgery* **2017**, *162*, 577–585. [CrossRef]
53. Zhou, T.; Prather, E.R.; Garrison, D.E.; Zuo, L. Interplay between ROS and antioxidants during ischemia-reperfusion injuries in cardiac and skeletal muscle. *Int. J. Mol. Sci.* **2018**, *19*, 417. [CrossRef] [PubMed]
54. Salin, M.L.; McCord, J.M. Superoxide dismutases in polymorphonuclear leukocytes. *J. Clin. Investig.* **1974**, *54*, 1005–1009. [CrossRef] [PubMed]
55. Ighodaro, O.M.; Akinloye, O.A. First line defence antioxidants-superoxide dismutase (SOD), catalase (CAT) and glutathione peroxidase (GPX): Their fundamental role in the entire antioxidant defence grid. *Alex. J. Med.* **2018**, *54*, 287–293. [CrossRef]
56. Mates, J.M.; Perez-Gomez, C.; Decastro, I.N. Antioxidant enzymes and human diseases. *Clin. Biochem.* **1999**, *32*, 595–603. [CrossRef]
57. Kolodziejczyk, L.; Siemieniuk, E.; Skrzydlewska, E. Antioxidant potential of rat liver in experimental infection with *Fasciola hepatica*. *Parasitol. Res.* **2005**, *96*, 367–372. [CrossRef]
58. Kolli, V.K.; Abraham, P.; Isaac, B. Alteration in antioxidant defense mechanisms in the small intestines of methotrexate treated rat may contribute to its gastrointestinal toxicity. *Cancer Ther.* **2007**, *5*, 501–510.
59. Akinrinmade, F.J.; Akinrinde, A.S.; Soyemi, O.O.; Oyagbemi, A.A. Antioxidant potential of the methanol extract of *Parquetina nigrescens* mediates protection against intestinal ischemia-reperfusion injury in rats. *J. Diet. Suppl.* **2016**, *13*, 420–432. [CrossRef]
60. Tas, U.; Ayan, M.; Sogut, E.; Kuloglu, T.; Uysal, M.; Tanriverdi, H.I.; Senel, U.; Ozyurt, B.; Sarsilmaz, M. Protective effects of thymoquine and melatonin on intestinal ischemia-reperfusion injury. *Saudi J. Gastroenterol.* **2015**, *21*, 284–289. [CrossRef]
61. Yilmaz, A.S.; Badak, B.; Erkasap, N.; Ozkurt, M.; Colak, E. The effect of antioxidant Astaxanthin on intestinal ischemia-reperfusion damage in rats. *J. Investig. Surg.* **2023**, *36*, 2182930. [CrossRef]
62. Nisari, M.; Yay, A.; Ertekin, T.; Nisari, M.; Al, Ö.; Ceylan, D.; Önder, G.; Kavutcu, M. Evaluation of protective effects of melatonin on free radical metabolism in rat kidney during ischemia-reperfusion. *Ukr. J. Nephrol. Dial.* **2019**, *4*, 20–29. [CrossRef]
63. Zhang, X.; Zhou, X.; Zhang, Q.; Zhu, F. The preventive effects of dex medetomidine against intestinal ischemia-reperfusion injury in Wistar rats. *Iran J. Basic Med. Sci.* **2015**, *18*, 604–609. [PubMed]
64. Céspedes, M.E.; Rodriguez, J.C.; Campanioni, M. Enzimas que participan como barreras fisiológicas para eliminar los radicales libres: Catalasa. *Rev. Cubana Investig. Biomed.* **1996**, *15*, 39–47.
65. Keskin Çimen, F.; Çimen, O.; Altuner, D.; Çekiç, A.B.; Kurt, N.; Süleyman, H. Effect of rutin on experimentally induced small intestinal ischemia-reperfusion injury in rats: A biochemical and histopathological evaluation. *J. Surg. Med.* **2021**, *5*, 26–30. [CrossRef]
66. Lin, H.; Zhang, X.; Wang, D.; Liu, J.; Yuan, L.; Liu, J.; Wang, C.; Sun, J.; Chen, J.; Li, H.; et al. Anwulignan improves intestinal ischemia-reperfusion injury. *J. Pharmacol. Exp. Ther.* **2021**, *378*, 222–234. [CrossRef]
67. Durgun, C.; Deveci, E. Gallic acid treatment protects intestinal tissue against ischaemia-reperfusion. *Folia Morphol.* **2023**, *82*, 633–640. [CrossRef]
68. Durgun, C.; Aşır, F. Daidzein alleviated the pathologies in intestinal tissue against ischemia-reperfusion. *Eur. Rev. Med. Pharmacol. Sci.* **2023**, *27*, 1487–1493. [CrossRef]
69. García, O.H.; Pereira, N.; Flores, R.M. Enzimas generadoras de especies reactivas del oxígeno: Mieloperoxidasa. *Rev. Cubana Inv. Bioméd.* **1998**, *17*, 190–197.
70. Chen, S.; Chen, H.; Du, Q.; Shen, J. Targeting myeloperoxidase (MPO)-mediated oxidative stress and inflammation for reducing brain ischemia injury: Potential application of natural compounds. *Front. Physiol.* **2020**, *11*, 433. [CrossRef]
71. Liu, Q.; Liu, Y.; Shi, J.; Gao, M.; Liu, Y.; Cong, Y.; Li, Y.; Wang, Y.; Yu, M.; Lu, Y.; et al. Entire peroxidation reaction system of myeloperoxidase correlates with progressive low-density lipoprotein modifications via reactive aldehydes in atherosclerotic patients with hypertension. *Cell Physiol. Biochem.* **2018**, *50*, 1245–1254. [CrossRef]
72. Deng, Y.; Feng, S.; Xia, Q.; Gong, S.; Feng, G. A novel reaction-based fluorescence probe for rapid imaging of HClO in live cells, animals, and injured liver tissues. *Talanta* **2020**, *215*, 120901. [CrossRef]
73. Tanyeli, A.; Güzel, D.; Ekinci Akdemir, F.N.; Eraslan, E.; Güler, M.C. The role of chlorogenic acid in alleviating intestinal ischemia/reperfusion-induced lung injury. *New Trend Med. Sci.* **2020**, *1*, 59–64.
74. Souza, D.G.; Lomez, E.S.; Pinho, V.; Pesquero, J.B.; Bader, M.; Pesquero, J.L.; Teixeira, M.M. Role of bradykinin B2 and B1 receptors in the local, remote, and systemic inflammatory responses that follow intestinal ischemia and reperfusion injury. *J. Immunol.* **2004**, *172*, 2542–2548. [CrossRef] [PubMed]

75. Pompermayer, K.; Amaral, F.A.; Fagundes, C.T.; Vieira, A.T.; Cunha, F.Q.; Teixeira, M.M. Effects of the treatment with glibenclamide, an ATP-sensitive potassium channel blocker, on intestinal ischemia and reperfusion injury. *Eur. Pharmacol.* **2007**, *556*, 215–222. [CrossRef] [PubMed]
76. Gregová, K.; Čikoš, Š.; Bilecová-Rabajdová, M.; Urban, P.; Varga, J.; Feterik, Š.; Veselá, J. Intestinal ischemia-reperfusion injury mediates expression of inflammatory cytokines in rats. *Gen. Physiol. Biophys.* **2015**, *34*, 95–99. [CrossRef]
77. Ucar, B.I.; Erikci, A.; Kosemehmetoglu, K.; Ozkul, C.; Iskit, A.B.; Ucar, G.; Zeren, S. Effects of endothelin receptor blockade and COX inhibition on intestinal I/R injury in a rat model: Experimental research. *Int. J. Surg.* **2020**, *83*, 89–97. [CrossRef]

antioxidants

MDPI

Article

Blood Progenitor Cell Mobilization Driven by TWEAK Promotes Neovascularization and Reduces Brain Damage in a Rat Model of Intracerebral Hemorrhage

Daniel Romaus-Sanjurjo [1,2,*,†], Esteban López-Arias [1,3,†], Cristina Rodríguez [4,5], Pablo Hervella [6], Mariña Rodríguez-Arrizabalaga [1,2], Manuel Debasa-Mouce [1], Juan Manuel Pías-Peleteiro [1,2,7], Ramón Iglesias-Rey [6], Pablo Aguiar [2,8,9], Ángeles Almeida [4,5], José Castillo [6], Alberto Ouro [1,2,*] and Tomás Sobrino [1,2]

1 NeuroAging Group Laboratory (NEURAL), Clinical Neurosciences Research Laboratory (LINC), Health Research Institute of Santiago de Compostela (IDIS), 15706 Santiago de Compostela, Spain; esteban.lopez.arias@sergas.es (E.L.-A.); marina.rodriguez.arrizabalaga@sergas.es (M.R.-A.); manuel.debasa@rai.usc.es (M.D.-M.); juan.manuel.pias.peleteiro@sergas.es (J.M.P.-P.); tomas.sobrino.moreiras@sergas.es (T.S.)

2 Centro de Investigación Biomédica en Red de Enfermedades Neurodegenerativas (CIBERNED), Instituto de Salud Carlos III, 28029 Madrid, Spain; pablo.aguiar.fernandez@sergas.es

3 Translational Stroke Laboratory Group (TREAT), Clinical Neurosciences Research Laboratory (LINC), Health Research Institute of Santiago de Compostela (IDIS), 15706 Santiago de Compostela, Spain

4 Institute of Biomedical Research of Salamanca (IBSAL), University Hospital of Salamanca, CSIC, University of Salamanca, 37007 Salamanca, Spain; c.rodriguez@usal.es (C.R.); aaparra@usal.es (Á.A.)

5 Institute of Functional Biology and Genomics (IBFG), CSIC, University of Salamanca, 37007 Salamanca, Spain

6 Neuroimaging and Biotechnology Laboratory (NOBEL), Clinical Neurosciences Research Laboratory (LINC), Health Research Institute of Santiago de Compostela (IDIS), 15706 Santiago de Compostela, Spain; pablo.hervella.lorenzo@sergas.es (P.H.); ramon.iglesias.rey@sergas.es (R.I.-R.); jose.antonio.castillo.sanchez@sergas.es (J.C.)

7 Department of Neurology, Hospital Clínico Universitario, Universidad de Santiago de Compostela, 15706 Santiago de Compostela, Spain

8 Molecular Imaging Biomarkers and Theragnosis Lab, Center for Research in Molecular Medicine and Chronic Diseases (CiMUS), University of Santiago de Compostela (USC), 15706 Santiago de Compostela, Spain

9 Nuclear Medicine Service and Molecular Imaging Group, Health Research Institute of Santiago de Compostela (FIDIS), 15706 Santiago de Compostela, Spain

* Correspondence: daniel.romaus.sanjurjo@sergas.es (D.R.-S.); alberto.ouro.villasante@sergas.es (A.O.); Tel.: +34-981951086 (D.R.-S. & A.O.)

† These authors have contributed equally to this work and share the first authorship.

Abstract: Non-traumatic intracerebral hemorrhage (ICH) is one of the most devastating and disabling forms of stroke; however, there are no effective pharmacological therapies available following the insult. Angiogenesis appears as a key step to overcoming the damage and promoting functional recovery. In this context, endothelial progenitor cells (EPCs) mobilization improves oxidative stress and promotes neovascularization, which has been linked to beneficial outcomes following both ischemic and hemorrhagic stroke. The TNF-like weak inducer of apoptosis (TWEAK), binding to its receptor Fn14, has been suggested as an inducer of EPCs differentiation, viability and migration to the injury site in a model of myocardial infarction. Here, we have performed a proof-of-concept preclinical study in a rat model of ICH where we report that a 50 µg/kg dose of rat recombinant TWEAK (rTWEAK) promotes blood progenitor cells mobilization, mainly EPCs. As soon as 72 h post-injury, brain neovascularization, and, importantly, long-term hematoma reduction and improved functional recovery is reported. In contrast, a higher dose of 150 µg/kg blocked those beneficial outcomes. Therefore, a low dose of rTWEAK treatment promotes neovascularization and reduces brain damage in a rat model of ICH.

Further clinical studies will be needed to demonstrate if rTWEAK could represent a new strategy to promote recovery following ICH.

Keywords: endothelial progenitor cells; intracerebral hemorrhage; neovascularization; TWEAK

1. Introduction

Non-traumatic intracerebral hemorrhage (ICH) results from the spontaneous rupture of blood vessels in the brain and represents one of the most devastating and disabling forms of stroke. It accounts for 10–15% of all cases of stroke, showing the highest mortality rate: more than one-third of patients will not survive the first year [1]. Currently, the lack of effective therapies following ICH prevents better functional outcomes [2].

ICH induces cerebral angiogenesis around hematoma from 4 to 7 days post-lesion [3,4], a fact that has been related to motor recovery following ICH [5]. However, the exact role of endothelium during angiogenesis and neuronal repair following cerebral hemorrhage remains unknown, although endothelial progenitor cells (EPCs) have been suggested as the main players during these processes after stroke [6,7]. EPCs are circulating endothelial cells with the capacity to differentiate into mature endothelial cells and self-renewing [7]. EPCs are mobilized from their niches to the bloodstream following stroke, reaching the damaged area and carrying out neovascularization and endothelial repair through self-differentiation, paracrine signaling and exosomes [8–10]. Importantly, several clinical studies have reported an improved long-term recovery in stroke patients who had higher numbers of circulating EPCs within the first week after both ischemic [11–13] and hemorrhagic [14,15] insults. Furthermore, it has been reported that EPC mobilization reduces oxidative stress in several conditions including hypoxia [16,17]. Therefore, EPCs are a feasible therapeutic target following ICH.

The TNF-like weak inducer of apoptosis (TWEAK) is a ligand of the TNF family that can be presented in two forms: as a transmembrane protein and as a soluble ligand (sTWEAK) following furin proteases activity [18]. TWEAK was initially discovered in cell death-related mechanisms [19], but subsequent achievements revealed that it controls other activities besides apoptosis, such as proliferation, migration, differentiation, angiogenesis, and inflammation [20]. Indeed, the acute inflammatory response has an important role in ICH as shown by the association between several inflammatory biomarkers and a poor outcome following the injury [21]. The binding of sTWEAK to its cellular surface receptor Fn14 triggers several signaling pathways, including the canonical NFκB pathway [20]. The TWEAK-Fn14 axis regulates several physiological processes, and it is particularly important in tissue repair following acute damage [22].

Interestingly, Sheng and colleagues [23] highlighted the relevance of the TWEAK-Fn14-NFκB axis in EPC differentiation, viability, migration to injured tissue and angiogenesis in an in vivo model of acute myocardial infarction. Therefore, TWEAK-mediated mobilization of EPCs could represent a new avenue to promote recovery following ICH. However, the use of TWEAK may be controversial. Several previous studies suggested detrimental effects of endogenous sTWEAK as well as TWEAK treatments in both in vitro and in vivo models of cerebral ischemia [24–27]. There are no preclinical studies addressing the relationship between TWEAK treatment and hemorrhagic stroke so far.

Altogether, the main goal of this proof-of-concept preclinical study was to assess the use of TWEAK as a treatment to provide brain tissue repair through EPCs-mediated neovascularization in a rat model of ICH.

2. Materials and Methods

2.1. Animals

All Experimental protocols were approved by the University Clinical Hospital of Santiago de Compostela Animal Care Committee (15010/2019/004), according to the European Union (EU) rules (86/609/CEE, 2003/65/CE and 2010/63/EU) and the ARRIVE guidelines. Male adult Sprague Dawley (SD) rats (300–350 g) were kept in day/night cycles of 12/12 h at a mean temperature of 22 $\pm$ 1 °C and humidity of 60 $\pm$ 5%, and they had water and food ad libitum.

2.2. ICH Rat Model

The ICH rat model was used as previously described [28,29]. Prior to surgery, animals were injected subcutaneously with buprenorphine dosed at 0.05–0.1 mg/kg. Anesthesia was maintained by inhalation of 4% sevoflurane in a N_2O/O_2 mixture (70/30), and body temperature was maintained at 37 $\pm$ 0.5 °C with a heating pad until animals completely recovered from anesthesia and displayed normal motor activity. Rats were placed in a stereotaxic frame (Stoelting Co., Wood Dale, IL, USA) under sevoflurane anesthesia. After drilling a small burr hole, 1 μL of saline containing 0.2 U/μL bacterial collagenase type VII (Sigma-Aldrich Corp, St. Louis, MO, USA) was injected into the right striatum (0.6 mm anterior to bregma, −3.0 mm lateral and 5.5 mm depth) using a Hamilton syringe with a 30 G needle. Injections took 10 min, and the needle was left for an additional 10 min before removal. The burr hole was filled with bone wax (Ethicon, Somerville, NJ, USA), the scalp incision was closed with sutures, and lidocaine was applied to the wound locally.

2.3. Experimental Groups

Three experimental groups (n = 6 per group) were designated: (1) a control group treated with saline (0.9% of NaCl); (2) 50 group, treated with 50 μg/kg of rat recombinant TWEAK (rTWEAK, #80154-R01H, Sino Biological, Beijing, China) dissolved in saline; and (3) 150 group, treated with 150 μg/kg of rTWEAK dissolved in saline. The concentrations of rTWEAK were selected taking previous work as a reference [30], but here we wanted to assess potential dose-dependent effects. All treatments were given as a single bolus (jugular) at two-timepoints: (1) 1 h after ICH, following the basal magnetic resonance imaging (MRI), and (2) 24 h after ICH induction. The required sample size was calculated from previous studies using the same model in order to be able to detect a 25% effect size on hematoma growth versus controls (2-tailed *t*-test) [28,31]. Six animals per group are required to detect this difference with a power ($1 - \beta$) of 0.8 and $\alpha = 0.05$. N was calculated using EPIDAT software version 4.2 (http://www.sergas.es/Saude-publica/EPIDAT-4-2, v4.2, accessed on 13 May 2025). Animals with hemorrhage located far from the basal ganglia (n = 2) were excluded from the study before treatment administration.

The experimental procedure was performed following several criteria derived from the STAIR (Stroke Therapy Academic Industry Roundtable) group guidelines for preclinical evaluation of stroke therapeutics [32]: (1) ICH hematoma was evaluated at 1 h, right before rTWEAK injections, by T2-weighted MRI to confirm ICH, as an index of the reliability of the hemorrhagic model; (2) animals were randomly assigned to treatment groups of the study; (3) researchers were blinded to treatment administration; (4) researchers were blinded to treatments during outcome assessment; and (5) temperature was controlled during the surgical period.

2.4. Magnetic Resonance Imaging Protocol

Based on a previous hematoma growth profile study [28,29], hematoma volumes were assessed basally (1 h after collagenase injection to induce ICH) and at 24 h, 7, 14, and 28 days after ICH induction by means of MRI conducted on a 9.4-T horizontal bore magnet system (Biospec 94/20USR, Bruker BioSpin, Ettlingen, Germany) with 20 cm-wide actively shielded gradient coils (440 mT/m), as previously described [28,29]. Before MRI acquisition, the animals were placed in a gas chamber containing 6% sevoflurane in a NO_2/O_2 mixture (70/30) until they were unconscious, and then they were positioned prone on the scanner bed. Rectal temperature was maintained at 37 ± 0.5 °C using a feedback-controlled heating pad. Radiofrequency transmission was achieved with a birdcage volume resonator, and the signal was detected using a four-element surface coil positioned over the head of the animal. Gradient-echo pilot scans were performed at the beginning of each imaging session for accurate positioning of the animal inside the magnet bore.

T2-weighted images were acquired using a Rapid Acquisition Relaxation Enhancement (RARE) sequence with the following acquisition parameters: echo time = 9.5 ms, 8 echos, rare factor = 4, repetition time = 3 s, number of averages = 2, field-of-view = 19.2×19.2 mm^2, image matrix = 192×192 (isotropic in-plane resolution of 0.1 mm^2/pixel), and 18 consecutive slices of 0.5 mm thickness. All images were processed using ImageJ (RasbandWS, ImageJ version 2.3, NIH, http://rsb.info.nih.gov/ij, 2.3v, accessed on 13 May 2025). The analyzed region of interest was the hematoma. Hematoma volumes (basal, 24 h and 7, 14, and 28 days), as well as edema volumes (24 h and 7, 14, and 28 days), were manually traced from T2-weighted images by a blind investigator.

Edema was firstly estimated by measuring the volumes of the affected (VLes) and contralateral (Vc) hemispheres and using the formula: edema (%) = $100 \times [(VLes - Vc)/Vc]$. Then, these values were normalized against those from the 24 h timepoint.

2.5. Bederson Scale

Following the STAIR criteria, animal models must show neurological and functional deficits in line with the produced lesion. The model of collagenase-induced hemorrhage primarily damages the striatum, producing a small forelimb paresis contralateral to the lesion. The neurological deficit was evaluated using a modified Bederson scale [33], ranging from 0 (asymptomatic) to 8 (severe deficit), which included the following items: spontaneous movement, spontaneous rotation, spontaneous flexing of the contralateral forelimb, edge detection, turn after tail suspension, and protection reflex.

Behavioral studies were performed at baseline (before surgery), as well as at 1, 7, and 28 days after ICH during the darkness cycle. An experienced blind investigator analyzed the behavioral tests.

2.6. Flow Cytometry Analysis of Blood Progenitor Cells

Blood samples were drawn from the tail vein before ICH (basal sample), and at days 1, 3, 7, 14, and 28 days after ICH. The samples were collected into K2EDTA tubes (BD Microtainer, BD, Franklin Lakes, NJ, USA), and then, erythrocytes were lysated using a commercial kit (FACS Lysing, #349202, BD Biosciences, USA). Immunofluorescence cell staining was performed with fluorescent conjugated antibodies anti-ckit (#567471, BD Biosciences, USA) and anti-sca-1 (#CL8934PE, Cederlane, Burlington, ON, Canada) [34]. Cell fluorescence was measured 15 min after staining by flow cytometry with BD FACS Aria II (BD,

Franklin Lakes, NJ, USA). Numbers of EPCs (ckit$^+$/sca1$^+$) were calculated using the FACS-Diva software (https://www.bdbiosciences.com/en-us/products/software/instrument-software/bd-facsdiva-software accessed on 13 May 2025), as previously described [34].

2.7. Tissue Processing

After the completion of the neuroimaging study, three animals per group at 28 days after ICH were euthanized by an overdose of anesthetic (sevoflurane 8%) and perfused with PBS and 4% formaldehyde. Brains were dissected out coronally in three parts and postfixed, in the same fixative solution, overnight at 4 °C. Brain blocks were rinsed with 0.1 M phosphate buffer and sequentially immersed in 10%, 20%, and 30% (*w*/*v*) sucrose in phosphate buffer until they sank. After cryoprotection, 20 µm-thick coronal sections were obtained with a freezing-sliding cryostat (Leica CM 1950 AgProtect; Leica Microsystems, Wetzlar, Germany).

2.8. Immunofluorescence Protocol

Sections were rinsed in 0.1 M phosphate buffer (PB) and incubated in 50 mM NH4Cl for 30 min. Then, a permeabilization protocol was carried out with 0.3% Triton X-100 (Sigma) in 0.1 M Tris/HCl (pH 8.0) for 10 min. Incubation in the primary antibody solution was carried out in $CaCl_2$-containing buffer (0.1 mM $CaCl_2$, 0.1 mM $MgCl_2$, 0.1 mM MnCl) and blocking solution, 0.05% (*v*/*v*) Triton X-100 (Sigma) and 2% (*v*/*v*) goat serum (Jackson Immunoresearch Laboratories, West Grove, PA, USA) [35]. Rabbit anti-Iba1 (#019-19741, 1:200, Wako Chemicals, Neuss, Germany) and anti-IB4 (#L2140, 1:50, Sigma) primary antibodies were used. Sections were incubated for 2 h at room temperature with fluorophore-conjugated secondary antibodies (1:500, Jackson Immunoresearch Laboratories). Nuclei were stained with the commercial monomeric cyanine nucleic acid stain TO-PRO-3 (far-red fluorescence; Molecular Probes T3605, Invitrogen) for 10 min. After rinsing with PB, sections were mounted with Fluoromount (Sigma) aqueous mounting medium. Sections were examined with a spectral laser confocal microscope (Leica TSC-SL; Leica Microsystems) with three lasers: multiline Argon (488 nm), Helium-Neon (543 nm), and Helium-Neon (633 nm), and equipped with Å~ 40, Å~ 63 (1.4) HCX PL Apo oil immersion objectives for high-resolution imaging.

2.9. Immunofluorescence Quantifications

To quantify the intensity of each immunofluorescence (IF) signal in perilesional cortical regions, the area occupied by IB4+ vessels and Iba1+ was estimated using ImageJ software. All values were normalized against control values. The experimenter was blinded during quantifications.

2.10. Statistical Analyses

Data were presented as mean ± S.E.M. Normality of the data was determined by the Shapiro–Wilk normality test. The results of each experiment (lesion volume, EPCs numbers, immunofluorescence, and Bederson's score) were analyzed by a one-way ANOVA (for normally distributed data) or a Kruskal–Wallis test (for non-normally distributed data). Correlation analysis was assessed with the Pearson correlation coefficient test. In the figures significant values were represented by different numbers of asterisks (vs. 150 µg/kg TWEAK treatment group) or pounds (vs Control group): *(#) $p < 0.05$; **(##) $p < 0.01$; ***(###) $p < 0.001$; ****(####) $p < 0.0001$. Statistical analysis was carried out using Prism 8 (GraphPad software, La Jolla, CA, USA).

3. Results

3.1. rTWEAK Decreases Long-Term Hematoma Volume After ICH Induction

The intraparenchymal injection of collagenase caused an intracerebral hematoma with similar size in all animals at the basal timepoint (Figure 1A–A″,F). The 50 µg/kg dose of rTWEAK showed decreased hematoma at long-term compared with both controls and the 150 µg/kg TWEAK treatment group, although differences were statistically significant at 28 days post-injury only vs. the 150 µg/kg TWEAK treatment group (Kruskal–Wallis test, $p = 0.040$) (Figure 1B–E″,G). In order to investigate the effects of a subacute injection of the treatment (at 24 h), we also analyzed the reduction in brain damage in relation to this timepoint. Here, the long-term reduction in the 50 µg/kg dose is even clearer compared to both controls (Kruskal–Wallis test, $p = 0.132$) and the 150 µg/kg dose (Kruskal–Wallis test, $p = 0.048$) at 28 days post-ICH (Figure 1B–E″,H). Edema was reduced in all experimental groups 7 days post-damage (Figure 1I); there was also a reduction in the volume of the ipsilateral hemisphere compared to the contralateral hemisphere (negative values) at 14 and 28 days, which was bigger in the controls than in the 50 and 150 µg/kg TWEAK treatment groups, but this was not statistically significant (Figure 1I).

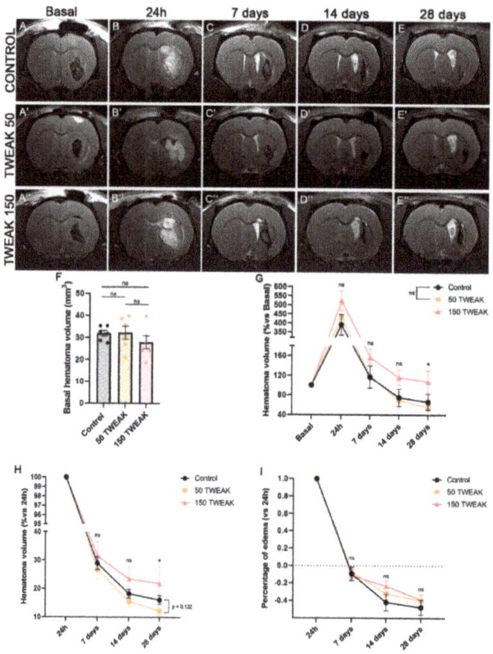

Figure 1. Treatment with 50 µg/kg of rTWEAK promotes a reduction in hematoma in the long term. **(A–E″)** Analysis of hematoma volume was performed by T2-weighted magnetic resonance image. Saline (control) or rTWEAK (50 µg/kg and 150 µg/kg) treatments were administered at 1 and 24 h after collagenase injection. **(F)** Basal hematoma volumes. **(G)** Percentage of hematoma expansion from basal timepoint. **(H)** Percentage of hematoma reduction from the 24 h timepoint. **(I)** Analysis of edema evolution from the 24 h timepoint. In all graphics, results are expressed as the mean ± SEM and analyzed by one-way ANOVA or Kruskal–Wallis tests; differences from 150 group vs. 50 group are denoted as * $p < 0.05$; non-significant results are denoted as "ns". Six rats per group were used.

3.2. rTWEAK Promotes and Maintains Long-Term Blood Progenitor Cell Mobilization

Our analysis demonstrates that only the 50 µg/kg treatment increased the levels of circulating blood progenitor cells, mainly EPCs, at different post-ICH timepoints (Figure 2). Such elevated numbers of EPCs were statistically significant as soon as 72 h post-injury (Kruskal–Wallis test, vs. Control: $p = 0.009$), and at 7 (One-way ANOVA test, vs. Control: $p = 0.013$; vs. 150: $p = 0.045$), 14 (One-way ANOVA test, vs. Control: $p = 0.007$; vs. 150: $p = 0.0004$), and 28 days (Kruskal–Wallis test, vs. Control: $p = 0.004$; vs. 150: $p = 0.010$) (Figure 2A). Moreover, the peak of circulating EPCs in the 50 µg/kg TWEAK treatment group was reached at 7 days post-injury (Figure 2A) and this correlates with lower hematoma volumes at this timepoint (Figure 2B).

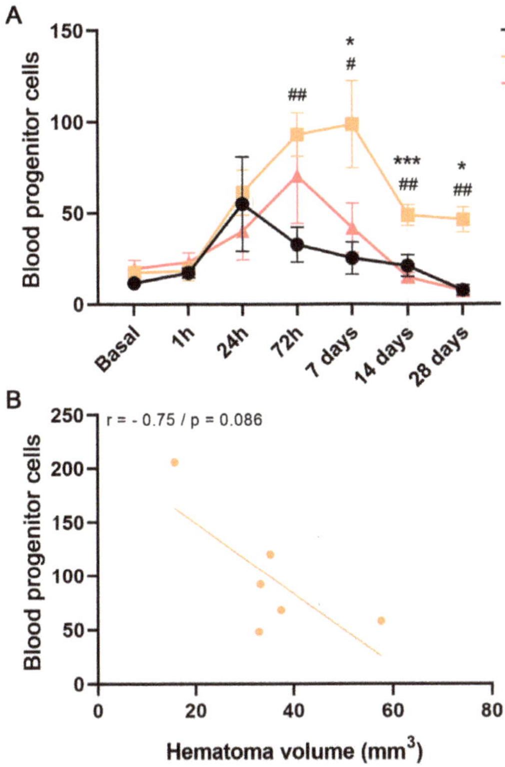

Figure 2. (**A**) Time course of blood progenitor cells numbers from blood samples (250.000 cells counted in each one). Circulating cells were determined by the expression of the surface antigens ckit$^+$/sca1$^+$ using flow cytometry: we first gated sca1$^+$ peripheral blood cells and then examined the resulting population for dual expression of c-kit. Stats at each timepoint are controls (#) and 150 (*) vs. 50 group. Results are expressed as the mean ± SEM and analyzed by one-way ANOVA or Kruskal–Wallis tests (*(#) $p < 0.05$; ## $p < 0.01$; *** $p < 0.001$); non-significant results are denoted as "ns". (**B**) Negative correlation between the number of blood progenitor cells and hematoma volume at 7 days post-injury (Pearson correlation's coefficient, r = −0.75; $p = 0.086$). Six rats per group were used.

3.3. rTWEAK Enhanced Cortical Neovascularization

We performed immunohistochemical analysis targeting the vascular cell marker isolectin-B4 (IB4), which represents a suitable index of vascularization [32,33]. Given that IB4 also labels microglial cells, we used the microglia-specific marker Iba1 to distinguish microglial cells from endothelial cells (Figure 3A–E). Regarding IB4+ cells, we observed that only the 50 μg/kg TWEAK treatment group had increased vascular density in cortical areas at 28 days post-injury, as revealed by the enhanced IB4 staining indicating vascular repair, and so, neovascularization (One-way ANOVA test, vs. Control: $p = 0.0571$; vs. 150: $p = 0.001$) (Figure 3B,E and Figure 4). Moreover, the 150 μg/kg TWEAK treatment group also displayed statistically significant differences compared to controls (One-way ANOVA test, $p = 0.016$). Iba1 staining displayed a 10% increase in the 150 μg/kg TWEAK treatment group compared to controls, but without statistical significance (Figure 3C,E).

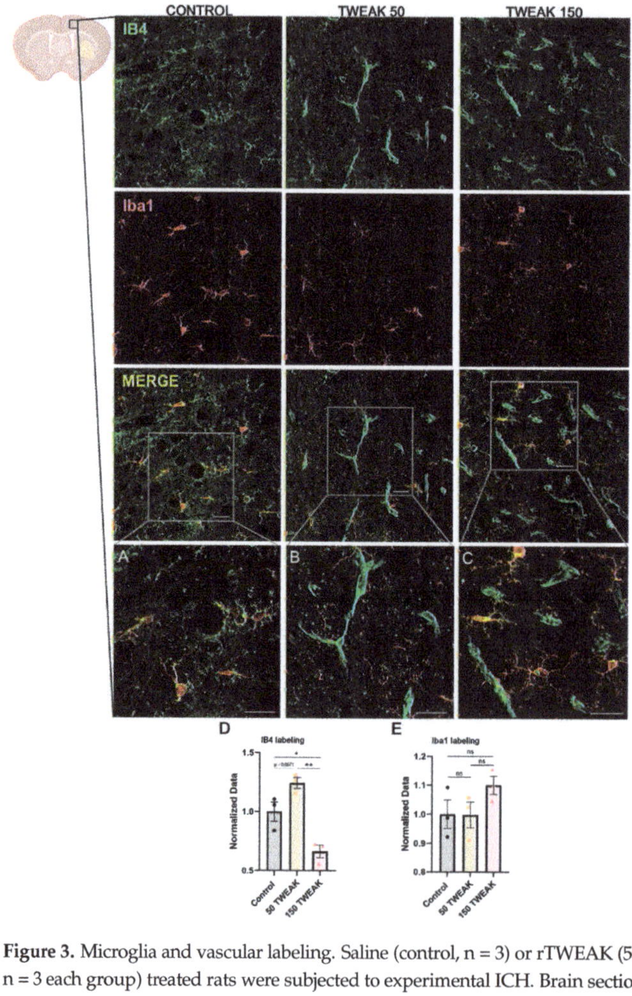

Figure 3. Microglia and vascular labeling. Saline (control, n = 3) or rTWEAK (50 μg/kg and 150 μg/kg, n = 3 each group) treated rats were subjected to experimental ICH. Brain sections were co-stained with the vascular endothelial cell marker IB4 and the microglia-specific marker Iba1 on day 28 after experimental ICH. Scale bars: 50 μm. (**A–C**) Detail from the cortical area (gray box) at higher magnification. Scale bars: 25 μm. Quantification of IB4 (**D**) and Iba1 (**E**) immunoreactivity in perilesional cortical regions. Results are expressed as the mean ± SEM and analyzed by one-way ANOVA test (* $p < 0.05$); (** $p < 0.001$); non-significant results are denoted as "ns". Three rats per group were used.

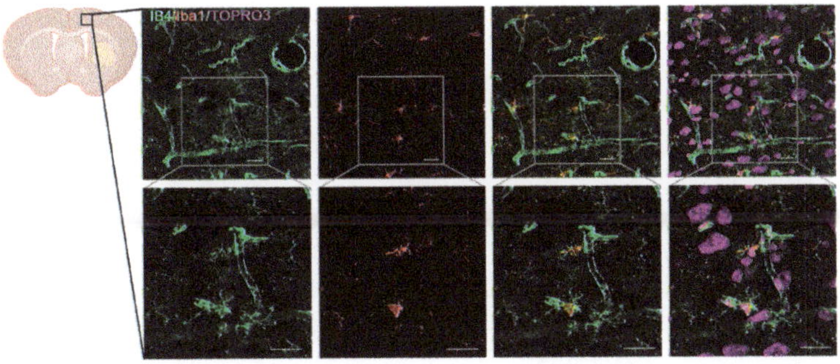

Figure 4. Neovascularization after ICH is increased only by the 50 μg/kg rTWEAK treatment. Brain sections from the 50 group were stained with the vascular endothelial cell marker IB4, the far-red fluorescent nuclear dye TO-PRO3 and the microglia-specific marker Iba1 on day 28 after experimental ICH. Scale bars: 50 μm. Gray box: Detail at higher magnification. Scale bars: 25 μm. Three rats per group were used.

3.4. The Effect of rTWEAK Treatments on Neurological Recovery

We used the modified Bederson scale to assess any beneficial effect of rTWEAK treatments on the neurological deficits caused by the hemorrhagic lesion. Results showed that scores were close to 0 at baseline, as expected for healthy subjects (Figure 5A); however, both rTWEAK treatments showed higher deficit at 48 h (Figure 5A), in agreement with the larger hematoma volume seen at 24 h. Therefore, we analyzed the effects of a subacute injection (24 h) and observed that the 50 μg/kg dose, but not 150 μg/kg dose, induced a relevant neurological recovery at post-ICH timepoints compared to both other groups, especially at 28 days (Kruskal–Wallis test, vs. controls: $p = 0.1688$; vs. 150: $p = 0.012$) post-injury (Figure 5B).

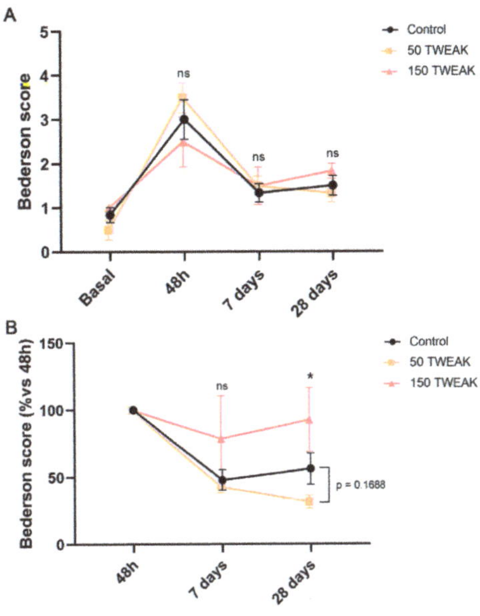

Figure 5. The 50 μg/kg rTWEAK treatments improved long-term neurological recovery after ICH. Neurological deficit was evaluated by the Bederson scale. (**A**) Bederson scores were obtained in the

control and rats treated with the 50 µg/kg dose or the 150 µg/kg dose at 1 day before surgery (baseline) and 48 h, 7, and 28 days afterwards. (**B**) Analysis of neurological recovery from a 48 h timepoint. Results are expressed as the mean ± SEM and analyzed by the Kruskal–Wallis test (* $p < 0.05$); non-significant results are denoted as "ns". Six rats per group were used.

4. Discussion

In this study, we show that a 50 µg/kg dose of rTWEAK induces smaller long-term lesion volumes, mobilizes higher numbers of circulating blood progenitor cells, mainly EPCs, and enhances neovascularization. Thus, our study represents the first proof-of-concept study assessing the therapeutic and dose-effect of TWEAK treatments in an animal model of ICH. Remarkably, our results suggest a direct effect of this treatment on EPCs-mediated vascularization. Here, we discuss the implications and possible mechanisms underlying this TWEAK-mediated response following ICH.

The role of the TWEAK-Fn14 axis as an in vitro and in vivo inducer of growth, proliferation, and migration of mature and progenitor endothelial cells is well-known, and it acts in a dose-dependent manner [23,25,36–40]. Intriguingly, our experiments showed that the rTWEAK treatment of 50 µg/kg mobilizes progenitor cells to the blood flow, likely EPCs, in a significant way, whereas the 150 µg/kg concentration had no effect on EPCs, likely because of the saturation of the Fn14 receptor. Moreover, several previous studies also showed that TWEAK can promote angiogenesis in mature and progenitor endothelial cells both in vitro and in vivo [23,36,37,39]. Our experimental group treated with a 50 µg/kg dose of TWEAK showed a higher degree of neovascularization in immunohistochemical analysis at day 28 post-injury, which agrees with previous studies. Based on the important role of EPCs in angiogenesis and neovascularization [7], it is plausible that a low dose of TWEAK induces EPCs-mediated neovascularization, given that this outcome was not seen in the high-dose group, where no significant EPCs mobilization was seen. Future studies should confirm whether TWEAK-mediated neovascularization is achieved through EPCs mobilization and/or angiogenic factors.

Addition to modulating angiogenesis and neovascularization, many studies have addressed the beneficial roles of EPCs following stroke such as reducing inflammation and promoting neuronal survival [7]. Indeed, higher numbers of circulating EPCs within the first week were associated with an improved long-term recovery in patients who suffered from both ischemic [11–13] and hemorrhagic [14,15] stroke. Here, we observed a higher and sustained EPCs mobilization and neovascularization after the administration of the 50 µg/kg dose, which was reflected in a beneficial long-term outcome both on lesion volume and on the neurological recovery of animals compared to control counterparts. Furthermore, peak levels of circulating EPCs in the 50 µg/kg TWEAK treatment group were reached at 7 days post-injury and were correlated with lower hematoma volumes. This result aligns with a previous clinical study of our group, in which hemorrhagic stroke patients with good functional outcome showed higher EPC levels at day 7, and a correlation was found between increased levels of EPCs and smaller ICH residual volume at 6 months [15]. Based on this, we proposed an indirect effect of TWEAK on reducing ICH damage through EPCs. As previously discussed, EPCs can promote angiogenesis and the repair of damaged vessels as well as trigger neovascularization. Moreover, a protective role of EPCs has been suggested by maintaining the integrity of the blood–brain barrier (BBB) following both ischemic [41] and hemorrhagic [15] stroke. Overall, our results highlight the positive role of increasing EPCs following stroke likely by restoring and protecting vascular integrity.

Results in rodent models of ischemic stroke showed that the blockage of the TWEAK/Fn14 axis results in beneficial effects [24–27]. Similarly, a few clinical studies reported a potential correlation between serum levels of sTWEAK and a poor functional outcome in ischemic stroke patients [42], as well as with the risk of developing early ICH growth [43]. Moreover, the ICH injury may not activate the same molecular pathways as the ischemic injury (e.g., the NFκB pathway [44]) [29,45], and this could explain the differences between previous ischemic studies and our results. Nevertheless, our strategy was not based on inhibiting TWEAK but on using it in a low dose given that several works indicated that the TWEAK/Fn14 axis can coordinate the inflammation and the response of progenitor cells in the context of acute tissue damage to promote tissue repair [46]. In this way, present results suggest that our hypothesis was partially right as the 50 μg/kg dose exhibited modest results compared to the control group regarding lesion, edema, and behavior, but it had a major impact on EPCs dynamics and angiogenesis. Remarkably, the second injection at 24 h post-injury appeared to be crucial in this TWEAK-mediated EPCs mobilization. Indeed, acute injection of rTWEAK at 1 h post-injury seems to slightly increase injury volumes at 24 h. Such results suggest that the subacute treatment is more efficient than the acute one, which may explain the statistically relevant differences when data are relativized to 24 h/48 h. Therefore, this indicates that activating the TWEAK/Fn14 axis following hemorrhagic stroke is not harmful per se, but it depends on the intensity and/or the timing. Further studies assessing lower doses than 50 μg/kg of TWEAK at different subacute/chronic timepoints would be necessary to find the best dose and time to apply the treatment.

TWEAK is a pro-inflammatory cytokine that controls other activities besides apoptosis, such as inflammation and oxidative stress [18,47–50]. A previous in vitro study reported the dose-dependent increase in pro-inflammatory cytokines released by astrocytes treated with TWEAK [51]. Similarly, we showed that only the 150 μg/kg TWEAK treatment group had an increase in microglia labeling on day 28 after ICH, suggesting increased neuroinflammation even in the chronic phase of the insult. Indeed, microglia plays vital roles in both tissue damage and repair processes after ICH, specifically the perihematomal activated microglia [52]. So, it is plausible that this increased inflammation seen in the 150 μg/kg TWEAK treatment group is linked to higher lesion volumes and sensorimotor deficit. Furthermore, excessive TWEAK-mediated activation increases reactive oxygen species in several cell cultures, including human umbilical vein endothelial cells [47], macrophages [48], and astrocytes [49]. Both neuroinflammation and oxidative damage are important causes of BBB disruption, as they alter the architecture of the neurovascular unit (NVU) and they exacerbate the brain injury following ICH as well [53]. Our data reported that a 150 μg/kg dose of TWEAK increased the hematoma volume compared to the control and the 50 μg/kg groups at all timepoints after ICH. Several in vivo studies showed glial cells as the main targets of endogenous TWEAK that trigger BBB dysfunction after cerebral ischemia and ICH [25–27,52,54,55]. Based on our data, we hypothesize that the 150 μg/kg dose is harmful enough to act on and activate NVU-forming glial cells, resulting in bigger lesion volumes and poorer animal behavior. Undoubtedly, further studies are mandatory to elucidate the exact impact of TWEAK on glial cells and BBB dysfunction following ICH.

There are several limitations in this study. We used the IB4 marker to assess angiogenesis as it is widely used as a well-known index of neovascularization [35,56]. Although additional assays assessing angiogenesis would have provided further information on this process, our proof-of-concept study fully supports the assumption that a 50 μg/kg dose of TWEAK promotes angiogenesis in vivo following ICH. This result agrees with previous studies showing that TWEAK activates the Hippo-YAP signaling [57], a positive regulator of angiogenesis [58], and promotes EPCs differentiation, viability, migration to injured tissue and angiogenesis in an in vivo model of acute myocardial infarction [23]. We cannot exclude the possibility of EPC-derived secretome/exosomes having a role during the neovascularization seen in this study [7,59], and future studies are needed to decipher the exact impact of these exosomes during this process. We characterized blood progenitor cells by studying the surface expression of both sca1 and ckit antibodies as previously described [34]. Although we did not determine the co-expression of those markers with CD31, a mature endothelial marker, ~90% of sca-1^+ cells are also $CD31^+$ [34], and so the majority of these cells are EPCs. Importantly, our results agree with those from hemorrhagic stroke patients, showing a correlation between increased levels of EPCs and smaller ICH residual volume at 6 months [15], similar to what we report here. Finally, the sample size may be considered a limitation as the 50 μg/kg dose exhibited modest results compared to the control group regarding lesion, edema, and behavior, although such differences are close to the statistical significance at day 28. However, this is a proof-of-concept preclinical study to assess the use of TWEAK as a treatment to provide brain tissue repair through EPCs-mediated neovascularization in a rat model of ICH, and present results suggest that our hypothesis is correct, as we observed a major impact on EPCs dynamics and angiogenesis.

In conclusion, we found that a 50 μg/kg dose of rTWEAK mobilizes higher numbers of circulating EPCs, enhances neovascularization, and induces smaller lesion volumes. Remarkably, our results suggest a direct effect of this treatment on EPC-mediated vascularization. However, further regulatory preclinical and clinical studies should be conducted to clarify whether rTWEAK may be able to be a therapeutic target in hemorrhagic stroke.

Author Contributions: Conceptualization and design, D.R.-S., E.L.-A., A.O. and T.S.; methodology, D.R.-S., E.L.-A., C.R., P.H., M.R.-A., M.D.-M. and R.I.-R.; data analysis, D.R.-S., E.L.-A., C.R., P.H., M.R.-A., M.D.-M., J.M.P.-P., P.A., Á.A., J.C., A.O. and T.S.; writing the draft, D.R.-S. and T.S.; funding acquisition, D.R.-S., Á.A., J.C. and T.S. All authors have contributed to editing the manuscript. All authors have read and agreed to the published version of the manuscript.

Funding: This study was partially supported by grants from the Xunta de Galicia (IN607A2022/07), Instituto de Salud Carlos III (ISCIII) (PI22/00938; PI21/00727; RD21/0006/0005) and CIBERNED (CB22/05/00067). This project has also received funding from the European Union's Horizon 2020 research and innovation program under the Marie Skłodowska-Curie grant agreement (No. 101066444). R. Iglesias-Rey from the Miguel Servet Program of Instituto de Salud Carlos III and co-financed by the EU (CP22/00061). Furthermore, this study was also supported by grants from the INTERREG Atlantic Area (EAPA_791/2018_NEUROATLANTIC project), INTER-REG V A España Portugal (POCTEP) (0624_2IQBIONEURO_6_E), and the European Regional Development Fund (ERDF).

Institutional Review Board Statement: The animal study protocol was approved by the University Clinical Hospital of Santiago de Compostela Animal Care Committee (15010/2019/004), according to the European Union (EU) rules (86/609/CEE, 2003/65/CE and 2010/63/EU) and the ARRIVE guidelines.

Informed Consent Statement: Not applicable.

Data Availability Statement: Data are contained within the article.

Conflicts of Interest: The authors declare no conflicts of interest. The funders had no role in the design of the study; in the collection, analyses, or interpretation of data; in the writing of the manuscript; or in the decision to publish the results.

Abbreviations

The following abbreviations are used in this manuscript:

BBB	Blood–brain barrier
EPCs	Endothelial progenitor cells
ICH	Non-traumatic intracerebral hemorrhage
IF	Immunofluorescence
MRI	Magnetic resonance imaging
rTWEAK	Recombinant TWEAK
PB	Phosphate buffer
RARE	Rapid Acquisition Relaxation Enhancement
STAIR	Stroke Therapy Academic Industry Roundtable
TWEAK	TNF-like weak inducer of apoptosis

References

1. Carhuapoma, L.; Murthy, S.; Shah, V.A. Outcome Trajectories after Intracerebral Hemorrhage. *Semin. Neurol.* **2024**, *44*, 298–307. [CrossRef] [PubMed]
2. Seiffge, D.J.; Fandler-Höfler, S.; Du, Y.; Goeldlin, M.B.; Jolink, W.M.; Klijn, C.J.; Werring, D.J. Intracerebral haemorrhage—Mechanisms, diagnosis and prospects for treatment and prevention. *Nat. Rev. Neurol.* **2024**, *20*, 708–723. [CrossRef] [PubMed]
3. Tang, T.; Liu, X.J.; Zhang, Z.Q.; Zhou, H.J.; Luo, J.K.; Huang, J.F.; Yang, Q.D.; Li, X.Q. Cerebral angiogenesis after collagenase-induced intracerebral hemorrhage in rats. *Brain Res.* **2007**, *1175*, 134–142. [CrossRef] [PubMed]
4. Yang, A.L.; Zhou, H.J.; Tang, T.; Luo, J.K.; Cui, H.J. Temporal profile of angiogenesis and expression of extracellular matrix-related genes in rat brains following experimental intracerebral hemorrhage. *Sci. Prog.* **2022**, *105*, 368504221115509. [CrossRef]
5. Hua, Y.; Schallert, T.; Keep, R.F.; Wu, J.; Hoff, J.T.; Xi, G. Behavioral tests after intracerebral hemorrhage in the rat. *Stroke* **2002**, *33*, 2478–2484. [CrossRef]
6. Pías-Peleteiro, J.; Campos, F.; Perez-Mato, M.; Lopez-Arias, E.; Rodriguez-Yanez, M.; Castillo, J.; Sobrino, T. Endothelial Progenitor Cells as a Therapeutic Approach for Intracerebral Hemorrhage. *Curr. Pharm. Des.* **2017**, *23*, 2238–2251. [CrossRef]
7. Custodia, A.; Ouro, A.; Sargento-Freitas, J.; Aramburu-Núñez, M.; Pías-Peleteiro, J.M.; Hervella, P.; Rosell, A.; Ferreira, L.; Castillo, J.; Romaus-Sanjurjo, D. Unraveling the potential of endothelial progenitor cells as a treatment following ischemic stroke. *Front. Neurol.* **2022**, *13*, 940682. [CrossRef]
8. Banno, K.; Yoder, M.C. Tissue regeneration using endothelial colony-forming cells: Promising cells for vascular repair. *Pediatr. Res.* **2018**, *83*, 283–290. [CrossRef]
9. Hayakawa, K.; Chan, S.J.; Mandeville, E.T.; Park, J.H.; Bruzzese, M.; Montaner, J.; Arai, K.; Rosell, A.; Lo, E.H. Protective Effects of Endothelial Progenitor Cell-Derived Extracellular Mitochondria in Brain Endothelium. *Stem Cells* **2018**, *36*, 1404–1410. [CrossRef]
10. Yan, F.; Liu, X.; Ding, H.; Zhang, W. Paracrine mechanisms of endothelial progenitor cells in vascular repair. *Acta Histochem.* **2022**, *124*, 151833. [CrossRef]
11. Sobrino, T.; Hurtado, O.; Moro, M.A.; Rodri, M.; Castellanos, M.; Brea, D.; Moldes, O.; Blanco, M.; Arenillas, J.F.; Leira, R. The increase of circulating endothelial progenitor cells after acute ischemic stroke is associated with good outcome. *Stroke* **2007**, *38*, 2759–2764. [CrossRef] [PubMed]
12. Sobrino, T.; Pérez-Mato, M.; Brea, D.; Rodríguez-Yáñez, M.; Blanco, M.; Castillo, J. Temporal profile of molecular signatures associated with circulating endothelial progenitor cells in human ischemic stroke. *J. Neurosci. Res.* **2012**, *90*, 1788–1793. [CrossRef]
13. Xue, L.; Chen, H.; Zhang, T.; Chen, J.; Geng, Z.; Zhao, Y. Changes in serum vascular endothelial growth factor and endostatin concentrations associated with circulating endothelial progenitor cells after acute ischemic stroke. *Metab. Brain Dis.* **2017**, *32*, 641–648. [CrossRef]
14. Paczkowska, E.; Gołąb-Janowska, M.; Bajer-Czajkowska, A.; Machalińska, A.; Ustianowski, P.; Rybicka, M.; Kłos, P.; Dziedziejko, V.; Safranow, K.; Nowacki, P.; et al. Increased circulating endothelial progenitor cells in patients with haemorrhagic and ischaemic stroke: The role of endothelin-1. *J. Neurol. Sci.* **2013**, *325*, 90–99. [CrossRef] [PubMed]
15. Pías-Peleteiro, J.; Pérez-Mato, M.; López-Arias, E.; Rodríguez-Yáñez, M.; Blanco, M.; Campos, F.; Castillo, J.; Sobrino, T. Increased Endothelial Progenitor Cell Levels are Associated with Good Outcome in Intracerebral Hemorrhage. *Sci. Rep.* **2016**, *6*, 28724. [CrossRef] [PubMed]
16. Tousoulis, D.; Andreou, I.; Antoniades, C.; Tentolouris, C.; Stefanadis, C. Role of inflammation and oxidative stress in endothelial progenitor cell function and mobilization: Therapeutic implications for cardiovascular diseases. *Atherosclerosis* **2008**, *201*, 236–247. [CrossRef]

17. Halurkar, M.S.; Wang, J.; Chen, S.; Bihl, J.C. EPC-EXs improve astrocyte survival and oxidative stress through different uptaking pathways in diabetic hypoxia condition. *Stem Cell Res. Ther.* **2022**, *13*, 91. [CrossRef]
18. Trebing, J.; Arana, J.A.; Salzmann, S.; Wajant, H. Analyzing the signaling capabilities of soluble and membrane TWEAK. *Methods Mol. Biol.* **2014**, *1155*, 31–45.
19. Chicheportiche, Y.; Bourdon, P.R.; Xu, H.; Hsu, Y.-M.; Scott, H.; Hession, C.; Garcia, I.; Browning, J.L. TWEAK, a new secreted ligand in the tumor necrosis factor family that weakly induces apoptosis. *J. Biol. Chem.* **1997**, *272*, 32401–32410. [CrossRef]
20. Winkles, J.A. The TWEAK-Fn14 cytokine-receptor axis: Discovery, biology and therapeutic targeting. *Nat. Rev. Drug Discov.* **2008**, *7*, 411–425. [CrossRef]
21. Bader, E.R.; Pana, T.A.; Barlas, R.S.; Metcalf, A.K.; Potter, J.F.; Myint, P.K. Elevated inflammatory biomarkers and poor outcomes in intracerebral hemorrhage. *J. Neurol.* **2022**, *269*, 6330–6341. [CrossRef] [PubMed]
22. Wang, S.; Li, L.; Cook, C.; Zhang, Y.; Xia, Y.; Liu, Y. A potential fate decision landscape of the TWEAK/Fn14 axis on stem and progenitor cells: A systematic review. *Stem Cell Res. Ther.* **2022**, *13*, 270. [CrossRef]
23. Sheng, Z.; Ju, C.; Li, B.; Chen, Z.; Pan, X.; Yan, G.; He, Y.; Yao, Y.; Ma, G. TWEAK promotes endothelial progenitor cell vasculogenesis to alleviate acute myocardial infarction via the Fn14-NF-κB signaling pathway. *Exp. Ther. Med.* **2018**, *16*, 4019–4029. [CrossRef] [PubMed]
24. Potrovita, I.; Zhang, W.; Burkly, L.; Hahm, K.; Lincecum, J.; Wang, M.Z.; Maurer, M.H.; Rossner, M.; Schneider, A.; Schwaninger, M. Tumor necrosis factor-like weak inducer of apoptosis-induced neurodegeneration. *J. Neurosci.* **2004**, *24*, 8237–8244. [CrossRef]
25. Polavarapu, R.; Gongora, M.C.; Winkles, J.A.; Yepes, M. Tumor necrosis factor-like weak inducer of apoptosis increases the permeability of the neurovascular unit through nuclear factor-kappa B pathway activation. *J. Neurosci.* **2005**, *25*, 10094–10100. [CrossRef]
26. Yepes, M.; Brown, S.A.; Moore, E.G.; Smith, E.P.; Lawrence, D.A.; Winkles, J.A. A soluble Fn14-Fc decoy receptor reduces infarct volume in a murine model of cerebral ischemia. *Am. J. Pathol.* **2005**, *166*, 511–520. [CrossRef]
27. Zhang, X.; Winkles, J.A.; Gongora, M.C.; Polavarapu, R.; Michaelson, J.S.; Hahm, K.; Burkly, L.; Friedman, M.; Li, X.-J.; Yepes, M. TWEAK-Fn14 pathway inhibition protects the integrity of the neurovascular unit during cerebral ischemia. *J. Cereb. Blood Flow. Metab.* **2007**, *27*, 534–544. [CrossRef]
28. Rodríguez, J.A.; Sobrino, T.; López-Arias, E.; Ugarte, A.; Sánchez-Arias, J.A.; Vieites-Prado, A.; de Miguel, I.; Oyarzabal, J.; Páramo, J.A.; Campos, F. CM352 Reduces Brain Damage and Improves Functional Recovery in a Rat Model of Intracerebral Hemorrhage. *J. Am. Heart Assoc.* **2017**, *6*, e006042. [CrossRef] [PubMed]
29. Gómez-Lado, N.; López-Arias, E.; Iglesias-Rey, R.; Díaz-PlatasSantiago, L.; Medín-AguerreAnxo, S.; Fernández-FerreiroAdrián, A.; Posado-FernándezLara, A.; García-VarelaManuel, L.; Rodríguez-Pérez, M.; Campos, F. [18F]-FMISO PET/MRI Imaging Shows Ischemic Tissue around Hematoma in Intracerebral Hemorrhage. *Mol. Pharm.* **2020**, *17*, 4667–4675. [CrossRef]
30. Dogra, C.; Changotra, H.; Wedhas, N.; Qin, X.; Wergedal, J.E.; Kumar, A. TNF-related weak inducer of apoptosis (TWEAK) is a potent skeletal muscle-wasting cytokine. *FASEB J.* **2007**, *21*, 1857–1869. [CrossRef]
31. da Silva-Candal, A.; Vieites-Prado, A.; Gutiérrez-Fernández, M.; Rey, R.I.; Argibay, B.; Mirelman, D.; Sobrino, T.; Rodríguez-Frutos, B.; Castillo, J.; Campos, F. Blood glutamate grabbing does not reduce the hematoma in an intracerebral hemorrhage model but it is a safe excitotoxic treatment modality. *J. Cereb. Blood Flow. Metab.* **2015**, *35*, 1206–1212. [CrossRef]
32. Philip, M.; Benatar, M.; Fisher, M.; Savitz, S.I. Methodological quality of animal studies of neuroprotective agents currently in phase II/III acute ischemic stroke trials. *Stroke* **2009**, *40*, 577–581. [CrossRef] [PubMed]
33. Bederson, J.B.; Pitts, L.H.; Tsuji, M.; Nishimura, M.C.; Davis, R.L.; Bartkowski, H. Rat middle cerebral artery occlusion: Evaluation of the model and development of a neurologic examination. *Stroke* **1986**, *17*, 472–476. [CrossRef] [PubMed]
34. Fadini, G.P.; Sartore, S.; Schiavon, M.; Albiero, M.; Baesso, I.; Cabrelle, A.; Agostini, C.; Avogaro, A. Diabetes impairs progenitor cell mobilisation after hindlimb ischaemia-reperfusion injury in rats. *Diabetologia* **2006**, *49*, 3075–3084. [CrossRef] [PubMed]
35. Rodríguez, C.; Sobrino, T.; Agulla, J.; Bobo-Jiménez, V.; Ramos-Araque, M.E.; Duarte, J.J.; Gómez-Sánchez, J.C.; Bolaños, J.P.; Castillo, J.; Almeida, Á. Neovascularization and functional recovery after intracerebral hemorrhage is conditioned by the Tp53 Arg72Pro single-nucleotide polymorphism. *Cell Death Differ.* **2017**, *24*, 144–154. [CrossRef]
36. Lynch, C.N.; Wang, Y.C.; Lund, J.K.; Chen, Y.W.; Leal, J.A.; Wiley, S.R. TWEAK induces angiogenesis and proliferation of endothelial cells. *J. Biol. Chem.* **1999**, *274*, 8455–8459. [CrossRef]
37. Wiley, S.R.; Cassiano, L.; Lofton, T.; Davis-Smith, T.; Winkles, J.A.; Lindner, V.; Liu, H.; Daniel, T.O.; Smith, C.A.; Fanslow, W.C. A novel TNF receptor family member binds TWEAK and is implicated in angiogenesis. *Immunity* **2001**, *15*, 837–846. [CrossRef]
38. Harada, N.; Nakayama, M.; Nakano, H.; Fukuchi, Y.; Yagita, H.; Okumura, K. Pro-inflammatory effect of TWEAK/Fn14 interaction on human umbilical vein endothelial cells. *Biochem. Biophys. Res. Commun.* **2002**, *299*, 488–493. [CrossRef]
39. Jakubowski, A.; Browning, B.; Lukashev, M.; Sizing, I.; Thompson, J.S.; Benjamin, C.D.; Hsu, Y.-M.; Ambrose, C.; Zheng, T.S.; Burkly, L.C. Dual role for TWEAK in angiogenic regulation. *J. Cell Sci.* **2002**, *115*, 267–274. [CrossRef]

40. Donohue, P.J.; Richards, C.M.; Brown, S.A.; Hanscom, H.N.; Buschman, J.; Thangada, S.; Hla, T.; Williams, M.S.; Winkles, J.A. TWEAK is an endothelial cell growth and chemotactic factor that also potentiates FGF-2 and VEGF-A mitogenic activity. *Arter. Thromb. Vasc. Biol.* **2003**, *23*, 594–600. [CrossRef]
41. Martí-Fàbregas, J.; Crespo, J.; Delgado-Mederos, R.; Martínez-Ramírez, S.; Peña, E.; Marín, R.; Dinia, L.; Jiménez-Xarrié, E.; Fernández-Arcos, A.; Pérez-Pérez, J.; et al. Endothelial progenitor cells in acute ischemic stroke. *Brain Behav.* **2013**, *3*, 649–655. [CrossRef] [PubMed]
42. da Silva-Candal, A.; Pérez-Mato, M.; Rodríguez-Yáñez, M.; López-Dequidt, I.; Pumar, J.M.; Ávila-Gómez, P.; Sobrino, T.; Campos, F.; Castillo, J.; Hervella, P. The presence of leukoaraiosis enhances the association between sTWEAK and hemorrhagic transformation. *Ann. Clin. Transl. Neurol.* **2020**, *7*, 2103–2114. [CrossRef] [PubMed]
43. da Silva-Candal, A.; López-Dequidt, I.; Rodriguez-Yañez, M.; Ávila-Gómez, P.; Pumar, J.M.; Castillo, J.; Sobrino, T.; Campos, F.; Iglesias-Rey, R.; Hervella, P. sTWEAK is a marker of early haematoma growth and leukoaraiosis in intracerebral haemorrhage. *Stroke Vasc. Neurol.* **2021**, *6*, 528–535. [CrossRef]
44. Shih, R.H.; Wang, C.Y.; Yang, C.M. NF-kappaB Signaling Pathways in Neurological Inflammation: A Mini Review. *Front. Mol. Neurosci.* **2015**, *8*, 77. [CrossRef]
45. Xi, G.; Keep, R.F.; Hoff, J.T. Mechanisms of brain injury after intracerebral haemorrhage. *Lancet Neurol.* **2006**, *5*, 53–63. [CrossRef]
46. Burkly, L.C.; Michaelson, J.S.; Hahm, K.; Jakubowski, A.; Zheng, T.S. TWEAKing tissue remodeling by a multifunctional cytokine: Role of TWEAK/Fn14 pathway in health and disease. *Cytokine* **2007**, *40*, 1–16. [CrossRef] [PubMed]
47. Liu, H.; Peng, H.; Xiang, H.; Guo, L.; Chen, R.; Zhao, S.; Chen, W.; Chen, P.; Lu, H.; Chen, S. TWEAK/Fn14 promotes oxidative stress through AMPK/PGC-1α/MnSOD signaling pathway in endothelial cells. *Mol. Med. Rep.* **2018**, *17*, 1998–2004. [CrossRef]
48. Madrigal-Matute, J.; Fernandez-Laso, V.; Sastre, C.; Llamas-Granda, P.; Egido, J.; Martin-Ventura, J.L.; Zalba, G.; Blanco-Colio, L.M. TWEAK/Fn14 interaction promotes oxidative stress through NADPH oxidase activation in macrophages. *Cardiovasc. Res.* **2015**, *108*, 139–147. [CrossRef]
49. Samidurai, M.; Tarale, P.; Janarthanam, C.; Estrada, C.G.; Gordon, R.; Zenitsky, G.; Jin, H.; Anantharam, V.; Kanthasamy, A.G.; Kanthasamy, A. Tumor Necrosis Factor-Like Weak Inducer of Apoptosis (TWEAK) Enhances Activation of STAT3/NLRC4 Inflammasome Signaling Axis through PKCδ in Astrocytes: Implications for Parkinson's Disease. *Cells* **2020**, *9*, 1831. [CrossRef]
50. Tarín, C.; Fernández-Laso, V.; Sastre, C.; Madrigal-Matute, J.; Gómez, M.; Zaragoza, C.; Egido, J.; Burkly, L.C.; Martín-Ventura, J.L.; Blanco-Colio, L.M. Tumor necrosis factor-like weak inducer of apoptosis or Fn14 deficiency reduce elastase perfusion-induced aortic abdominal aneurysm in mice. *J. Am. Heart Assoc.* **2014**, *3*, e000723. [CrossRef]
51. Saas, P.; Boucraut, J.; Walker, P.R.; Quiquerez, A.-L.; Billot, M.; Desplat-Jego, S.; Chicheportiche, Y.; Dietrich, P.-Y. TWEAK stimulation of astrocytes and the proinflammatory consequences. *Glia* **2000**, *32*, 102–107. [CrossRef] [PubMed]
52. Bi, R.; Fang, Z.; You, M.; He, Q.; Hu, B. Microglia Phenotype and Intracerebral Hemorrhage: A Balance of Yin and Yang. *Front. Cell Neurosci.* **2021**, *15*, 765205. [CrossRef] [PubMed]
53. Shao, L.; Chen, S.; Ma, L. Secondary Brain Injury by Oxidative Stress After Cerebral Hemorrhage: Recent Advances. *Front. Cell Neurosci.* **2022**, *16*, 853589. [CrossRef]
54. Zhang, Y.; Khan, S.; Liu, Y.; Wu, G.; Yong, V.W.; Xue, M. Oxidative Stress Following Intracerebral Hemorrhage: From Molecular Mechanisms to Therapeutic Targets. *Front. Immunol.* **2022**, *13*, 847246. [CrossRef]
55. Zheng, Y.; Li, R.; Fan, X. Targeting Oxidative Stress in Intracerebral Hemorrhage: Prospects of the Natural Products Approach. *Antioxidants* **2022**, *11*, 1811. [CrossRef] [PubMed]
56. Wälchli, T.; Mateos, J.M.; Weinman, O.; Babic, D.; Regli, L.; Hoerstrup, S.P.; Gerhardt, H.; Schwab, M.E.; Vogel, J. Quantitative assessment of angiogenesis, perfused blood vessels and endothelial tip cells in the postnatal mouse brain. *Nat. Protoc.* **2015**, *10*, 53–74. [CrossRef]
57. Tong, W.; Zhu, L.; Han, P.; Bai, Y.; Wang, T.; Chen, D.; Li, Z.; Chi, H.; Deng, X.; Zhang, Y.; et al. TWEAK is an activator of Hippo-YAP signaling protecting against hepatic Ischemia/ reperfusion injury. *Int. Immunopharmacol.* **2024**, *143*, 113567. [CrossRef]
58. Kim, J.; Kim, Y.H.; Kim, J.; Park, D.Y.; Bae, H.; Lee, D.H.; Kim, K.H.; Hong, S.P.; Jang, S.P.; Kubota, Y.; et al. YAP/TAZ regulates sprouting angiogenesis and vascular barrier maturation. *J. Clin. Investig.* **2017**, *127*, 3441–3461. [CrossRef]
59. Rosell, A.; Morancho, A.; Navarro-Sobrino, M.; Martínez-Saez, E.; Hernández-Guillamon, M.; Lope-Piedrafita, S.; Barceló, V.; Borrás, F.; Penalba, A.; García-Bonilla, L.; et al. Factors secreted by endothelial progenitor cells enhance neurorepair responses after cerebral ischemia in mice. *PLoS ONE* **2013**, *8*, e73244. [CrossRef]

antioxidants

MDPI

Article

The Inhibition of Prolyl Endopeptidase (PREP) by KYP-2047 Treatment to Reduce Myocardial Ischemia/Reperfusion Injury

Laura Cucinotta [1,†], Nicoletta Palermo [2,†], Alessio Ardizzone [1], Anna Paola Capra [1], Michela Campolo [1], Emanuela Esposito [1], Giovanna Casili [1,*] and Marika Lanza [1]

[1] Department of Chemical, Biological, Pharmaceutical and Environmental Sciences, University of Messina, Viale Ferdinando Stagno D'Alcontres, 31, 98166 Messina, Italy

[2] Department of Biomedical and Dental Sciences and Morphofunctional Imaging, University of Messina, Via Consolare Valeria, 1, 98125 Messina, Italy

* Correspondence: gcasili@unime.it

† These authors contributed equally to this work.

Abstract: Myocardial ischemia–reperfusion injury (MI/R) is a negative and adverse cardiovascular outcome following myocardial ischemia, cardiac surgery, or circulatory arrest. Prolyl endopeptidase (PREP) appears to be involved in inflammatory responses, so it could be a possible therapeutic target for counteracting ischemia injury. This study aimed to investigate the role of PREP inhibitor, KYP-2047 (4-phenylbutanoyl-l-prolyl-2(S)-cyanopyrolidine), in the modulation of molecular and biochemical processes involved in MI/R. MI/R was induced through coronary artery occlusion (15 min), followed by reperfusion (2 h). KYP-2047 was intraperitoneally administrated at doses of 2.5 mg/kg and 5 mg/kg 24 h before the surgical procedures. The hearts were removed and processed for analysis. KYP-2047 treatment limited ischemic myocardial-induced histological damage and neutrophil accumulation, limiting inflammation, fibrosis, and apoptosis processes. Additionally, KYP-2047 was able to modulate p-38 and p-ERK expression, suggesting an improving role in recovering cardiac function. These findings highlighted the protective effects of KYP-2047 pretreatment in MI/R injury, suggesting PREP as a potential target therapy for the pathogenesis of MI/R. Although the molecular mechanisms underlying the action of KYP-2047 are still to be explored, these results suggested that the regulation of NF-κB, apoptosis, and MAPK pathways by KYP-2047 treatment could preventatively limit the damage caused by MI/R.

Keywords: myocardial ischemia/reperfusion injury (MI/R); prolyl endopeptidase; KYP-2047; MAPK; NF-κB

1. Introduction

Cardiovascular diseases cause approximately one-third of fatalities worldwide. In the 21st century, ischemic heart disease represents the most common cardiovascular disease and is recognized as a significant disease for sustainable development [1]. Myocardial ischemia–reperfusion injury (MI/R) can lead to adverse cardiovascular events after myocardial ischemia, circulatory arrest or cardiac surgery and remains a challenging entity in cardiovascular medicine [2]. Vascular, metabolic, and neurohormonal factors interact and take part in causing a deficit to perfusion without the typical chest pain [3]. Comprehending these processes is essential for identifying various clinical manifestations and creating focused therapies [4]. Ischemia–reperfusion (I/R) refers to a condition where tissue is initially deprived of oxygen and nutrients (ischemia) due to a reduction or blockage in blood flow, followed by the restoration of blood flow (reperfusion). I/R damage is caused by complex molecular and cellular processes that are the result of the convergence of different biological pathways [5]. Interestingly, following MI/R, macrophages penetrate damaged cardiac tissue and modify their polarization phenotype to react to acute inflammation and chronic fibrotic remodeling [6]. Moreover, recent evidence showed that microvascular abnormalities, including compromised angiogenesis, are part of the pathogenesis of MI/R; therefore, vasopromotion to enhance collateral circulation is an important therapeutic avenue in the treatment of MI/R injury [7]. To date, there is no effective treatment for reperfusion injury, and research is increasingly focusing on finding an efficient preventive approach. Although there are many successful animal studies on how to prevent reperfusion injury, clinical translation has not always been satisfactory [8,9]. There is no pharmacological treatment even if animal models have shown positive results; this may be explained by variations between preclinical animal MI/R models and the clinical scenario in patients, including comorbidities, age, and cotreatments [10]. A lack of particular biomarkers for properly diagnosing MI/R and a limited understanding of the underlying pathophysiology might be other reasons. New molecules strongly involved in angiogenesis and inflammation have been recently evaluated in various inflammatory models. The release of proinflammatory and pro-angiogenic chemicals is facilitated by the proteolytic enzyme prolyl endopeptidase (PREP), which is a member of the serine protease family [11]. PREP is expressed in different body tissues and the cells of the renin–angiotensin system, and PREP has a significant role in peptide regulation, participating in processing angiotensin II. However, there is evidence that PREP plays a role in the digestion of thymosin β4 to generate the tetrapeptide Ac-SDKP, which increases angiogenesis and decreases fibrosis and apoptosis [12]. Considering the involvement of PREP in inflammatory and pro-angiogenic processes, PREP inhibitors may represent new therapeutic approaches. Interestingly, KYP-2047 (4-phenylbutanoyl-l-prolyl-2(S)-cyanopyrolidine) represents the most selective and potent inhibitor, having a good ability to reach PREP intracellularly [13]. KYP-2047 causes a conformational stabilization of PREP's active site by regulating protein–protein interactions that modulate inflammation and oxidative stress [14]. It has been demonstrated that PREP inhibition has substantial potential in being able to reduce the level of inflammation, and moreover, our previous studies have demonstrated the ability of KYP-2047 to reduce MI/R damage in organs such as the intestine and kidneys, which makes PREP inhibition an interesting therapeutic approach for MI/R [15–18]. Based on this evidence, in the present study, we investigated the preventive effects of KYP-2047 in an in vivo model of MI/R.

2. Materials and Methods

2.1. Materials

KYP-2047 (Sigma, CAS No.: SML020) was purchased from Sigma-Aldrich (Milan, Italy). All other chemicals used in this study were of the highest commercial grade available. All the stock solutions were prepared in non-pyrogenic saline (0.9% NaCl, B. Braun Melsungen AG, Berlin, Germany).

2.2. Animals

Male adult CD1 mice (25–30 g; Envigo, Milan, Italy) were accommodated in stainless steel cages and kept on a 12 h light/12 h dark cycle at an ambient temperature of 22 °C ± 1 °C. The animals were 6–8 weeks old and had free access to standard rodent chow and water ad libitum. All efforts were made to reduce animal pain. Animal care was in conformity with current legislation for the protection of animals used for scientific purposes (D.Lgs 2014/26 and EU Directive 2010/63).

2.3. Myocardial I/R Surgery

All mice were anesthetized with a mixture of ketamine and xylazine, under sterile conditions. Myocardial ischemia–reperfusion injury was induced by occlusion of the left anterior descending artery (LAD) as described before by Di Paola et al. [19]. Briefly, after anesthesia, the body temperature was maintained at 37 ± 1 °C with the support of a heating pad during the surgery. In brief, the pericardium was removed after thoracotomy at the fifth intercostal space, and a 6-0 silk thread was placed around the LAD approximately 1–2 mm below its origin. After 15 min, to allow the reperfusion of the previously ischemic myocardium, the ligation was released. The duration of reperfusion was predetermined at 2 h. The identical procedure was performed on sham-operated animals, except the left anterior descending coronary artery was not tied. After surgery, mice were allowed to equilibrate under a heating lamp under observation for at least 6 h. The choice of the occlusion time and consequently the type of experimental model were chosen in the report of the literature to maximize the reproducibility of functional myocardial damage while minimizing mortality in animals. KYP-2047 was administrated to animals at doses of 2.5 and 5 mg/kg 24 h before the surgical procedures. The dose and route of administration of KYP-2047 were chosen based on previous studies [11,15,18]. Hearts were excised for histological analysis to determine the size of ischemic injury.

2.4. Experimental Groups

To evaluate the effect of KYP-2047 in vivo, the animals were divided into the following groups at random:

- Sham: Mice were subjected to surgery, except for coronary artery occlusion shock, and were kept under anesthesia for the duration of the experiment (N = 8).
- Sham + KYP-2047 2.5 mg/kg group: Mice were subjected to surgery, except for coronary artery occlusion shock, and were kept under anesthesia for the duration of the experiment. KYP-2047 (2.5 mg/kg 0.001% DMSO i.p) was administered 24 h before the surgical procedures (N = 8).
- Sham + KYP-2047 5 mg/kg group: Mice were subjected to surgical procedures, except for coronary artery occlusion shock, and were kept under anesthesia for the duration of the experiment. KYP-2047 (5 mg/kg 0.001% DMSO i.p) was administered 24 h before the surgical procedures (N = 8).
- Ischemia/Reperfusion: Mice were subjected to coronary artery occlusion (15 min), followed by reperfusion (2 h) plus administration of saline (N = 8).
- Ischemia/Reperfusion + KYP-2047 2.5 mg/kg group: Mice were subjected to coronary artery occlusion (15 min), followed by reperfusion (2 h) plus administration of saline. KYP-2047 was administered intraperitoneally (2.5 mg/kg 0.001% DMSO i.p) 24 h before surgical procedures (N = 8).
- Ischemia/Reperfusion + KYP-2047 5 mg/kg group: Mice were subjected to coronary artery occlusion (15 min), followed by reperfusion (2 h) plus administration of saline. KYP-2047 was administered intraperitoneally (5 mg/kg 0.001% DMSO i.p) 24 h before surgical procedures (N = 8).

The doses of KYP-2047 (2.5 and 5 mg/kg) were based on previous in vivo studies performed in our laboratories. The Sham groups treated with KYP-2047 at both doses showed neither toxicity nor improvement compared to the Sham group; therefore, their results are not shown.

2.5. Histological Analysis

Hearts were collected 6 h after reperfusion. The whole heart was removed and was fixed in 10% (*w*/*v*) PBS-buffered formaldehyde solution (Bio-Optica Milano S.p.A., Milan, Italy) for 24 h at room temperature, dehydrated by graded ethanol, and embedded in paraffin (Bio-Optica Milano S.p.A., Milan, Italy) as described before [20]. Then, 7 mm slices were cut from paraffin-embedded tissue. After deparaffinization, sections were stained with hematoxylin/eosin (H&E) staining to evaluate histological damage. Data were analyzed in a double-double-blind manner, that is, analyses by the pathologist who sampled hearts, performed the sectioning, and examined the pathological images. The score scale-point was chosen based on a previous study [19], using the following criteria: 0, no damage; 1 (minor), focal swelling and necrosis of the myocytes; 2 (severe), necrosis with evidence of neutrophil infiltration in the myocytes; 3 (major), necrosis with massive neutrophil infiltration. Every piece was viewed at a magnification of ×10 and ×20 (100 µm and 50 µm scale bar), and morphological changes were evaluated by two blinded investigators. All sections were evaluated using a Nikon Eclipse Ci-L microscope (Nikon Europe B.V; Stroombaan, The Netherland).

2.6. Masson's Trichrome

To determine the degree of fibrosis collagen accumulation, cardiac tissue sections were stained with Masson trichrome according to the manufacturer's protocol (Bio-Optica, Milan, Italy) as previously described [17,21]. Images were shown at 2.5×, 10×, and 20× magnification (200 µm, 100 µm, and 50 µm scale bar, respectively), using a Nikon Eclipse Ci-L microscope.

2.7. Toluidine Blue Staining

The number of mast cells and their degranulation in heart tissue were evaluated using toluidine blue (Bio-Optica, Milan, Italy) as previously described [22]. Briefly, after deparaffinizing, sections were soaked in water for 5 min, moved to toluidine blue for 3 min, and then blotted carefully. Sections were placed in absolute alcohol, cleared in xylene, and finally fixed on glass slides using Eukitt (Bio-Optica, Milan, Italy). Images were shown at 2.5×, 10×, 20×, and 40× magnification (200 µm, 100 µm, 50 µm, and 20 µm scale bar, respectively). The number of metachromatic stained mast cells was determined by counting in five high-power fields (40×) per section by using a Nikon Eclipse Ci-L microscope.

2.8. Immunohistochemistry

The immunohistochemistry analysis was performed as described in previous work [23]. The heart sections (7 µm) were incubated overnight with the primary antibody at room temperature. The used antibodies were anti-mast cell tryptase (1:100, Santa Cruz Biotechnology, Dallas, TX, USA, sc-59587) anti-nitrotyrosine (1:100, Merck-Millipore, Burlington, MA, USA, 06-284), anti-VEGF (Santa Cruz Biotechnology, Dallas, TX, USA, sc-7269; 1:100), and anti-CD34 (Santa Cruz Biotechnology, Dallas, TX, USA, sc-74499; 1:100). The slices were rinsed with PBS and then incubated with a secondary antibody for 1 h at room temperature. After incubation, the staining agent (brown DAB) was used together with the Nuclear Fast Red counterstain. Then, the sections were observed using a Nikon Eclipse Ci-L microscope. The percentage area of immunoreactivity (determined by the number of positive pixels) was expressed as a percentage of the total tissue area (red staining) within five random fields at 2.5×, 10×, and 20× magnification (200 µm, 100 µm, and 50 µm scale bar, respectively), after being quantified using ImageJ software version 1.54.

2.9. Terminal Deoxynucleotidyl Transferase-Mediated UTP End Labeling (TUNEL) Assay

The TUNEL staining was performed using a cell death detection kit following the manufacturer's instructions (Roche, Basel, Switzerland, Catalog: 12156792910), as previously described [24]. The sections, after being deparaffinized and hydrated, were permeabilized with 0.1 M citrate buffer and then incubated in the TUNEL reaction at 37 °C for 60 min in the dark. For TUNEL staining, 2.5×, 10×, and 20× magnification (200 μm, 100 μm, and 50 μm scale bar, respectively) were shown.

2.10. Western Blot

The heart tissues were suspended in two distinct buffers to extract the cytosolic and nuclear fractions, as previously described [25]. Cytosolic lysates from the samples were utilized for SDS-PAGE, and then membranes were incubated overnight with the following primary antibodies: anti-IκB-α (1:500; Santa Cruz Biotechnology sc-1643), anti-IL-18 (1:500; Santa Cruz Biotechnology sc-7954,), anti-p-p38 MAPK (Thr180/Tyr182) (1:500; Cell Signaling, Danvers, MA, USA, 9211S), anti-p-ERK (1:500; Santa Cruz Biotechnology sc-7383), Then, membranes were incubated with peroxidase-conjugated bovine anti-mouse secondary antibody (1:1000, Jackson ImmunoResearch, West Grove, PA, USA) for 1 h at room temperature. Signals were evaluated via a chemiluminescence (ECL) detection system reagent according to the manufacturer's instructions). The expression of the protein bands was quantified by densitometry with Bio-Rad ChemiDoc TMXRS + software 6.1 (Bio-Rad, Milan, Italy) and standardized to β-actin (1:500; Santa Cruz Biotechnology sc-47778) or ERK 1/2 (1:500; Santa Cruz Biotechnology sc-514302).

2.11. ELISA Assay

An ELISA kit was used to detect the levels of p65 (Cusabio, Catalog: CSB-E08789m) on cytosolic and nuclear tissue lysates according to the manufacturer's protocols. Briefly, the samples (100 μL) were added to anti-NF-κBp65-coated well plates and incubated at 37 °C for 2 h. Subsequently, 100 μL of the horseradish peroxidase (HRP) was added to each well and incubated for 1 h at 37 °C. The plates were washed with washing buffer 1X, and TMB (3,3′5,5′ tetramethyl-benzidine) substrate solution (90 μL) was added and incubated for 15 min at 37 °C. Finally, the stop solution (50 μL) was added, and the concentrations of p65 were determined spectrophotometrically at an absorbance of 450 nm and interpolated with a standard curve.

2.12. Statistical Analysis

Experimental data are expressed as mean ± standard deviation (SD) of N observations, in which N represents the number of animals studied. One-way ANOVA analysis of variance followed by the Bonferroni post hoc test for multiple comparisons was used to analyze the results, and only a *p*-value less than 0.05 was considered significant. Data are representative of a minimum of three independent experiments.

3. Results

3.1. Effects of KYP-2047 on Histological Assessment

H&E staining was performed to evaluate the morphology of myocardial cells. Histological examination showed tissue damage and necrosis with neutrophil infiltration in the ischemic reperfused heart (Figure 1(B,B1)) compared to the treatment (Figure 1(C,C1) and 1(D,D1); see histological score in Figure 1E). In Sham mice, myocardial tissue structure assumed the typical normal architecture (Figure 1(A,A1); see histological score in Figure 1E). The myocardial tissue in the MI/R group showed a disordered arrangement of myocardial fibers and a large number of inflammatory cell infiltrations; instead, in the MI/R + KYP-2047 group, cardiomyocytes were arranged in a more orderly manner with a decrease in necrosis; furthermore, the degree and severity of cell necrosis were significantly lower after pretreatment with KYP-2047 5 mg/kg.

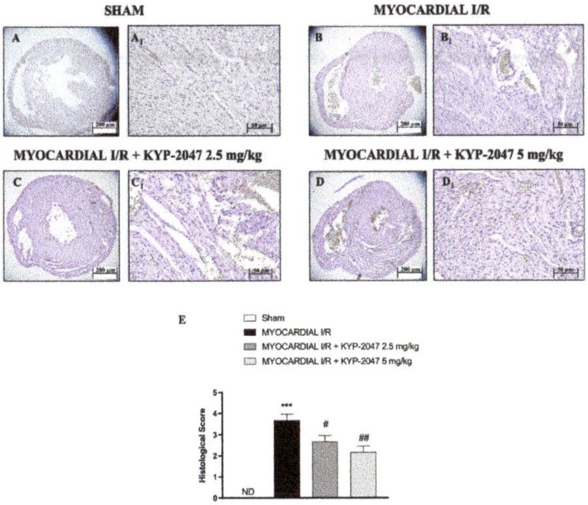

Figure 1. KYP-2047 reduced the severity and the degree of cell necrosis. H&E staining of Sham group (**A**,**A1**), Myocardial I/R group (**B**,**B1**), Myocardial I/R + KYP-2047 2.5 mg/kg group (**C**,**C1**), Myocardial I/R + KYP-2047 5 mg/kg group (**D**,**D1**); see histological score (**E**). Here, 2.5× and 20× magnification is shown (200 μm and 50 μm scale bar, respectively). Data are expressed as mean ± SD of N = 8 mice/group. (ND) Not detectable. *** $p < 0.001$ vs. Sham; # $p < 0.05$ vs. MI/R; ## $p < 0.01$ vs. MI/R.

3.2. Role of KYP-2047 Pretreatment in Reducing Fibrosis

Masson's trichrome staining was used to assess mouse heart tissue. Red staining indicates healthy tissue, while blue staining indicates the area of fibrotic scarring. The data showed an increased level of collagen deposition in MI/R (Figure 2(B,B1)) because of the normal thrombus that formed in the tissue. However, KYP-2047 at doses of 2.5 and 5 mg/kg was not capable of preventing collagen deposition (Figure 2(C,C1) and Figure 2(D,D1), respectively).

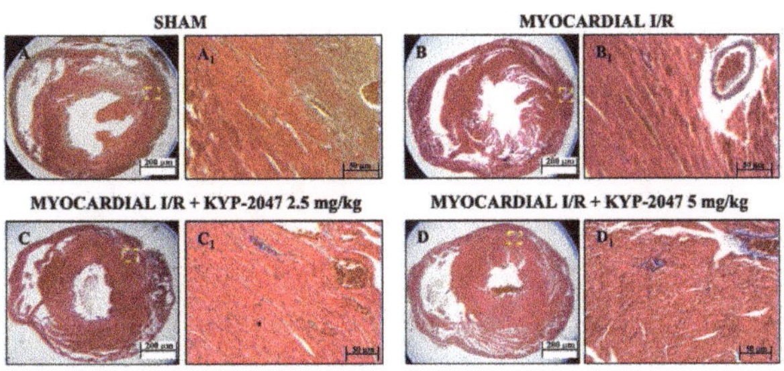

Figure 2. Inhibition of PREP by KYP-2047 prevented collagen deposition. Masson's trichrome staining of Sham group (**A**,**A1**), Myocardial I/R group (**B**,**B1**), Myocardial I/R + KYP-2047 2.5 mg/kg group (**C**,**C1**), Myocardial I/R + KYP-2047 5 mg/kg group (**D**,**D1**). Red parts index cardiomyocytes and blue parts index fibrosis. Magnification 2.5×, scale bar 200 μm (**A–D**); magnification 20×, scale bar 50 μm (**A1–D1**).

3.3. Effect of KYP-2047 on Myocardial Injury: Mast Cell Staining and Tryptase Evaluation

The presence of mast cells in myocardial tissue was evaluated by toluidine blue staining. The data showed an increase in mast cell (MC) infiltration in the heart tissues collected from mice subjected to MI/R (Figure 3B), compared to Sham mice (Figure 3A; see percentage of total tissue area in Figure 3E). However, both doses, 2.5 mg/kg and 5 mg/kg, prevented MC infiltration in heart tissues (Figures 3C and 3D, respectively) as shown by mast cell density (Figure 3E). On the other hand, the levels of tryptase (Figure 3F–I; see percentage of total tissue area in Figure 3J), evaluated by immunohistochemistry, increased following the pretreatment with the highest dose of KYP-2047 (see Figure 3I; see percentage of total tissue area in Figure 3J).

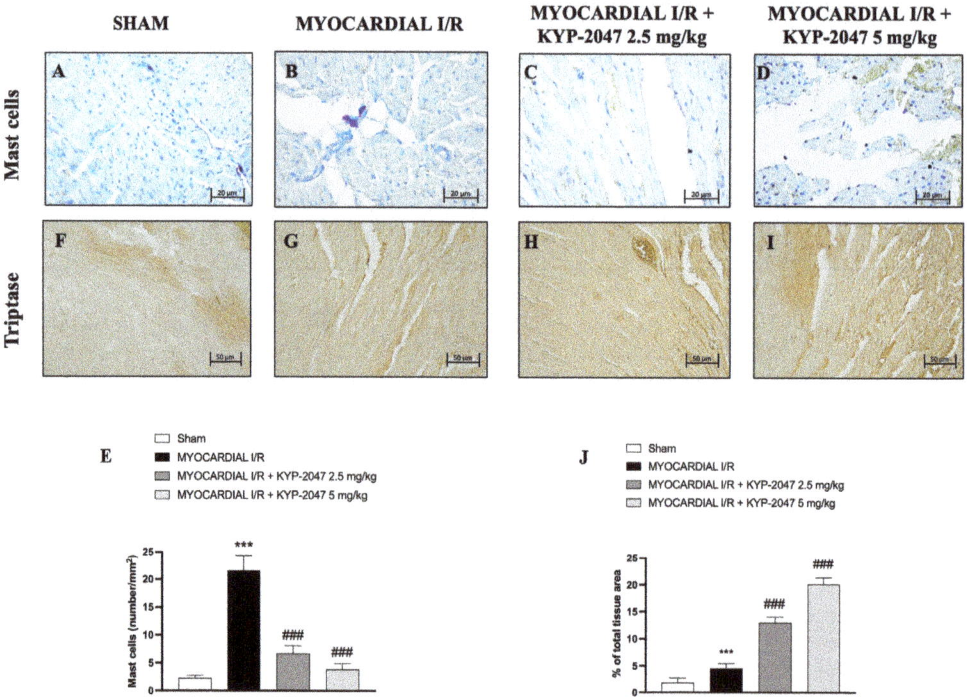

Figure 3. KYP-2047 reduced mast cell infiltration in heart samples. Toluidine blue staining of Sham group (**A**), Myocardial I/R group (**B**), Myocardial I/R + KYP-2047 2.5 mg/kg group (**C**), Myocardial I/R + KYP-2047 5 mg/kg group (**D**). Mast cell graph (number/mm^2) (**E**). Immunohistochemical evaluation of tryptase. Sham group (**F**), Myocardial I/R group (**G**), Myocardial I/R + KYP-2047 2.5 mg/kg group (**H**), Myocardial I/R + KYP-2047 5 mg/kg group (**I**). See percentage of total tissue area (**J**). Magnification 40×, scale bar 20 μm (**A–D**); magnification 20×, scale bar 50 μm (**F–I**). Data are expressed as mean ± SD of N = 8 mice/group. *** $p < 0.001$ vs. Sham; ### $p < 0.001$ vs. MI/R.

3.4. Effect of KYP-2047 on Angiogenesis in Myocardial I/R

Vascular endothelial growth factor (VEGF) expression is regulated by hypoxia and cytokines; specifically, it represents a specific endothelial cell mitogen and plays an important role in myocardial angiogenesis and vascular leakage. In heart tissue collected from mice subjected to MI/R, an increase in positive staining for VEGF was observed through immunohistochemistry analysis (Figure 4B; see percentage of total tissue area in Figure 4E), compared to control mice (Figure 4A; see percentage of total tissue area in Figure 4E).

Furthermore, an increase in positive cells for CD34 in the MI/R group (Figure 4G; see percentage of total tissue area in Figure 4J), an index of the ability to stimulate angiogenesis after injury, was also observed. The data suggest that KYP-2047 at the dose of 5 mg/kg was able to reduce both VEGF- and C34-positive cells, as shown in Figure 4C,D (see percentage of total tissue area in Figure 4E) and Figure 4H,I (see percentage of total tissue area in Figure 4J), respectively.

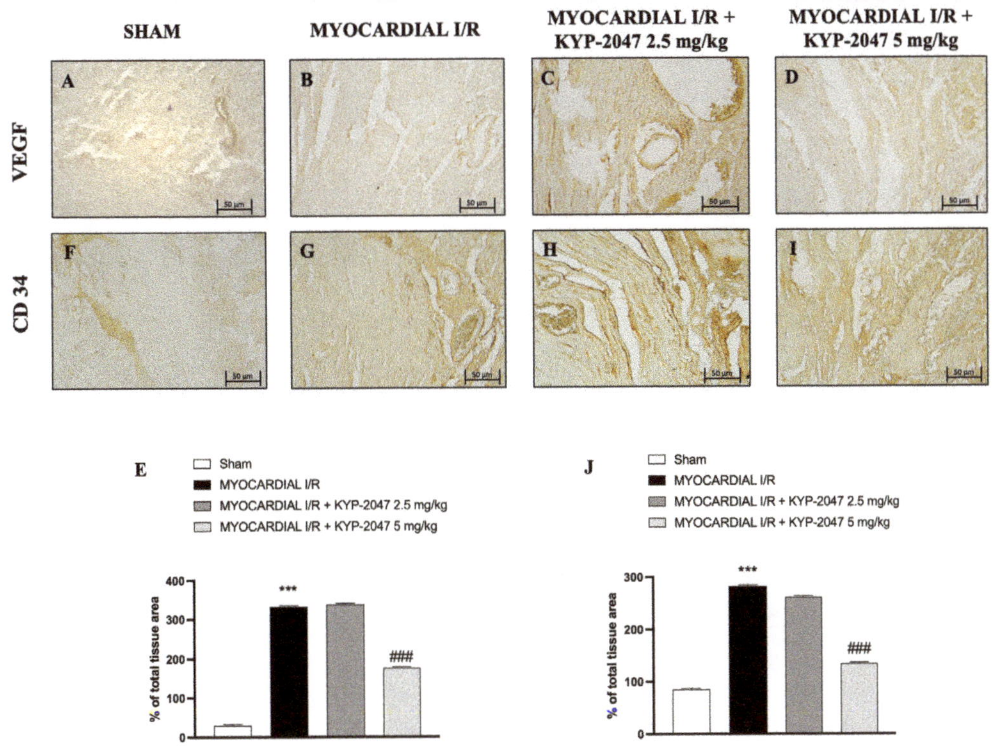

Figure 4. KYP-2047 treatments reduced myocardial angiogenesis. Immunohistochemistry of VEGF: Sham group (**A**), Myocardial I/R group (**B**), Myocardial I/R + KYP-2047 2.5 mg/kg group (**C**), Myocardial I/R + KYP-2047 5 mg/kg group (**D**); see percentage of total tissue area (**E**). Immunohistochemistry of CD34: Sham group (**F**), Myocardial I/R group (**G**), Myocardial I/R + KYP-2047 2.5 mg/kg group (**H**), Myocardial I/R + KYP-2047 5 mg/kg group (**I**); see percentage of total tissue area (**J**). Magnification 20×, scale bar 50 µm. Data are expressed as mean ± SD of N = 8 mice/group. *** $p < 0.001$ vs. Sham; ### $p < 0.001$ vs. MI/R.

3.5. *Effect of KYP-2047 on Nitrosative Stress and DNA Damage*

Nitrosative stress is closely associated with cardiovascular disease. Therefore, nitrotyrosine content, an established index of protein nitration and nitrative stress, was determined by immunohistochemistry. Compared with the control group (Figure 5A), MI/R increased nitrotyrosine content (Figure 5B), whereas the pretreatment with KYP-2047 reduced the nitrotyrosine-positive staining in heart tissue (Figure 5C,D). Furthermore, Western blot analysis showed a basal expression of IκB-α in control mice, while in mice subjected to MI/R, IκB-α expression in heart samples significantly decreased, due to the increased IκB-α cytosolic degradation (Figure 5(F,F2)). At the same time, nuclear NF-κBp65 levels were significantly increased in the MI/R group compared to Sham animals (Figure 5H).

The inhibition of nuclear translocation of NF-κBp65 by IκBα phosphorylation blockade could provide an effective approach to the attenuation of MI/R injury. In fact, pretreatment with KYP-2047, at both doses, significantly reduced nuclear NF-κBp65 levels (Figure 5H). In contrast, cytoplasmic NF-κBp65 levels were reduced in the MI/R group, and treatments with KYP-2047 effectively restored these levels. Considering that IL-18 is a proinflammatory cytokine responsive to NF-κB, its expression was evaluated by Western blot analysis. The results showed increased IL-18 levels in mice that underwent MI/R compared to control mice; treatment with KYP-2047 significantly reduced IL-18 levels (Figure 5(F,F1)).

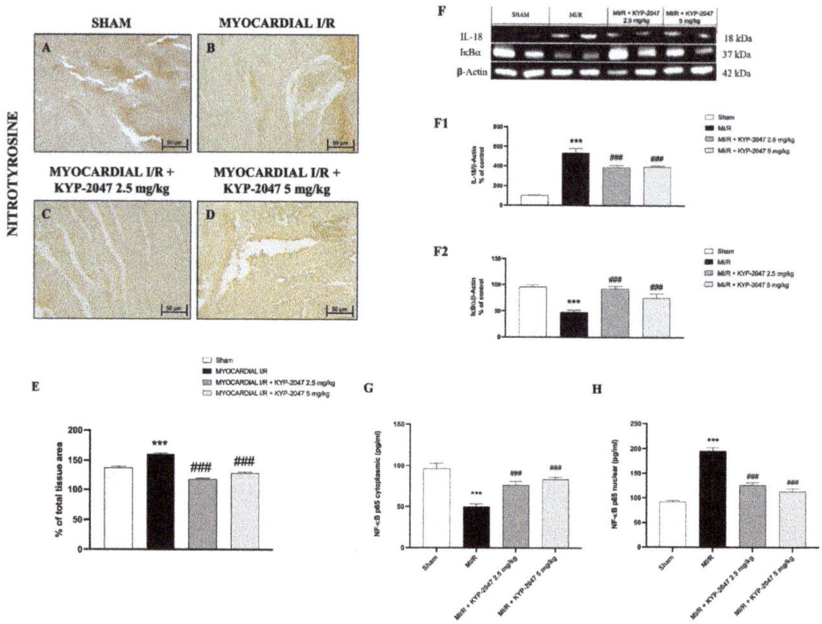

Figure 5. KYP-2047 treatments reduced nitrotyrosine content and modulated the NF-κBp65 pathway. Immunohistochemistry of nitrotyrosine: Sham group (**A**), Myocardial I/R group (**B**), Myocardial I/R + KYP-2047 2.5 mg/kg group (**C**), Myocardial I/R + KYP-2047 5 mg/kg group (**D**); see percentage of total tissue area (**E**). Images are shown at 20× magnification, scale bar 50 μm. Western blot analysis of IL-18 (**F,F1**) and IκB-α (**F,F2**) is shown. Actin (in (**F**)) was used as a loading control. Representative blots of three experiments are presented. ELISA assay of NF-κBp65 levels on cytosolic (**G**) and nuclear (**H**) tissue lysates is shown. Data are expressed as mean ± SD of N = 8 mice/group. *** $p < 0.001$ vs. Sham; ### $p < 0.001$ vs. Myocardial I/R (MI/R).

3.6. *Effect of KYP-2047 on Apoptosis*

The TUNEL assay was performed to evaluate apoptosis and whether pretreatment with KYP-2047 affected cardiomyocyte I/R injury. In hearts from MI/R injury mice (Figure 6(B,B1); see positive cells in Figure 6E), the TUNEL assay showed an intense upregulation in apoptotic cells as compared to the Sham group (Figure 6(A,A1); see positive cells in Figure 6E), whereas treatment with KYP-2047 at both doses, 2.5 mg/kg and 5 mg/kg, showed a reduction in the apoptosis process (Figure 6(C,C1) and Figure 6(D,D1), respectively; see positive cells in Figure 6E).

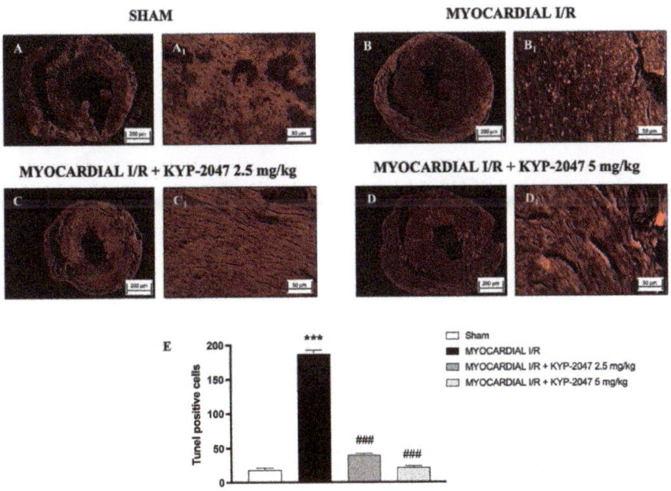

Figure 6. KYP-2047 reduced apoptosis process. Images of TUNEL assay are shown: Sham group (**A**,**A1**), Myocardial I/R group (**B**,**B1**), Myocardial I/R + KYP-2047 2.5 mg/kg group (**C**,**C1**), Myocardial I/R + KYP-2047 5 mg/kg group (**D**,**D1**). Count of TUNEL-positive cells (**E**). Here, 2.5× and 20× magnification is shown (200 µm and 50 µm scale bar, respectively). Data are expressed as mean ± SD of N = 8 mice/group. *** $p < 0.001$ vs. Sham; ### $p < 0.001$ vs. MI/R.

3.7. Role of KYP-2047 in MAPK Pathway During MI/R

Numerous protein kinase families are activated by myocardial ischemia–reperfusion. Among the principal protein kinase pathways linked to myocardial ischemia, there are MAP kinases, ERK 1/2, JNK 1/2, and p38 MAPKa/b. In this study, pretreatment with KYP-2047 was able to reduce p-38 expression compared to MI/R damage, suggesting an improving role in recovering cardiac function (Figure 7A). Erk 1/2 belongs to the family of serine–threonine kinases known as mitogen-activated protein kinases (MAPKs). In the context of ischemia–reperfusion, the ERK 1/2 cascade can be triggered, which can mediate cellular protection. In our study, ERK 1/2 levels were slightly reduced, but not significantly in the MI/R group compared to the control, while pretreatment with KYP-2047 at the dose of 2.5 mg/kg significantly increased ERK 1/2 phosphorylation, suggesting its cardioprotective role (Figure 7B).

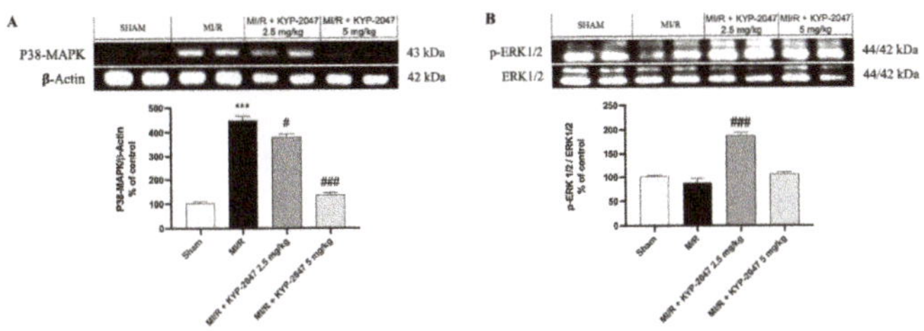

Figure 7. Inhibition of PREP by KYP-2047 prevented p38 activation and induced ERK1/2 phosphorylation. Western blot analysis of p38 (**A**) and Erk1/2 (**B**) phosphorylation. Whole myocardial lysate of indicated groups was processed for analysis of P-p38 and pERK1/2. Actin (in (**A**)) and total ERK1/2 (in (**B**)) were used as loading controls. Representative blots of three experiments are presented. Data are expressed as mean ± SD of N = 8 mice/group. *** $p < 0.001$ vs. Sham; # $p < 0.05$ vs. MI/R; ### $p < 0.001$ vs. MI/R.

4. Discussion

Myocardial ischemia–reperfusion injury is characterized by the death of cardiomyocytes due to reactive oxygen species (ROS) accumulation, calcium overload, and inflammation during the restoration of perfusion and simultaneous reoxygenation [26]. In its traditional form, tissue hypoxia is brought on by an embolus that obstructs the arterial blood supply, severely unbalancing the supply and demand for metabolism processes [27]. ROS overproduction, oxidative/nitrosative stress, and inflammatory reactions are some of the intricate and systematic networks at the base of the complex mechanisms of MI/R injury [28]. Moreover, apoptosis and necrosis of cardiomyocytes occur when there is cardiac ischemia, resulting in extensive myocardial tissue damage. Due to the limited proliferative capacity of myocardial cells, damaged areas of heart tissue cannot be effectively repaired or regenerated [27]. By restoring coronary artery blood flow to the ischemic tissue, timely reperfusion can effectively prevent or delay the progression of the disease and cell death.

Therefore, given the effects due to damage from MI/R, to evaluate whether inflammation, vascular alterations, and the apoptosis process involved in the pathophysiology of MI/R can be prevented, in this study, the protective effect of KYP-2047, a selective inhibitor of PREP, a serine protease involved in the release of pro-angiogenic molecules, was investigated in MI/R damage.

Inflammation contributes to the pathophysiology of cardiac IR injury; particularly, the coronary endothelium is associated with MI/R injury by activating the immune system through the expression of chemokines, cytokines, and adhesion molecules [5]. Immune cells participate in the pathogenesis of MI/R injury by triggering inflammatory responses such as monocytes, dendritic cells, and neutrophils accumulating at the damaged site [29]. Neutrophil activation and leukocyte infiltration lead to further cytokine secretion, oxidative stress, and protease release, exacerbating myocardial injury and death [30]. Pretreatment with KYP-2047 at the dose of 5 mg/kg significantly reduced the severity and the degree of cell necrosis, resulting in a better architectural state of the myocardial tissue compared to the injured one. Heart tissue was more compact and better organized with a reduced site of damage.

Furthermore, following the initial phase of ischemic insult, there is an increase in ROS as a result of oxidative stress and neutrophil clogging, and there is an obstruction of normal blood flow in capillaries and microcapillaries in a process known as the "no-reflow" phenomenon [31]. ROS generation partially contributes to mast cell degranulation, which mediates I/R, through a bilateral process [32]. Particularly, many recent studies have demonstrated the role of MCs in I/R damage such as in the heart and in the brain [33]. From bone marrow tissue, mast cells travel via the circulatory system to the target tissue, where they finish maturing and differentiating [34]. Through degranulation and the release of tryptase, chymase, and histamine, mast cells function as immediate reactors in the early stages of I/R occurrence [35]. Strong stimulation, such as myocardial ischemia, activates myocardial cells and releases cytotoxic mediators such as IL-6, TNF-α, and IL-1β [36]. The protective effect of KYP-2047, at the dose of 2.5 mg/kg and 5 mg/kg, consisted in slowing down MC degranulation, although immunohistochemistry analysis showed that KYP-2047 was not able to reduce tryptase release in the damage site. In both healthy and pathological circumstances, ROS and reactive nitrogen species (RNS) play a crucial role as intracellular and intercellular signal molecules in preserving proper homeostasis. Because of ischemic damage, in addition to hypoxia and oxidative stress, there is also nitrosative stress [37]. The formation and scavenging pathways of RNS overlap with those of ROS, which are involved in oxidative stress. These pathways are reciprocally regulated by ROS and nitric oxide (NO) [38,39]. Tyrosine nitration is the main characteristic of nitrosative stress, which causes cell membrane damage, lipid peroxidation, DNA strand breaks, the inactivation of functioning enzymes, and the activation of cascade signal responses that lead to cell death. So, high levels of ROS and RNS can damage DNA and lead cells to death. In this research, the role of KYP-2047 in preventing the increase in nitrotyrosine, a specific marker of the peroxynitrite-induced tyrosine nitration process, was confirmed in protecting cells from death. As a natural host defense mechanism, blood vessel formation in response to tissue ischemia aims to preserve tissue perfusion, which is essential for physiologic organ function. Neoangiogenesis after tissue ischemia has been associated with peripheral blood circulating progenitor cells derived from bone marrow [40,41]. In this context, CD34+ cells play paracrine functions through angiogenesis and direct incorporation into the growing vascular system. These functions include immunomodulatory, anti-inflammatory, and anti-apoptosis roles aimed at the formation of microcirculation [42–44]. In hypoxic conditions, other effects occur during MI/R injury: increased vascular permeability, inflammation, endothelial cell activation, an imbalance between vasodilatory and vasoconstrictor factors, and the activation of the complement and coagulation systems [27]. VEGF is an important angiogenesis factor acting exclusively on endothelial cells [45]. After damage, it plays an important role in promoting blood vessel growth and remodeling processes [46]. Thus, after myocardial damage, there were high levels of CD34+ and VEGF+ cells, as confirmed by immunohistochemistry analysis. Pretreatment with KYP-2047 at the highest dose was able to reduce VEGF levels because of the reduced damage and therefore the reduced necessity to create new vessels.

It is known that NF-κB promotes oxidative-stress-induced necrosis and I/R injury [47]. Thus, myocardial protection may be provided through inhibition of the NF-κB pathway [48–52]. In fact, NF-κB is maintained in an inactive form in the cytoplasm due to its binding to IκBα, preventing its translocation into the nucleus. Nevertheless, phosphorylation-induced proteolytic degradation of IκBα occurs during the activation of NF-κB signaling [53]. In this study, the results confirmed that NF-κB was activated in the heart after MI/R, while pretreatment with KYP-2047 significantly reduced the nuclear translocation of NF-κB; on the other hand, the expression of IκBα was increased even at the lowest dose of KYP-2047. Furthermore, it is known that the binding of IL18 to its receptor and the activation of NF-κB mediates the activity of IL18, leading to the production and release of numerous cytokines, chemokines, and cell adhesion molecules. Here, it was confirmed that KYP-2047 reduced both the downregulation of NF-κB and the levels of IL-18 proinflammatory cytokines.

The role of NF-κB in myocardial I/R results not only in the release of proinflammatory factors but also in promoting apoptosis of cardiomyocytes [54]. Programmed cell death has been linked to numerous heart pathologies, including myocardial ischemia through tissue damage and malfunctions, although reperfusion can prevent cell death that follows ischemia [29]. In this study, it was confirmed that pretreatment with KYP-2047 reduced the apoptosis process compared to the MI/R group.

Phosphorylation at the end of the cascade, composed of MAPK kinase (MKK) and MKK kinase (MEKK), controls p38 activity.

Myocardial ischemia leads to the activation of several protein kinase pathways, including MAPKs. In particular, phosphorylation at the end of the MAPK cascade, composed of MAPK kinase (MKK) and MKK kinase (MEKK) controls the activity of p38, an important pro-apoptotic mediator in cardiac myocytes [55–58]. The apoptosis process is also linked to the activation of ERK1/2 phosphorylates substrates in the cytoplasm or nucleus [59]. In the literature, the role of ERK1/2 is controversial; while some research has indicated that ERK1/2 expression and activation might exacerbate I/R, other research has suggested that

ERK1/2 activity may protect against MI/R [60–62]. Although our study demonstrated that the pretreatment with KYP-2047 at the highest dose had a protective role and promoted the repair of damaged tissue, by inhibiting the activation of p38 MAPK, we did not observe significant changes in ERK1/2 expression at this dose. However, at lower doses of KYP-2047, we still observed a protective effect, suggesting that the activation of survival kinases such as ERK1/2 may exert a protective action against cardiac cells and reduce apoptosis as confirmed by the TUNEL assay.

There are no certain data on the possible PREP mechanisms of action; therefore, it would be interesting to provide an extracellular mechanism of action of PREP in the myocardial context, although ours could be only a hypothesis. In fact, since PREP is able to hydrolyze and activate short peptides, we could hypothesize that it is involved in the activation of atrial natriuretic peptides (ANPs), which are overexpressed following stress; specifically, ANPs are rapidly secreted from cardiomyocytes during ischemia brought on by coronary artery occlusion, playing an important role in regulating blood pressure and volume through its natriuretic and vasodilatory effects [63–66]. Therefore, PREP could promote the activations of ANPs, contributing to the exacerbation of ischemic damage; however, additional experiments would be needed to confirm our hypothesis.

5. Conclusions

In conclusion, this study highlighted the ability of KYP-2047 to reduce the harmful consequences of MI/R injury, suggesting PREP as a potential target therapy for the pathogenesis of MI/R. Although the molecular mechanisms underlying the action of KYP-2047 are still to be investigated, as MI/R is a complex interaction of different pathways, these findings indicated that the modulation of NF-κB, apoptosis, and MAPK pathways was able to increase cell survival, also improving cardiac function. Therefore, PREP's multifaceted mechanism may provide more comprehensive protection against MI/R injury compared to many existing single-target drugs. The use of KYP-2047 could be particularly useful for patients with risk factors for myocardial ischemia or those undergoing cardiac procedures [67]. However, the clinical translation of drugs for MI/R injury remains a significant challenge, with many promising treatments failing to demonstrate efficacy in human trials. Additionally, further investigations are needed to define how long the protective therapy must be applied to fully prevent myocardial damage and to thoroughly assess its safety profile in clinical settings.

Author Contributions: Conceptualization, G.C. and L.C.; methodology, L.C. and N.P.; software, A.A. and A.P.C.; validation, E.E. and M.C.; formal analysis, M.L.; investigation, G.C. and M.L.; resources, E.E.; data curation, A.A.; writing—original draft preparation, N.P. and G.C.; writing—review and editing, G.C.; visualization, E.E.; supervision, G.C.; funding acquisition, E.E. All authors have read and agreed to the published version of the manuscript.

Funding: This research received no external funding.

Institutional Review Board Statement: The study was approved by the University of Messina review board for the care of animals (499/2018). All animal experiments were carried out in agreement with European Union regulations (2010/63/EU amended by Regulation 2019/1010).

Informed Consent Statement: Not applicable.

Data Availability Statement: The data presented in this study are available on request from the corresponding author.

Conflicts of Interest: The authors declare no conflicts of interest.

Abbreviations

The following abbreviations are used in this manuscript:

MI/R	Myocardial ischemia–reperfusion injury
PREP	Prolyl endopeptidase
LAD	Left anterior descending artery
H&E	Hematoxylin/eosin
TUNEL	Terminal deoxynucleotidyl transferase-mediated UTP end labeling
MCs	Mast cells
VEGF	Vascular endothelial growth factor
MAPKs	Mitogen-activated protein kinases
ROS	Reactive oxygen species
RNS	Reactive nitrogen species
NO	Nitric oxide

References

1. Khan, M.A.; Hashim, M.J.; Mustafa, H.; Baniyas, M.Y.; Al Suwaidi, S.; AlKatheeri, R.; Alblooshi, F.M.K.; Almatrooshi, M.; Alzaabi, M.E.H.; Al Darmaki, R.S.; et al. Global Epidemiology of Ischemic Heart Disease: Results from the Global Burden of Disease Study. *Cureus* **2020**, *12*, e9349. [CrossRef]
2. Sagris, M.; Apostolos, A.; Theofilis, P.; Ktenopoulos, N.; Katsaros, O.; Tsalamandris, S.; Tsioufis, K.; Toutouzas, K.; Tousoulis, D. Myocardial Ischemia-Reperfusion Injury: Unraveling Pathophysiology, Clinical Manifestations, and Emerging Prevention Strategies. *Biomedicines* **2024**, *12*, 802. [CrossRef]
3. Theofilis, P.; Antonopoulos, A.S.; Sagris, M.; Papanikolaou, A.; Oikonomou, E.; Tsioufis, K.; Tousoulis, D. Silent Myocardial Ischemia: From Pathophysiology to Diagnosis and Treatment. *Biomedicines* **2024**, *12*, 259. [CrossRef] [PubMed]
4. Frank, A.; Bonney, M.; Bonney, S.; Weitzel, L.; Koeppen, M.; Eckle, T. Myocardial ischemia reperfusion injury: From basic science to clinical bedside. *Semin. Cardiothorac. Vasc. Anesth.* **2012**, *16*, 123–132. [CrossRef] [PubMed]
5. Turer, A.T.; Hill, J.A. Pathogenesis of myocardial ischemia-reperfusion injury and rationale for therapy. *Am. J. Cardiol.* **2010**, *106*, 360–368. [CrossRef]
6. Shen, S.C.; Xu, J.; Cheng, C.; Xiang, X.J.; Hong, B.Y.; Zhang, M.; Gong, C.; Ma, L.K. Macrophages promote the transition from myocardial ischemia reperfusion injury to cardiac fibrosis in mice through GMCSF/CCL2/CCR2 and phenotype switching. *Acta Pharmacol. Sin.* **2024**, *45*, 959–974. [CrossRef]
7. Liu, X.; Fan, B.; Huang, S.; Wang, M.; Teng, H.; Wang, X.; Shi, M.; Li, T.; Zhao, Y.; Wang, L. Design and synthesis of matrine derivatives for anti myocardial ischemia-reperfusion injury by promoting angiogenesis. *Bioorg. Med. Chem.* **2024**, *108*, 117776. [CrossRef]
8. Fernandez Rico, C.; Konate, K.; Josse, E.; Nargeot, J.; Barrère-Lemaire, S.; Boisguérin, P. Therapeutic Peptides to Treat Myocardial Ischemia-Reperfusion Injury. *Front. Cardiovasc. Med.* **2022**, *9*, 792885. [CrossRef]
9. Kasama, S.; Toyama, T.; Hatori, T.; Sumino, H.; Kumakura, H.; Takayama, Y.; Ichikawa, S.; Suzuki, T.; Kurabayashi, M. Effects of intravenous atrial natriuretic peptide on cardiac sympathetic nerve activity and left ventricular remodeling in patients with first anterior acute myocardial infarction. *J. Am. Coll. Cardiol.* **2007**, *49*, 667–674. [CrossRef]
10. Heusch, G.; Gersh, B.J. The pathophysiology of acute myocardial infarction and strategies of protection beyond reperfusion: A continual challenge. *Eur. Heart J.* **2017**, *38*, 774–784. [CrossRef]
11. Cucinotta, L.; Mannino, D.; Casili, G.; Repici, A.; Crupi, L.; Paterniti, I.; Esposito, E.; Campolo, M. Prolyl oligopeptidase inhibition ameliorates experimental pulmonary fibrosis both in vivo and in vitro. *Respir. Res.* **2023**, *24*, 211. [CrossRef] [PubMed]
12. Garcia-Horsman, J.A. The role of prolyl oligopeptidase, understanding the puzzle. *Ann. Transl. Med.* **2020**, *8*, 983. [CrossRef]
13. Toppila, M.; Hytti, M.; Korhonen, E.; Ranta-Aho, S.; Harju, N.; Forsberg, M.M.; Kaarniranta, K.; Jalkanen, A.; Kauppinen, A. The Prolyl Oligopeptidase Inhibitor KYP-2047 Is Cytoprotective and Anti-Inflammatory in Human Retinal Pigment Epithelial Cells with Defective Proteasomal Clearance. *Antioxidants* **2023**, *12*, 1279. [CrossRef] [PubMed]
14. Etelainen, T.; Kulmala, V.; Svarcbahs, R.; Jantti, M.; Myohanen, T.T. Prolyl oligopeptidase inhibition reduces oxidative stress via reducing NADPH oxidase activity by activating protein phosphatase 2A. *Free Radic. Biol. Med.* **2021**, *169*, 14–23. [CrossRef] [PubMed]
15. Casili, G.; Ardizzone, A.; Basilotta, R.; Lanza, M.; Filippone, A.; Paterniti, I.; Esposito, E.; Campolo, M. The protective role of prolyl oligopeptidase (Pop) inhibition in kidney injury induced by renal ischemia–reperfusion. *Int. J. Mol. Sci.* **2021**, *22*, 11886. [CrossRef]

16. Scuderi, S.A.; Casili, G.; Filippone, A.; Lanza, M.; Basilotta, R.; Giuffrida, R.; Munao, S.; Colarossi, L.; Capra, A.P.; Esposito, E.; et al. Beneficial effect of KYP-2047, a propyl-oligopeptidase inhibitor, on oral squamous cell carcinoma. *Oncotarget* **2021**, *12*, 2459–2473. [CrossRef]
17. Casili, G.; Scuderi, S.A.; Lanza, M.; Filippone, A.; Basilotta, R.; Mannino, D.; Campolo, M.; Esposito, E.; Paterniti, I. The protective role of prolyl oligopeptidase (POP) inhibition in acute lung injury induced by intestinal ischemia-reperfusion. *Oncotarget* **2021**, *12*, 1663.
18. Filippone, A.; Casili, G.; Ardizzone, A.; Lanza, M.; Mannino, D.; Paterniti, I.; Esposito, E.; Campolo, M. Inhibition of prolyl oligopeptidase prevents consequences of reperfusion following intestinal ischemia. *Biomedicines* **2021**, *9*, 1354. [CrossRef]
19. Di Paola, R.; Fusco, R.; Gugliandolo, E.; D'Amico, R.; Campolo, M.; Latteri, S.; Carughi, A.; Mandalari, G.; Cuzzocrea, S. The antioxidant activity of pistachios reduces cardiac tissue injury of acute ischemia/reperfusion (I/R) in diabetic streptozotocin (STZ)-induced hyperglycaemic rats. *Front. Pharmacol.* **2018**, *9*, 51.
20. Filippone, A.; Scuderi, S.A.; Basilotta, R.; Lanza, M.; Casili, G.; Bova, V.; Paterniti, I.; Esposito, E. BAY-117082-driven NLRP3 inflammasome inhibition resolves nitro-glycerine (NTG) neuronal damage in in vivo model of migraine. *Biomed. Pharmacother.* **2022**, *156*, 113851.
21. Sridharan, D.; Pracha, N.; Dougherty, J.A.; Akhtar, A.; Alvi, S.B.; Khan, M. A one-stop protocol to assess myocardial fibrosis in frozen and paraffin sections. *Methods Protoc.* **2022**, *5*, 13. [CrossRef]
22. Zhou, J.; Wang, Y.; Zhu, P.; Sun, H.; Mou, Y.; Duan, C.; Yao, A.; Lv, S.; Wang, C. Distribution and characteristics of telocytes as nurse cells in the architectural organization of engineered heart tissues. *Sci. China Life Sci.* **2014**, *57*, 241–247. [CrossRef]
23. Filippone, A.; Cucinotta, L.; Bova, V.; Lanza, M.; Casili, G.; Paterniti, I.; Campolo, M.; Cuzzocrea, S.; Esposito, E. Inhibition of LRRK2 Attenuates Depression-Related Symptoms in Mice with Moderate Traumatic Brain Injury. *Cells* **2023**, *12*, 1040. [CrossRef]
24. Campolo, M.; Casili, G.; Lanza, M.; Filippone, A.; Cordaro, M.; Ardizzone, A.; Scuderi, S.A.; Cuzzocrea, S.; Esposito, E.; Paterniti, I. The inhibition of mammalian target of rapamycin (mTOR) in improving inflammatory response after traumatic brain injury. *J. Cell. Mol. Med.* **2021**, *25*, 7855–7866.
25. Ardizzone, A.; Mannino, D.; Capra, A.P.; Repici, A.; Filippone, A.; Esposito, E.; Campolo, M. New insights into the mechanism of Ulva pertusa on colitis in mice: Modulation of the pain and immune system. *Mar. Drugs* **2023**, *21*, 298. [CrossRef]
26. Zhao, T.; Wu, W.; Sui, L.; Huang, Q.; Nan, Y.; Liu, J.; Ai, K. Reactive oxygen species-based nanomaterials for the treatment of myocardial ischemia reperfusion injuries. *Bioact. Mater.* **2022**, *7*, 47–72.
27. Eltzschig, H.K.; Eckle, T. Ischemia and reperfusion—From mechanism to translation. *Nat. Med.* **2011**, *17*, 1391–1401.
28. Shen, Y.; Liu, X.; Shi, J.; Wu, X. Involvement of Nrf2 in myocardial ischemia and reperfusion injury. *Int. J. Biol. Macromol.* **2019**, *125*, 496–502.
29. Liu, Y.; Li, L.; Wang, Z.; Zhang, J.; Zhou, Z. Myocardial ischemia-reperfusion injury; Molecular mechanisms and prevention. *Microvasc. Res.* **2023**, *149*, 104565.
30. Marchant, D.J.; Boyd, J.H.; Lin, D.C.; Granville, D.J.; Garmaroudi, F.S.; McManus, B.M. Inflammation in myocardial diseases. *Circ. Res.* **2012**, *110*, 126–144.
31. Vrints, C.J. Pathophysiology of the no-reflow phenomenon. *Acute Card. Care* **2009**, *11*, 69–76. [CrossRef]
32. Zhao, W.; Gan, X.; Su, G.; Wanling, G.; Li, S.; Hei, Z.; Yang, C.; Wang, H. The interaction between oxidative stress and mast cell activation plays a role in acute lung injuries induced by intestinal ischemia–reperfusion. *J. Surg. Res.* **2014**, *187*, 542–552. [CrossRef] [PubMed]
33. Yang, M.-Q.; Ma, Y.-Y.; Tao, S.-F.; Ding, J.; Rao, L.-H.; Jiang, H.; Li, J.-Y. Mast cell degranulation promotes ischemia–reperfusion injury in rat liver. *J. Surg. Res.* **2014**, *186*, 170–178. [CrossRef]
34. Collington, S.J.; Williams, T.J.; Weller, C.L. Mechanisms underlying the localisation of mast cells in tissues. *Trends Immunol.* **2011**, *32*, 478–485. [CrossRef] [PubMed]
35. Xiong, W.; Yao, M.; Zhou, R.; Qu, Y.; Yang, Y.; Wang, Z.; Song, N.; Chen, H.; Qian, J. Oxytocin ameliorates ischemia/reperfusion-induced injury by inhibiting mast cell degranulation and inflammation in the rat heart. *Biomed. Pharmacother.* **2020**, *128*, 110358. [CrossRef] [PubMed]
36. Yu, X.; Sun, X.; Zhao, M.; Hou, Y.; Li, J.; Yu, J.; Hou, Y. Propofol attenuates myocardial ischemia reperfusion injury partly through inhibition of resident cardiac mast cell activation. *Int. Immunopharmacol.* **2018**, *54*, 267–274. [CrossRef]
37. Wang, F.; Yuan, Q.; Chen, F.; Pang, J.; Pan, C.; Xu, F.; Chen, Y. Fundamental mechanisms of the cell death caused by nitrosative stress. *Front. Cell Dev. Biol.* **2021**, *9*, 742483. [CrossRef]
38. Espey, M.G.; Miranda, K.M.; Feelisch, M.; Fukuto, J.; Grisham, M.B.; Vitek, M.P.; Wink, D.A. Mechanisms of cell death governed by the balance between nitrosative and oxidative stress. *Ann. N. Y. Acad. Sci.* **2000**, *899*, 209–221. [CrossRef]

39. Maes, M.; Galecki, P.; Chang, Y.S.; Berk, M. A review on the oxidative and nitrosative stress (O&NS) pathways in major depression and their possible contribution to the (neuro) degenerative processes in that illness. *Progress Neuro-Psychopharmacol. Biol. Psychiatry* **2011**, *35*, 676–692.
40. Kalka, C.; Masuda, H.; Takahashi, T.; Kalka-Moll, W.M.; Silver, M.; Kearney, M.; Li, T.; Isner, J.M.; Asahara, T. Transplantation of ex vivo expanded endothelial progenitor cells for therapeutic neovascularization. *Proc. Natl. Acad. Sci. USA* **2000**, *97*, 3422–3427. [CrossRef]
41. Bozdag-Turan, I.; Turan, R.G.; Turan, C.H.; Ludovicy, S.; Akin, I.; Kische, S.; Arsoy, N.S.; Schneider, H.; Ortak, J.; Rehders, T. Relation between the frequency of CD34+ bone marrow derived circulating progenitor cells and the number of diseased coronary arteries in patients with myocardial ischemia and diabetes. *Cardiovasc. Diabetol.* **2011**, *10*, 107. [CrossRef]
42. Xie, J.; Jiang, L.; Wang, J.; Yin, Y.; Wang, R.; Du, L.; Chen, T.; Ni, Z.; Qiao, S.; Gong, H. Multilineage contribution of CD34+ cells in cardiac remodeling after ischemia/reperfusion injury. *Basic. Res. Cardiol.* **2023**, *118*, 17. [PubMed]
43. Rai, B.; Shukla, J.; Henry, T.D.; Quesada, O. Angiogenic CD34 stem cell therapy in coronary microvascular repair—A systematic review. *Cells* **2021**, *10*, 1137. [CrossRef] [PubMed]
44. Hassanpour, M.; Salybekov, A.A.; Kobayashi, S.; Asahara, T. CD34 positive cells as endothelial progenitor cells in biology and medicine. *Front. Cell Dev. Biol.* **2023**, *11*, 1128134.
45. Leung, D.W.; Cachianes, G.; Kuang, W.-J.; Goeddel, D.V.; Ferrara, N. Vascular endothelial growth factor is a secreted angiogenic mitogen. *Science* **1989**, *246*, 1306–1309.
46. Ramakrishnan, S.; Anand, V.; Roy, S. Vascular endothelial growth factor signaling in hypoxia and inflammation. *J. Neuroimmune Pharmacol.* **2014**, *9*, 142–160. [CrossRef]
47. Guo, X.; Hong, S.; He, H.; Zeng, Y.; Chen, Y.; Mo, X.; Li, J.; Li, L.; Steinmetz, R.; Liu, Q. NFκB promotes oxidative stress-induced necrosis and ischemia/reperfusion injury by inhibiting Nrf2-ARE pathway. *Free Radic. Biol. Med.* **2020**, *159*, 125–135.
48. Kim, J.W.; Jin, Y.C.; Kim, Y.M.; Rhie, S.; Kim, H.J.; Seo, H.G.; Lee, J.H.; Ha, Y.L.; Chang, K.C. Daidzein administration in vivo reduces myocardial injury in a rat ischemia/reperfusion model by inhibiting NF-kB activation. *Life Sci.* **2009**, *84*, 227–234. [CrossRef]
49. Gao, H.-K.; Yin, Z.; Zhang, R.-Q.; Zhang, J.; Gao, F.; Wang, H.-C. GSK-3β inhibitor modulates TLR2/NF-κB signaling following myocardial ischemia-reperfusion. *Inflamm. Res.* **2009**, *58*, 377–383.
50. Fischer, U.M.; Antonyan, A.; Bloch, W.; Mehlhorn, U. Impact of antioxidative treatment on nuclear factor kappa-B regulation during myocardial ischemia–reperfusion. *Interact. Cardiovasc. Thorac. Surg.* **2006**, *5*, 531–535. [CrossRef]
51. Zhang, H.-L.; Xu, M.; Wei, C.; Qin, A.-P.; Liu, C.-F.; Hong, L.-Z.; Zhao, X.-Y.; Liu, J.; Qin, Z.-H. Neuroprotective effects of pioglitazone in a rat model of permanent focal cerebral ischemia are associated with peroxisome proliferator-activated receptor gamma-mediated suppression of nuclear factor-κB signaling pathway. *Neuroscience* **2011**, *176*, 381–395. [CrossRef]
52. Onai, Y.; Suzuki, J.-i.; Kakuta, T.; Maejima, Y.; Haraguchi, G.; Fukasawa, H.; Muto, S.; Itai, A.; Isobe, M. Inhibition of IκB phosphorylation in cardiomyocytes attenuates myocardial ischemia/reperfusion injury. *Cardiovasc. Res.* **2004**, *63*, 51–59. [CrossRef] [PubMed]
53. Tuntipopipat, S.; Muangnoi, C.; Chingsuwanrote, P.; Parengam, M.; Chantravisut, P.; Charoenkiatkul, S.; Svasti, S. Anti-inflammatory activities of red curry paste extract on lipopolysaccharide-activated murine macrophage cell line. *Nutrition* **2011**, *27*, 479–487. [CrossRef] [PubMed]
54. Dong, P.; Liu, K.; Han, H. The role of NF-κB in myocardial ischemia/reperfusion injury. *Curr. Protein Pept. Sci.* **2022**, *23*, 535–547. [PubMed]
55. Armstrong, S.C. Protein kinase activation and myocardial ischemia/reperfusion injury. *Cardiovasc. Res.* **2004**, *61*, 427–436. [CrossRef]
56. Chang, L.; Karin, M. Mammalian MAP kinase signalling cascades. *Nature* **2001**, *410*, 37–40. [CrossRef]
57. Romero-Becerra, R.; Santamans, A.M.; Folgueira, C.; Sabio, G. p38 MAPK pathway in the heart: New insights in health and disease. *Int. J. Mol. Sci.* **2020**, *21*, 7412. [CrossRef]
58. See, F.; Kompa, A.; Krum, H. p38 MAP kinase as a therapeutic target in cardiovascular disease. *Drug Discov. Today Ther. Strateg.* **2004**, *1*, 149–154. [CrossRef]
59. Kong, T.; Liu, M.; Ji, B.; Bai, B.; Cheng, B.; Wang, C. Role of the extracellular signal-regulated kinase 1/2 signaling pathway in ischemia-reperfusion injury. *Front. Physiol.* **2019**, *10*, 1038. [CrossRef]
60. Yue, T.-L.; Wang, C.; Gu, J.-L.; Ma, X.-L.; Kumar, S.; Lee, J.C.; Feuerstein, G.Z.; Thomas, H.; Maleeff, B.; Ohlstein, E.H. Inhibition of extracellular signal–regulated kinase enhances ischemia/reoxygenation–induced apoptosis in cultured cardiac myocytes and exaggerates reperfusion injury in isolated perfused heart. *Circ. Res.* **2000**, *86*, 692–699. [CrossRef]
61. Shimizu, N.; Yoshiyama, M.; Omura, T.; Hanatani, A.; Kim, S.; Takeuchi, K.; Iwao, H.; Yoshikawa, J. Activation of mitogen-activated protein kinases and activator protein-1 in myocardial infarction in rats. *Cardiovasc. Res.* **1998**, *38*, 116–124.

62. Iannelli, A.; de Sousa, G.; Zucchini, N.; Saint-Paul, M.C.; Gugenheim, J.; Rahmani, R. Anti-apoptotic pro-survival effect of clotrimazole in a normothermic ischemia reperfusion injury animal model. *J. Surg. Res.* **2011**, *171*, 101–107. [CrossRef] [PubMed]
63. McGrath, M.F.; de Bold, A.J. Determinants of natriuretic peptide gene expression. *Peptides* **2005**, *26*, 933–943. [CrossRef]
64. Nakayama, T. The Genetic Contribution of the Natriuretic Peptide System to Cardiovascular Diseases. *Endocr. J.* **2005**, *52*, 11–21. [CrossRef] [PubMed]
65. Cicilini, M.A.; Ramos, P.S.; Vasquez, E.C.; Cabral, A.M. Heart prolyl endopeptidase activity in one-kidney, one clip hypertensive rats. *Braz. J. Med. Biol. Res.* **1994**, *27*, 2821–2830. [PubMed]
66. Schulz, I.; Zeitschel, U.; Rudolph, T.; Ruiz-Carrillo, D.; Rahfeld, J.-U.; Gerhartz, B.; Bigl, V.; Demuth, H.-U.; Roßner, S. Subcellular localization suggests novel functions for prolyl endopeptidase in protein secretion. *J. Neurochem.* **2005**, *94*, 970–979. [CrossRef]
67. Kakavand, H.; Aghakouchakzadeh, M.; Coons, J.C.; Talasaz, A.H. Pharmacologic Prevention of Myocardial Ischemia–Reperfusion Injury in Patients With Acute Coronary Syndrome Undergoing Percutaneous Coronary Intervention. *J. Cardiovasc. Pharmacol.* **2021**, *77*, 430–449. [CrossRef]

antioxidants

MDPI

Article

Intermittent Fasting Protects Against the Progression from Acute Kidney Injury to Chronic Kidney Disease

Yoonjoo Jang [1,2], Young Suk Kim [2], Seo Rin Kim [1,2], Dong Won Lee [1,2], Soo Bong Lee [1,2] and Il Young Kim [1,2,*]

1 Department of Internal Medicine, Pusan National University School of Medicine, Yangsan 50612, Republic of Korea; kim.seorin@pusan.ac.kr (S.R.K.)

2 Research Institute for Convergence of Biomedical Science and Technology, Pusan National University Yangsan Hospital, Yangsan 50612, Republic of Korea

* Correspondence: iykim@pusan.ac.kr

Abstract: Acute kidney injury (AKI) is a major but often underestimated risk factor for the development of chronic kidney disease (CKD). Exploring innovative approaches to prevent this progression is critical. Intermittent fasting (IF), recognized for its metabolic and anti-inflammatory benefits, may offer protective effects in this context. Using a unilateral ischemia-reperfusion injury (UIRI) model in male C57BL/6 mice, we evaluated the impact of IF on tubulointerstitial fibrosis and tubular epithelial–mesenchymal transition (EMT) over 8 weeks. Mice in the IF group followed a 5:2 regimen, fasting for 24 h twice weekly. Four groups were studied: control, IF, UIRI, and IF + UIRI. The UIRI group exhibited increased fibrosis and EMT, both of which were significantly attenuated in the IF + UIRI group. IF also reduced levels of TGF-β1, phosphorylated NF-κB p65, inflammatory cytokines, and F4/80-positive macrophages, along with markers of oxidative stress. These findings highlight IF's ability to mitigate fibrosis and EMT through reductions in inflammation and oxidative stress during AKI-to-CKD progression. Our study suggests that IF may serve as a promising dietary strategy to prevent AKI from advancing into CKD.

Keywords: acute kidney injury; chronic kidney disease; epithelial–mesenchymal transition; intermittent fasting; tubulointerstitial fibrosis

1. Introduction

Acute kidney injury (AKI) denotes a medical condition characterized by a swift deterioration in kidney function, often associated with significant morbidity and mortality [1,2]. Historically, AKI was considered a reversible condition. However, recent studies suggest that kidney recovery following AKI is often incomplete, with persistent structural impairment that may result in the development of chronic kidney disease (CKD) [2]. Both epidemiological and experimental research shows that the intensity and length of AKI episodes are predictive of future CKD development [3]. As a result, the progression from AKI to CKD has emerged as a central focus of kidney disease research. Unfortunately, there are currently no treatments that can successfully halt the advancement of AKI to CKD.

The progression from AKI to CKD involves a complex and not fully understood pathophysiology [4]. However, increasing evidence highlights the roles of tubular epithelial cell (TEC) damage, interstitial inflammation, fibrosis, and endothelial dysfunction as key contributors to this process [4]. Various factors, including ischemia, sepsis, inflammation, and exposure to nephrotoxic agents, can trigger AKI [5]. When compensatory mechanisms fail to repair the damage, the healing process becomes impaired (maladaptive repair), leading to defective angiogenesis, cell cycle disruption, epithelial–mesenchymal transition (EMT) in TECs, interstitial tissue expansion, and inflammatory cell infiltration in the injured kidney [6,7]. TECs are particularly crucial in the progression from AKI to CKD, responding to injury by secreting inflammatory mediators and signaling molecules that drive tissue inflammation and fibrosis in the interstitium. Moreover, TECs are thought to drive this transition through EMT [6,8]. Thus, TECs are not passive players but actively contribute to inflammation and fibrosis during the AKI-to-CKD progression.

Caloric restriction involves reducing daily caloric intake over an extended period. Studies in animals have shown that caloric restriction can improve health, extend lifespan, and reduce mortality rates [9]. However, caloric restriction is difficult to maintain and may increase the risk of malnutrition. Consequently, intermittent fasting (IF) has gained popularity as a more practical alternative and has received growing attention in recent years. IF consists of cycles of consumption and abstention from food (or significantly reduced calorie intake) and has become a widely adopted lifestyle approach [10]. Both animal and human studies have demonstrated the broad health benefits of IF, particularly in managing metabolic disorders, through mechanisms beyond simple caloric restriction [10]. Several clinical trials have indicated that IF may provide similar or even greater improvements in weight loss and insulin resistance compared to continuous caloric restriction, with better adherence to the regimen [11]. While preclinical studies consistently show that IF has strong disease-modifying effects across a range of persistent health issues, such as excessive weight gain, insulin resistance, heart-related disorders, malignancies, and neurodegenerative diseases [10], its impact on kidney health has been less thoroughly investigated. In this study, we explore whether IF can protect against kidney injury in a mouse model of AKI-to-CKD progression.

2. Materials and Methods

2.1. Animal Experimental Design

All procedures involving animals were conducted with approval from the Institutional Animal Care and Use Committee of Pusan National University (PNU-IACUC, L2023-023-A1C0) and in compliance with the standards set by the Korean Association for Laboratory Animals. Eight-week-old male C57BL/6 mice were obtained from Koatech Technology Corporation (Seoul, Republic of Korea) and were kept in an animal housing unit with a 12 h light/dark schedule at 22 °C, where they had unrestricted availability of food and water.

To create a murine model for the progression from AKI to CKD, UIRI was induced in mice without performing nephrectomy on the opposite side, following established protocols [12]. Briefly, the mice were anesthetized with isoflurane vapors, and an incision was made on the right flank to expose the right renal pedicle. Ischemia was induced by placing a microaneurysm clamp on the renal pedicle for 30 min, as indicated by a visible change in color from red to dark blue. Afterward, the clamp was released, and normal blood flow was confirmed by the restoration of the typical coloration. The kidney was repositioned, and the surgical site was sutured in two layers. In the sham surgery group, the same steps were followed, except the renal pedicle was left unclamped.

Following UIRI or sham surgeries, the mice were allocated into four groups ($n = 6$ per group) in a random manner (Figure 1A): (a) sham: free access to food without UIRI, (b) IF: IF without UIRI, (c) UIRI: free access to food with UIRI, and (d) IF + UIRI: IF with UIRI. Mice in the ad libitum groups were provided with unlimited access to food at all times, while those in the IF group followed a 5:2 diet regimen. The IF group and IF + UIRI group fasted for two non-consecutive days per week (Monday and Thursday) for 24 h each time (from 9 a.m. to 9 a.m.). Fasting for the IF and IF + UIRI groups commenced immediately after IRI or sham surgery on Monday, aligning with the start of the 5:2 IF regimen. After 8 weeks of either IF or ad libitum feeding, the mice were euthanized. Blood β-hydroxybutyrate (β-HB) and glucose levels were measured from blood samples obtained from the tail vein of fasted mice, using a Free-Style Optium Neo device (Abbott, CN, USA) after 8 weeks of either ad libitum feeding or IF. Furthermore, body weight and food intake were monitored and recorded on a weekly basis.

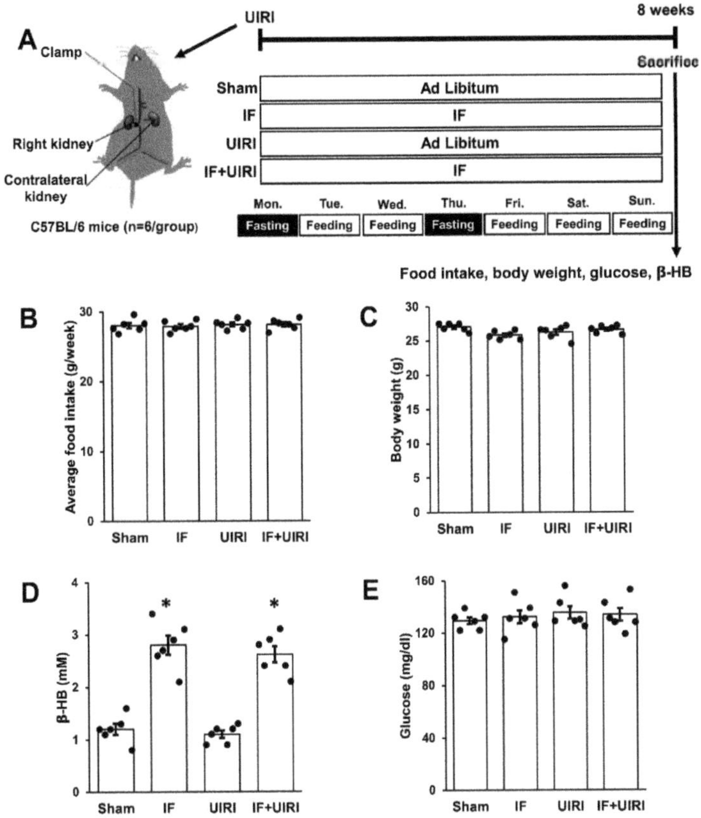

Figure 1. Effect of IF on metabolism. (**A**) Study setup: The ad libitum group had unrestricted food access throughout the day, whereas the IF group adhered to a 5:2 fasting schedule. In this regimen, the IF group fasted for a full day on two separate days each week, specifically on Monday and Thursday, from 9 a.m. to 9 a.m. (**B**) Mice subjected to IF for two months consumed food quantities comparable to those of the ad libitum group. (**C**) Body weight remained stable in the IF group. (**D**) The IF groups showed a marked increase in β-HB levels. (**E**) Blood glucose levels were similar between the IF and ad libitum groups. The measurements are shown as means ± SD (n = 6 per group; * $p < 0.05$ in comparison with sham and UIRI groups).

2.2. Histologic Examination

Paraffin-embedded kidney tissues were sliced into 3 μm thick sections for light microscopy analysis. As previously described [12], periodic acid-Schiff (PAS) and Masson's trichrome (MT) staining were employed to assess tubular injury and interstitial fibrosis, respectively. Stained tissue slides were visualized using a ZEISS Axioscan7 (Carl Zeiss, Jena, Germany) and images were captured with ZEN Lite software version 3.9 (Carl Zeiss) at a magnification of 20×. Tubular damage was assessed by an evaluator unaware of the experimental groups, who analyzed 10 high-power fields (HPFs) of the renal cortex from PAS-stained samples, scoring based on the following scale: 0 for no damage, 1 for less than 10% damage, 2 for 10–25%, 3 for 25–50%,

4 for 50–75%, and 5 for more than 75%. Tubular damage was identified by various signs, such as thickening of the tubular basement membrane, cast formation, shedding of tubular epithelial cells (TECs), loss of the brush border, dilation, and atrophy. For interstitial fibrosis, MT-stained sections were examined in 10 cortical high-power fields, with scoring based on the following criteria: 0 for no fibrosis, 1 for fibrosis affecting up to 25%, 2 for fibrosis involving 25–50%, and 3 for fibrosis affecting more than 50% [12].

2.3. Immunohistochemical Analysis

Immunohistochemical analysis was performed on 3 μm thick paraffin-embedded tissue slices. Following established protocols [13], the sections were first deparaffinized using xylene and gradually rehydrated through a series of ethanol solutions. Antigen retrieval was accomplished by heating in a microwave. Non-specific binding was blocked using normal horse serum (Vector Laboratories, CA, USA), after which the tissue samples were placed at 4 °C overnight and exposed to primary antibodies. Afterward, secondary antibodies (ImmPRESS™ HRP reagent kit, Vector Laboratories) were applied at 37 °C for 30 min. The immunoreaction was visualized using DAB, followed by counterstaining with hematoxylin. The primary antibodies included anti-F4/80 (Abcam, Cambridge, UK), anti-E-cadherin (Cell Signaling Technology, MA, USA), anti-TGF-β1 (Abcam), anti-8-OHdG (JalCA, Sizuoka, Japan), anti-vimentin (Abcam), anti-nitrotyrosine (Abcam), anti-phosphorylated NF-κB p65 (Santa Cruz, CA, USA), anti-4-HNE (JalCA), and anti-α-smooth muscle actin (SMA) (Abcam). Images of the stained slides were captured with a ZEISS Axioscan 7 and analyzed using ZEN Lite software. Ten high-power fields (HPFs) were randomly chosen for evaluation. Quantification of 8-OHdG, p-NF-κB p65, and F4/80-positive cells was performed, and semi-quantitative scoring for 4-HNE, vimentin, α-SMA, TGF-β1, E-cadherin, and nitrotyrosine was carried out using the following system: 0 for no staining, 1 for staining covering 1–25% of the area, 2 for staining covering 26–50% of the area, 3 for staining covering 51–75% of the area, and 4 staining covering more than 75% of the area [13].

2.4. Quantitative Real-Time Polymerase Chain Reaction (PCR) Analysis

Real-time PCR was conducted as outlined in previous studies [13], utilizing *GAPDH* as a reference gene along with target genes *IL-1β*, *TNF-α*, and *IL-6*. The amplification products were validated through a melting curve analysis, with temperature cycling at 95 °C for 15 s, then 60 °C for 15 s, followed by a concluding phase at 95 °C for 15 s. The relative gene expression changes were calculated using the $2^{-\Delta\Delta CT}$ formula. The sequences of primers are listed in Table 1.

Table 1. Primers used in this study for PCR (mouse).

Gene	Gene Accession Number	Forward	Reverse
GAPDH	NM_008084.4	5′-CATCACTGCCACCCAGAAGACTG-3′	5′-ATGCCAGTGAGCTTCCCGTTCAG-3′
IL-6	NM_031168.2	5′-TACCACTTCACAAGTCGGAGGC-3′	5′-CTGCAAGTGCATCATCGTTGTTC-3′
TNF-α	NM_013693.3	5′-GGTGCCTATGTCTCAGCCTCTT-3′	5′-GCCATAGAACTGATGAGAGGGAG-3′
IL-1β	NM_008361.4	5′-CCACAGACCTTCCAGGAGAATG-3′	5′-GTGCAGTTCAGTGATCGTACAGG-3′

2.5. Statistical Analysis

All statistical evaluations were performed using SPSS version 27 (SPSS, Inc., Chicago, IL, USA). The information was assessed using the Mann–Whitney U test or Kruskal–Wallis test, depending on the circumstances. A *p*-value below 0.05 was considered to indicate a significant result. The measurements are shown as mean ± standard deviation (SD).

3. Results

3.1. Effect of IF on Metabolism

Over the course of two months, the IF group consumed a quantity of food similar to that of the ad libitum control group, confirming that IF did not involve caloric restriction during the feeding periods (Figure 1B). Importantly, no changes in body weight were observed in the IF group (Figure 1C). However, the β-HB levels were elevated in the IF group, indicating a state of ketosis induced by the fasting regimen (Figure 1D). Blood glucose levels remained comparable between the IF and ad libitum control groups (Figure 1E).

3.2. Effect of IF on Kidney Pathology and Function During the Progression from AKI to CKD

Two months after UIRI, PAS staining showed significant tubular damage in the UIRI group, with noticeable dilation, atrophy, and cast formation compared to the sham group. These pathological alterations showed a marked reduction in the IF + UIRI group (Figure 2A,C). Similarly, MT staining revealed a marked increase in interstitial fibrosis in the UIRI group, whereas the IF + UIRI group exhibited a substantial reduction in fibrosis (Figure 2B,D). In line with these histological results, blood creatinine concentrations were higher in the UIRI group compared to the sham group, while the IF + UIRI group showed lower levels, suggesting that IF offers a protective effect on renal function during the progression from AKI to CKD (Figure 2E).

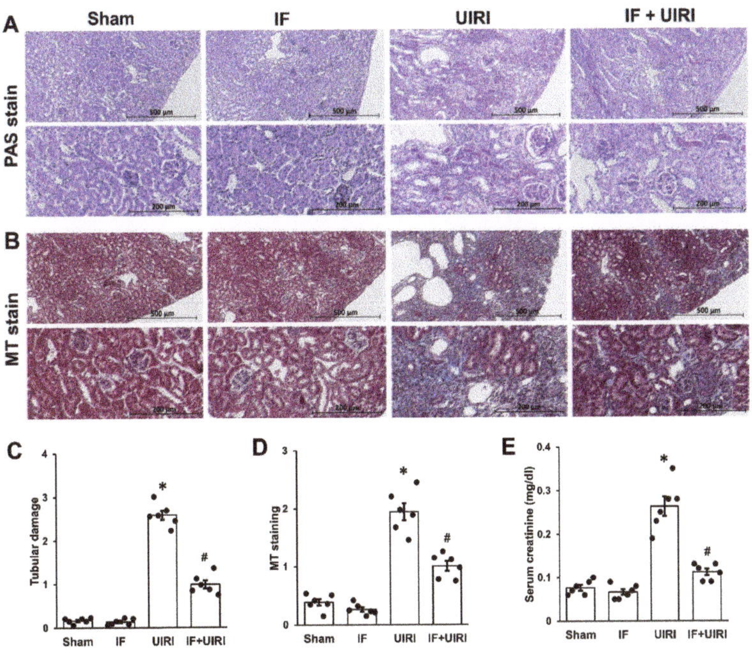

Figure 2. Effect of IF on kidney pathology and function during AKI-to-CKD progression. (**A**,**C**) Representative images stained with periodic acid-Schiff (PAS) reveal reduced tubular damage in the IF + UIRI group when contrasted with the UIRI group. (**B**,**D**) Masson's trichrome (MT) staining reveals significantly reduced tubulointerstitial fibrosis in the IF + UIRI group relative to the UIRI group. (**E**) The IF + UIRI group showed reduced serum creatinine concentrations in comparison to the UIRI group. The measurements are shown as means ± SD ($n = 6$ per group; * $p < 0.05$ vs. sham and IF groups; # $p < 0.05$ vs. UIRI group).

3.3. Effect of IF on Tubular EMT During the Progression from AKI to CKD

EMT in TECs is a known contributor to renal tubulointerstitial fibrosis [14]. Immunohistochemical analysis revealed a significant decrease in E-cadherin expression, an epithelial marker, in the UIRI group in relation to the sham group. However, this reduction was alleviated in the IF + UIRI group (Figure 3A). In contrast, the expression of mesenchymal markers, including α-SMA and vimentin, was elevated in the UIRI group in comparison with the sham group. These markers, however, showed a significant reduction in the IF + UIRI group relative to the UIRI group (Figure 3B,C).

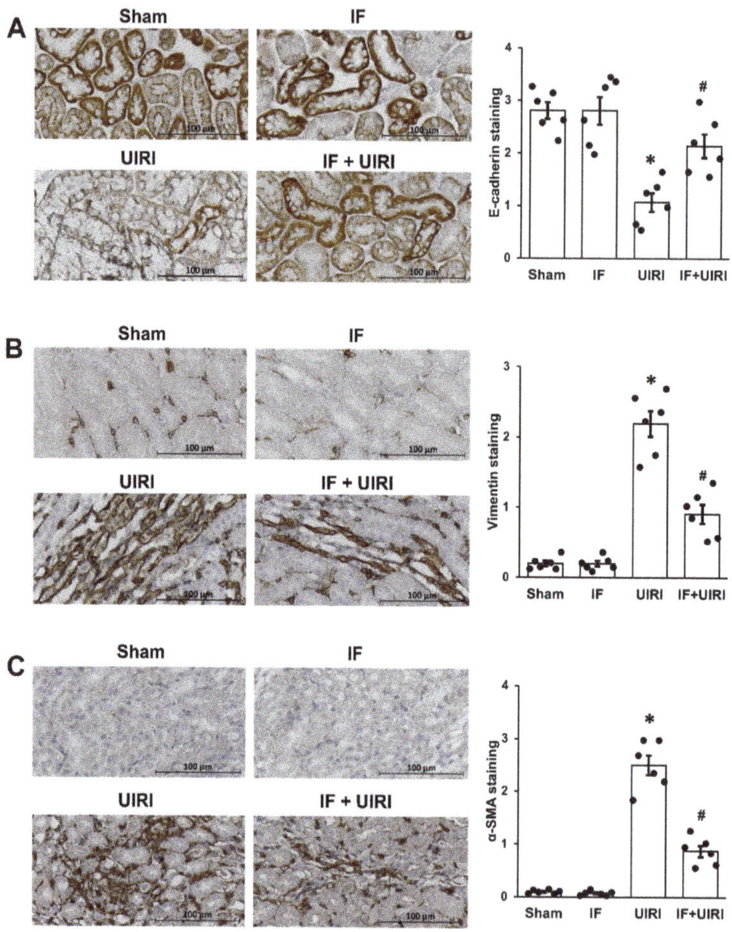

Figure 3. Effect of IF on tubular EMT during AKI-to-CKD progression. (**A**) Immunohistochemical analysis of E-cadherin revealed greater expression in the IF + UIRI group than in the UIRI group. (**B**,**C**) Immunohistochemical analysis of vimentin and α-SMA revealed reduced expression in the IF + UIRI group versus the UIRI group. The measurements are shown as means ± SD (n = 6 per group; * $p < 0.05$ vs. sham and IF groups; # $p < 0.05$ vs. UIRI group).

3.4. Effect of IF on Inflammation During the Progression from AKI to CKD

Inflammation is a key factor in tubular EMT and the development of kidney fibrosis [14]. Analysis of mRNA levels revealed that inflammatory mediators, such as *IL-6*, *IL-1β*, and *TNF-α*, were notably elevated in the UIRI group in contrast to the sham group. This increase was substantially reduced in the IF + UIRI group (Figure 4A). Additionally, the number of macrophages, identified by F4/80 staining in the interstitial region, was higher in the UIRI group than in the sham group, but this was notably reduced in the IF + UIRI group (Figure 4B). Considering the crucial roles of TGF-β and NF-κB in inflammation regulation [14], their expression levels were also examined. Immunohistochemical analysis revealed enhanced TGF-β1 and phosphorylated NF-κB p65 expression in the UIRI group, whereas these markers were considerably reduced in the IF + UIRI group (Figure 4C,D).

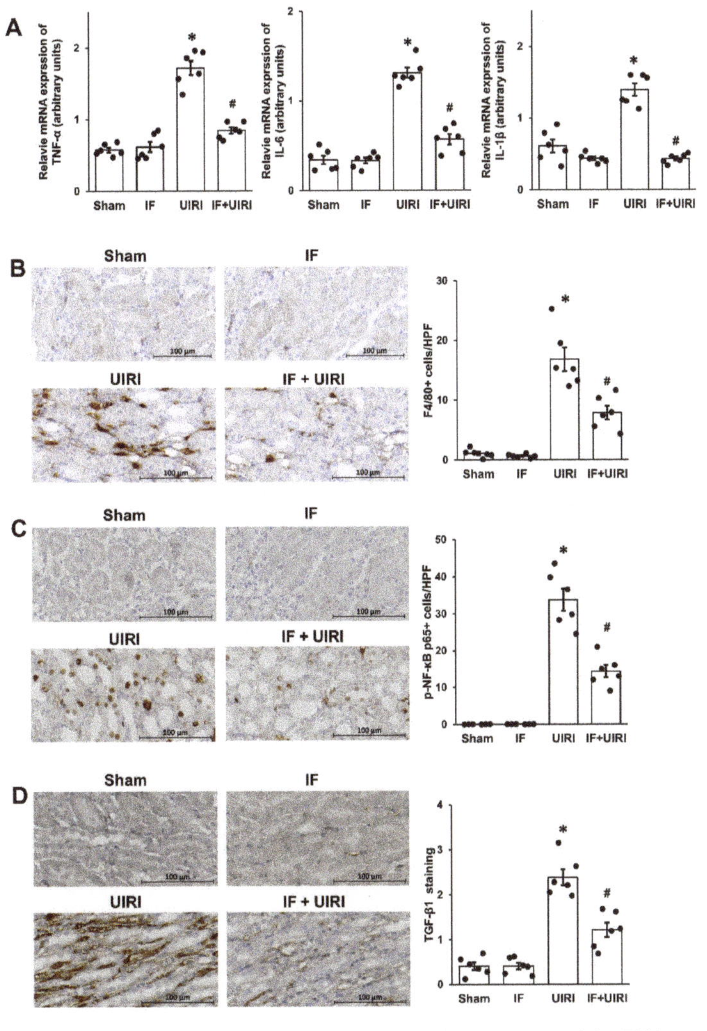

Figure 4. Effect of IF on inflammation during AKI-to-CKD progression. (**A**) mRNA expression of *TNF-α*, *IL-6*, and *IL-1β* was notably reduced in the IF + UIRI group relative to the UIRI group. (**B**) Immunohistochemical analysis revealed a decrease in F4/80-positive staining in the IF + UIRI group when assessed against the UIRI group. (**C,D**) Immunostaining demonstrated a reduction in phosphorylated NF-κB p65 and TGF-β1 levels in the IF + UIRI group, as compared to the UIRI group. The measurements are shown as means ± SD ($n = 6$ per group; * $p < 0.05$ vs. sham and IF groups; # $p < 0.05$ vs. UIRI group).

3.5. Effect of IF on Oxidative Stress During the Progression from AKI to CKD

Oxidative stress is a key driver of tubular EMT and renal fibrosis [14]. To assess the impact of IF, kidney tissues were stained for markers of oxidative damage: nitrotyrosine (protein), 4-HNE (lipid), and 8-OHdG (DNA). The levels of all three markers were elevated in the UIRI group, while these markers of oxidative damage were reduced in the IF + UIRI group, suggesting that IF helps alleviate oxidative stress during the progression from AKI to CKD (Figure 5A–C).

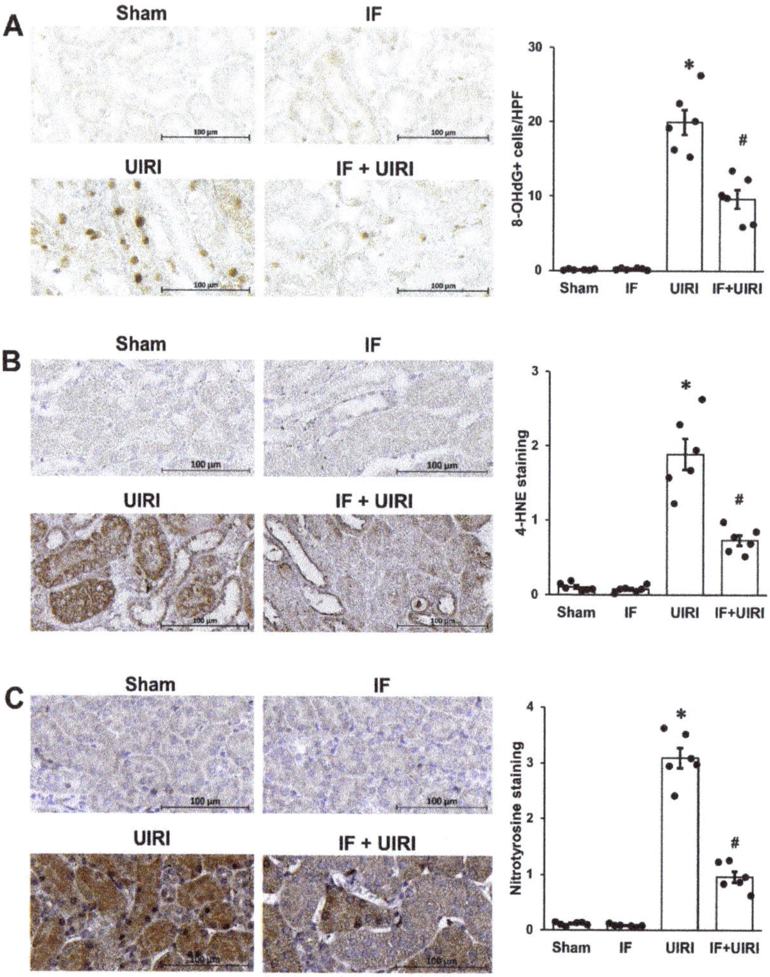

Figure 5. Effect of IF on oxidative stress during AKI-to-CKD progression. Immunohistochemical analysis revealed a decrease in oxidative stress markers, such as 8-OHdG (**A**), 4-HNE (**B**), and nitrotyrosine (**C**), in the IF + UIRI group in contrast to the UIRI group. The measurements are shown as means ± SD ($n = 6$ per group; * $p < 0.05$ vs. sham and IF groups; # $p < 0.05$ vs. UIRI group).

4. Discussion

In our study, we used the UIRI model without contralateral nephrectomy, which is widely accepted for investigating the progression from AKI to CKD [15]. Renal IRI is a key contributor to AKI in humans, triggering a pathological cascade that results in acute tubulointerstitial damage [16]. Following IRI, a repair mechanism is activated to restore the kidney's normal structure and function. However, in cases of severe injury, this can result in irreversible damage and progressive fibrosis [16]. Renal IRI is thus an important and valuable model for studying the transition from AKI to CKD. In our study, a mouse model of AKI-to-CKD progression was established, as evidenced by elevated serum creatinine levels and the onset of tubulointerstitial fibrosis. Notably, there was no significant difference in the degree of fibrosis in the left kidney (the kidney without IRI) among the four groups (MT staining score: sham, 0.21 ± 0.04; IF, 0.14 ± 0.02; UIRI, 0.13 ± 0.02; IF + UIRI, 0.13 ± 0.02, $p = 0.302$). The observed increase in serum creatinine in UIRI, despite the absence of contralateral nephrectomy, is thought to be due to the left kidney's inability to sufficiently compensate for overall renal function 8 weeks after IRI of the right kidney. In this model, IF was shown to enhance renal function, reduce tubulointerstitial fibrosis and EMT, and decrease inflammation and oxidative stress in this model. As far as we are aware, this investigation offers the first evidence demonstrating the positive effects of IF on the transition from AKI to CKD.

Numerous investigations have examined the potential advantages of IF for maintaining health and addressing diseases [10]. Some studies connect the positive outcomes of IF to reduced energy consumption, while others emphasize enhanced metabolic indicators and resistance to adverse conditions, even with comparable calorie intake [17]. In this research, mice in the IF groups showed weight patterns and food intake similar to those of the control groups throughout the observation period, ruling out energy limitation. These findings imply that the benefits of IF on the transition from AKI to CKD observed in this study were not dependent on lower calorie consumption.

Several previous studies have investigated the effects of dietary interventions on the progression of AKI to CKD. Rojas-Morales et al. conducted a study in which they induced fasting for 3 days prior to kidney IRI and evaluated the degree of kidney fibrosis 14 days later. They concluded that fasting for 3 days before IRI suppressed kidney fibrosis, primarily due to the inhibition of oxidative stress and mitochondrial dysfunction. Another study by the same researchers demonstrated that fasting for 3 days prior to RI improved kidney fibrosis 28 days post-IRI, and they suggested that this effect was related to reductions in inflammation and endoplasmic reticulum stress, in addition to oxidative stress and mitochondrial dysfunction.

Several previous studies have investigated the effects of dietary interventions on the progression of AKI to CKD. Rojas-Morales et al. conducted a study in which they induced fasting for 3 days prior to kidney IRI and evaluated the degree of kidney fibrosis 14 days later [18]. They concluded that fasting for 3 days before IRI suppressed kidney fibrosis, primarily due to the inhibition of oxidative stress and mitochondrial dysfunction. Another study by the same researchers demonstrated that fasting for 3 days prior to IRI improved kidney fibrosis 28 days post-IRI, and they suggested that this effect was related to reductions in inflammation and endoplasmic reticulum stress, in addition to oxidative stress and mitochondrial dysfunction [19]. Our current study has several differences compared to the two studies by Rojas-Morales et al. First, we investigated the effect of IF (5:2 regimen) initiated after IRI on the progression of AKI to CKD, whereas the studies by Rojas-Morales et al. implemented extreme fasting (complete fasting for 3 days) before IRI. This indicates differences not only in the type of dietary intervention regimens but also in their application timing before and after IRI. Notably, 3 days of extreme fasting can cause significant stress to both mice and humans, making it difficult to apply in clinical settings. In contrast, the 5:2 IF regimen is already in practical use and holds potential for application to AKI-to-CKD progression in humans. Second, while the two studies by Rojas-Morales et al. examined kidney fibrosis at 2 and 4 weeks post-IRI, our study extended the evaluation period to 8 weeks. This difference allowed us to study kidney fibrosis at a more advanced stage. Third, the studies by Morales et al. revealed that fasting suppressed kidney fibrosis after IRI by reducing oxidative stress, mitochondrial dysfunction, inflammation, and endoplasmic reticulum stress. In contrast, our study demonstrated that intermittent fasting not only reduces inflammation and oxidative stress but also suppresses EMT, highlighting a key difference in findings.

A significant finding from our research is the marked reduction in inflammation induced by IF in the AKI-to-CKD progression. Although this investigation did not fully clarify the processes responsible for IF's ability to reduce inflammation in this context, IF is widely recognized for its capacity to dampen inflammatory responses. Research in both human and animal models has shown that IF can alleviate inflammation in a variety of chronic inflammatory conditions, such as heart disease, metabolic disorders, neurological diseases, joint diseases, and different types of malignancies [20]. While these findings are compelling, the exact way through which IF reduces inflammation in the context of our investigation is not yet fully understood. One possible mechanism involves ketosis induced by IF. Higher levels of β-HB in mice undergoing IF suggest that this approach may lead to a state of ketosis. As a byproduct of liver fat metabolism, β-HB provides a substitute energy source when carbohydrates are scarce [21]. Beyond its metabolic role, β-HB plays an important role as a signaling molecule with the ability to influence inflammation by regulating forkhead box O1 (FOXO1) and peroxisome proliferator-activated receptor-gamma coactivator-1 alpha (PGC-1α) [21,22]. Further investigation is necessary to uncover the complex mechanisms through which IF impacts inflammation during the progression from AKI to CKD.

Additionally, our investigation has demonstrated that IF can decrease oxidative damage in a murine model of AKI-to-CKD progression. While we have not completely determined the precise mechanisms through which IF mitigates this transition, accumulating evidence points to IF's potential to attenuate oxidative damage. A comprehensive review of controlled clinical trials indicates that IF may reduce markers of oxidative harm in individuals with obesity [23]. Previous studies in both animal and human models have indicated that IF can lower indicators of oxidative damage in a variety of chronic disorders [20]. Although the exact biochemical mechanisms remain partially unknown, it is probable that PGC-1α and nuclear factor erythroid 2-related factor 2 (NRF2)—transcription factors sensitive to redox changes—contribute to IF's antioxidative properties [24]. Additionally, β-HB produced by IF has been shown to stimulate both FOXO1 and NRF2, which control genes that protect cells during the oxidative damage [25]. Further research is needed to uncover the intricate mechanisms through which IF influences oxidative stress in the transition from AKI to CKD.

Finally, our research has shown that IF reduces tubulointerstitial fibrosis and tubular EMT in a murine model of the progression from AKI to CKD. Tubulointerstitial fibrosis represents a crucial stage in the transition from AKI to CKD, marked by the stimulation of myofibroblasts, which are the key cells involved in the accumulation of interstitial extracellular matrix [26]. Although renal interstitial fibroblasts were previously thought to be the sole origin of myofibroblasts, increasing evidence indicates that injured TECs can undergo dedifferentiation, becoming a significant source of myofibroblasts [27]. Tubular EMT involves injured TECs losing epithelial markers and gaining mesenchymal characteristics, and it is recognized as a key mechanism underlying renal tubulointerstitial fibrosis [6]. In our study, the precise mechanism through which IF reduces tubulointerstitial fibrosis and tubular EMT remains unclear. However, accumulating evidence suggests that inflammation and oxidative stress work in tandem to induce EMT within the context of renal tubulointerstitial fibrosis. Notably, during inflammation associated with this fibrosis, TGF-β is recognized as the main factor driving tubular EMT, with NF-κB—activated by TGF-β—also playing a contributory role [14]. Under oxidative damage, reactive oxygen species are likewise implicated in tubular EMT [14]. As discussed, our findings show that IF mitigated both inflammation and oxidative stress throughout the transition from AKI to CKD. Given the well-established interactions between inflammation, oxidative stress, and tubular EMT, we propose that IF may reduce tubulointerstitial fibrosis and tubular EMT by alleviating inflammation and oxidative stress damage in the context of AKI-to-CKD progression.

5. Conclusions

The outcomes of this research are summarized in Figure 6. An increase in tubulointerstitial fibrosis and tubular EMT was observed as a result of enhanced inflammation and oxidative damage in a murine model of AKI-to-CKD progression. IF was shown to alleviate tubulointerstitial fibrosis following tubular EMT. This protective effect of IF seemed to be associated with decreased inflammation and oxidative damage. As a result, IF could represent a novel dietary strategy to prevent the progression from AKI to CKD. Further investigations are necessary to clarify the mechanisms through which IF exerts its beneficial influence on the transition from AKI to CKD.

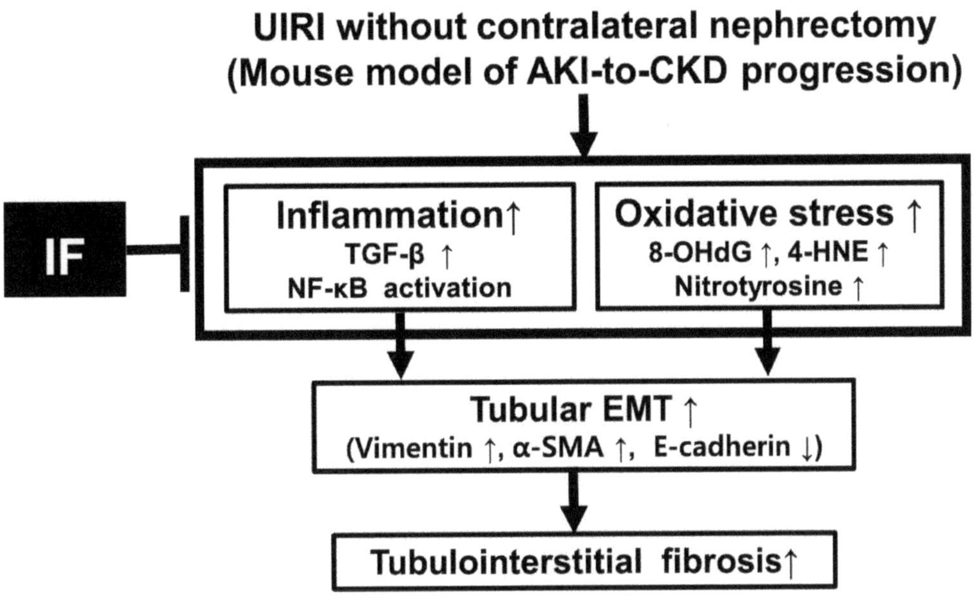

Figure 6. Summary of the protective effects of IF against tubulointerstitial fibrosis and tubular EMT in UIRI. This schematic highlights IF's ability to alleviate tubulointerstitial fibrosis and tubular EMT by suppressing oxidative damage and inflammation in a murine model of AKI-to-CKD progression.

Author Contributions: Conceptualization, Y.J. and I.Y.K.; methodology, I.Y.K. and S.B.L.; software, Y.S.K.; validation, D.W.L., S.R.K. and S.B.L.; formal analysis, Y.S.K., S.R.K. and I.Y.K.; investigation, Y.S.K. and I.Y.K.; resources, I.Y.K.; data curation, Y.S.K., I.Y.K. and D.W.L.; writing—original draft preparation, Y.J.; writing—review and editing, I.Y.K.; visualization I.Y.K.; supervision, S.B.L. and

D.W.L.; project administration, Y.S.K. and S.R.K.; funding acquisition, I.Y.K. All authors have read and agreed to the published version of the manuscript.

Funding: This work was supported by the National Research Foundation of Korea (NRF) grant funded by the Korea government (MSIT) (RS-2023-00251250).

Institutional Review Board Statement: All animal experiments received approval from the Pusan National University Institutional Animal Care and Use Committee (PNU-IACUC, L2023-023-A1C0) and were performed in accordance with the Guidelines for the Care and Use of Experimental Animals endorsed by the Korean Association for Laboratory Animals.

Informed Consent Statement: Not applicable.

Data Availability Statement: Data are contained within this article.

Conflicts of Interest: The authors declare no conflicts of interest. The funders had no role in the design of the study; in the collection, analyses, or interpretation of data; in the writing of the manuscript; or in the decision to publish the results.

References

1. Kellum, J.A.; Romagnani, P.; Ashuntantang, G.; Ronco, C.; Zarbock, A.; Anders, H.J. Acute Kidney Injury. *Nat. Rev. Dis. Primers* **2021**, *7*, 52. [CrossRef] [PubMed]
2. Kung, C.W.; Chou, Y.H. Acute Kidney Disease: An Overview of the Epidemiology, Pathophysiology, and Management. *Kidney Res. Clin. Pract.* **2023**, *42*, 686–699. [CrossRef] [PubMed]
3. Rifkin, D.E.; Coca, S.G.; Kalantar-Zadeh, K. Does Aki Truly Lead to Ckd? *J. Am. Soc. Nephrol.* **2012**, *23*, 979–984. [CrossRef] [PubMed]
4. Guzzi, F.; Cirillo, L.; Roperto, R.M.; Romagnani, P.; Lazzeri, E. Molecular Mechanisms of the Acute Kidney Injury to Chronic Kidney Disease Transition: An Updated View. *Int. J. Mol. Sci.* **2019**, *20*, 4941. [CrossRef] [PubMed]
5. Peerapornratana, S.; Manrique-Caballero, C.L.; Gomez, H.; Kellum, J.A. Acute Kidney Injury from Sepsis: Current Concepts, Epidemiology, Pathophysiology, Prevention and Treatment. *Kidney Int.* **2019**, *96*, 1083–1099. [CrossRef]
6. Sheng, L.; Zhuang, S. New Insights into the Role and Mechanism of Partial Epithelial-Mesenchymal Transition in Kidney Fibrosis. *Front. Physiol.* **2020**, *11*, 569322. [CrossRef]
7. Lovisa, S.; LeBleu, V.S.; Tampe, B.; Sugimoto, H.; Vadnagara, K.; Carstens, J.L.; Wu, C.C.; Hagos, Y.; Burckhardt, B.C.; Pentcheva-Hoang, T.; et al. Epithelial-to-Mesenchymal Transition Induces Cell Cycle Arrest and Parenchymal Damage in Renal Fibrosis. *Nat. Med.* **2015**, *21*, 998–1009. [CrossRef] [PubMed]
8. Wang, Z.; Zhang, C. From Aki to Ckd: Maladaptive Repair and the Underlying Mechanisms. *Int. J. Mol. Sci.* **2022**, *23*, 10880. [CrossRef] [PubMed]
9. Mattison, J.A.; Colman, R.J.; Beasley, T.M.; Allison, D.B.; Kemnitz, J.W.; Roth, G.S.; Ingram, D.K.; Weindruch, R.; de Cabo, R.; Anderson, R.M. Caloric Restriction Improves Health and Survival of Rhesus Monkeys. *Nat. Commun.* **2017**, *8*, 14063. [CrossRef]
10. de Cabo, R.; Mattson, M.P. Effects of Intermittent Fasting on Health, Aging, and Disease. *N. Engl. J. Med.* **2019**, *381*, 2541–2551. [CrossRef]
11. James, D.L.; Hawley, N.A.; Mohr, A.E.; Hermer, J.; Ofori, E.; Yu, F.; Sears, D.D. Impact of Intermittent Fasting and/or Caloric Restriction on Aging-Related Outcomes in Adults: A Scoping Review of Randomized Controlled Trials. *Nutrients* **2024**, *16*, 316. [CrossRef]
12. Kim, I.Y.; Park, Y.K.; Song, S.H.; Seong, E.Y.; Lee, D.W.; Bae, S.S.; Lee, S.B. Role of Akt1 in Renal Fibrosis and Tubular Dedifferentiation During the Progression of Acute Kidney Injury to Chronic Kidney Disease. *Korean J. Intern. Med.* **2021**, *36*, 962–974. [CrossRef] [PubMed]
13. Kim, D.K.; Kim, Y.S.; Kim, M.J.; Kim, S.R.; Lee, D.W.; Lee, S.B.; Kim, I.Y. Time-Restricted Feeding Protects against Renal Ischemia-Reperfusion Injury in Mice. *Int. J. Mol. Sci.* **2024**, *25*, 7652. [CrossRef] [PubMed]
14. Lopez-Novoa, J.M.; Nieto, M.A. Inflammation and Emt: An Alliance Towards Organ Fibrosis and Cancer Progression. *EMBO Mol. Med.* **2009**, *1*, 303–314. [CrossRef] [PubMed]
15. Le Clef, N.; Verhulst, A.; D'Haese, P.C.; Vervaet, B.A. Unilateral Renal Ischemia-Reperfusion as a Robust Model for Acute to Chronic Kidney Injury in Mice. *PLoS ONE* **2016**, *11*, e0152153. [CrossRef]
16. Dong, Y.; Zhang, Q.; Wen, J.; Chen, T.; He, L.; Wang, Y.; Yin, J.; Wu, R.; Xue, R.; Li, S.; et al. Ischemic Duration and Frequency Determines Aki-to-Ckd Progression Monitored by Dynamic Changes of Tubular Biomarkers in Iri Mice. *Front. Physiol.* **2019**, *10*, 153. [CrossRef]

17. Dwaib, H.S.; AlZaim, I.; Eid, A.H.; Obeid, O.; El-Yazbi, A.F. Modulatory Effect of Intermittent Fasting on Adipose Tissue Inflammation: Amelioration of Cardiovascular Dysfunction in Early Metabolic Impairment. *Front. Pharmacol.* **2021**, *12*, 626313. [CrossRef] [PubMed]
18. Rojas-Morales, P.; Leon-Contreras, J.C.; Aparicio-Trejo, O.E.; Reyes-Ocampo, J.G.; Medina-Campos, O.N.; Jimenez-Osorio, A.S.; Gonzalez-Reyes, S.; Marquina-Castillo, B.; Hernandez-Pando, R.; Barrera-Oviedo, D.; et al. Fasting Reduces Oxidative Stress, Mitochondrial Dysfunction and Fibrosis Induced by Renal Ischemia-Reperfusion Injury. *Free Radic. Biol. Med.* **2019**, *135*, 60–67. [CrossRef]
19. Rojas-Morales, P.; Tapia, E.; Leon-Contreras, J.C.; Gonzalez-Reyes, S.; Jimenez-Osorio, A.S.; Trujillo, J.; Pavon, N.; Granados-Pineda, J.; Hernandez-Pando, R.; Sanchez-Lozada, L.G.; et al. Mechanisms of Fasting-Mediated Protection against Renal Injury and Fibrosis Development after Ischemic Acute Kidney Injury. *Biomolecules* **2019**, *9*, 404. [CrossRef]
20. Mattson, M.P.; Allison, D.B.; Fontana, L.; Harvie, M.; Longo, V.D.; Malaisse, W.J.; Mosley, M.; Notterpek, L.; Ravussin, E.; Scheer, F.A.; et al. Meal Frequency and Timing in Health and Disease. *Proc. Natl. Acad. Sci. USA* **2014**, *111*, 16647–16653. [CrossRef] [PubMed]
21. Mierziak, J.; Burgberger, M.; Wojtasik, W. 3-Hydroxybutyrate as a Metabolite and a Signal Molecule Regulating Processes of Living Organisms. *Biomolecules* **2021**, *11*, 402. [CrossRef]
22. Kim, D.H.; Park, M.H.; Ha, S.; Bang, E.J.; Lee, Y.; Lee, A.K.; Lee, J.; Yu, B.P.; Chung, H.Y. Anti-Inflammatory Action of Beta-Hydroxybutyrate Via Modulation of Pgc-1alpha and Foxo1, Mimicking Calorie Restriction. *Aging* **2019**, *11*, 1283–1304. [CrossRef]
23. Mohr, A.E.; McEvoy, C.; Sears, D.D.; Arciero, P.J.; Sweazea, K.L. Impact of Intermittent Fasting Regimens on Circulating Markers of Oxidative Stress in Overweight and Obese Humans: A Systematic Review of Randomized Controlled Trials. *Adv. Redox Res.* **2021**, *3*, 100026. [CrossRef]
24. Lettieri-Barbato, D.; Minopoli, G.; Caggiano, R.; Izzo, R.; Santillo, M.; Aquilano, K.; Faraonio, R. Fasting Drives Nrf2-Related Antioxidant Response in Skeletal Muscle. *Int. J. Mol. Sci.* **2020**, *21*, 7780. [CrossRef] [PubMed]
25. Han, Y.M.; Ramprasath, T.; Zou, M.H. Beta-Hydroxybutyrate and Its Metabolic Effects on Age-Associated Pathology. *Exp. Mol. Med.* **2020**, *52*, 548–555. [CrossRef] [PubMed]
26. Wang, C.; Li, S.W.; Zhong, X.; Liu, B.C.; Lv, L.L. An Update on Renal Fibrosis: From Mechanisms to Therapeutic Strategies with a Focus on Extracellular Vesicles. *Kidney Res. Clin. Pract.* **2023**, *42*, 174–187. [CrossRef] [PubMed]
27. Grgic, I.; Duffield, J.S.; Humphreys, B.D. The Origin of Interstitial Myofibroblasts in Chronic Kidney Disease. *Pediatr. Nephrol.* **2012**, *27*, 183–193. [CrossRef]

antioxidants

MDPI

Article

Exercise-Intervened Circulating Extracellular Vesicles Alleviate Oxidative Stress in Cerebral Microvascular Endothelial Cells Under Hypertensive Plus Hypoxic Conditions

Smara Sigdel, Shuzhen Chen, Gideon Udoh and Jinju Wang *

Department of Biomedical Sciences, Joan C. Edwards School of Medicine, Marshall University, Huntington, WV 25755, USA; sigdels@marshall.edu (S.S.); chens@marshall.edu (S.C.); udoh3@marshall.edu (G.U.)
* Correspondence: wangjin@marshall.edu

Abstract: Our group has recently demonstrated that exercise intervention affects the release and function of bone marrow endothelial progenitor cell-derived extracellular vesicles (EVs) in transgenic hypertensive mice. Whether such an exercise regimen can impact circulating EVs (cEVs) remains unknown. In this study, we investigated the influence of exercise on cEV level and function. Transgenic hypertensive mice (Alb1-Ren) underwent 8-week treadmill exercise (10 m/min for 1 h, 5 days per week). Age- and sex-matched sedentary Alb1-Ren mice served as controls. cEVs were isolated from the blood of exercised and sedentary mice and are denoted as ET-cEV and nET-cEV, respectively. cEVs were labeled to determine their uptake efficiency and pathways. The functions of cEVs were assessed in an Angiotensin II (Ang II) plus hypoxia-injured cerebral microvascular endothelial cell (mBMEC) injury model. Cellular migration ability and oxidative stress were evaluated. We found that treadmill exercise stimulated cEV release, and ET-cEVs were more prone to be internalized by mBMECs. The ET-cEV internalization was mediated by macropinocytosis and endocytosis pathways. Functional studies showed that ET-cEVs can improve the compromised migration capability of mBMECs challenged by Ang II plus hypoxia. Additionally, ET-cEV treatment upregulated the expression of p-Akt/Akt in mBMECs. Compared to nET-cEVs, ET-cEVs significantly reduced ROS overproduction in Ang II plus hypoxia-injured mBMECs, associated with decreased Nox2 expression. All these findings suggest that exercise-intervened cEVs can protect cerebral microvascular endothelial cells against hypertensive and hypoxic injury.

Keywords: circulating extracellular vesicles; exercise; cerebral microvascular endothelial cells; hypertension; hypoxia

1. Introduction

Ischemic stroke is an occlusion in cerebral arteries, resulting in a loss of blood flow, oxygen, and nutrients. Stroke cases have been rising continuously over the years [1,2]. Every forty seconds, someone in the United States suffers from a stroke [3]. It is well recognized that hypertension is one of the major risk factors for ischemic stroke. Despite the benefits of anti-hypertensive therapy, the burden of brain disease, including stroke caused by hypertension, remains substantial [4]. Previous studies have demonstrated that hypertension can impair endothelial function, leading to cerebral supply issues [5,6]. Dysfunction of the endothelium in the brain microvasculature disrupts the balance between vasoconstriction and dilation, promotes leukocyte adhesion, encourages clotting, and prolongs inflammatory responses [7], which leads to exacerbated ischemic stroke damage and worsens outcomes in hypertensive individuals. Indeed, increasing evidence indicates that a cerebrovascular endothelium that is pre-emptively damaged may make an individual more prone to ischemic stroke [8].

Exercise is one of the well-known approaches to prevent and accelerate the recovery of ischemic stroke [9,10]. Exercise interventions have been shown to reduce blood pressure, improve insulin sensitivity, and alleviate pro-inflammatory cytokine levels [11]. Endothelial function may also be improved by exercise intervention, although the type and intensity of exercise could make a difference. It has been shown that moderate-intensity exercise can increase nitric oxide production, which might contribute to endothelial function improvement [12]. We have previously demonstrated that moderate-intensity exercise (10 m/min for 1 h, 5 days per week for 8 weeks) had better effects than low-intensity exercise (5 m/min for 1 h, 5 days per week for 8 weeks) on increasing the number of endothelial progenitor cells in the circulation in C57BL/6J mice [13]. Furthermore, our groups revealed that such an exercise regimen could reduce the cerebral infarct volume and raise microvessel density in middle cerebral artery occlusion-induced stroke in C57BL/6J mice [14]. Although great effort has been made in exercise and cerebrovascular disease research, the effects of and underlying mechanisms responsible for moderate-intensity exercise on the cerebrovasculature in the context of hypertension and ischemia have not been well understood.

Extracellular vesicles (EVs) are membranous particles released by most cell types in response to stimuli or as a part of cell physiology. EVs contain proteins, micro-RNA (miRNA), and lipids, all of which reflect the health status and type of cell they originate from. Yang et al. reported that lipid compositions could affect the size and functions of EVs derived from urine [15]. Increasing evidence suggests that the diverse cargoes of EVs could be carried throughout the blood and even past the blood–brain barrier to be taken up by cerebral cells, making them a crucial method of crosstalk within the body [16]. More recent data reveal that exercise can alter the cargo and functions of EVs. One study has shown that long-term preventative exercise downregulates exosomal miRNAs, such as miR-411-5p, which is associated with cardiovascular death in those with atrial fibrillation [17]. Bei and colleagues reported that a 3-week swimming regimen on C57BL/6 mice increased cEV levels by 1.85-fold. Furthermore, they found that these exercise-intervened cEVs exhibited an anti-apoptotic effect in H_2O_2-treated H9C2 cardiomyocytes [18]. Another group found that a 4-week swim exercise did not significantly change the number of cEVs but did change the functions of cEVs in protecting cardiomyocytes against hypoxia/reoxygenation injury. The underlying mechanism was related to the exosomal miR-342-5p. Importantly, the favorable cardioprotective effects and the rise of exosomal miR-342-5p were also observed in exercise-trained human volunteers [19]. Chaturvedi and colleagues showed that the heart and serum exosome concentrations were increased in db/db+ diabetic mouse models following 8 weeks of aerobic exercise. They noted significant increases in miR-29b and miR-455, with the latter being involved in the remodeling of extracellular matrices and fibrosis [20]. We have previously demonstrated that moderate exercise can alter the levels and miRNA profiles of EVs from bone marrow-derived endothelial progenitor cells in C57BL/6J mice [14]. More importantly, these EVs can effectively reduce the extent of cell damage and stroke size following ischemic stroke [14]. Besides the possible effects on EV-miR profiles, exercise intervention has also been shown to alter the protein profiles within EVs, impacting their composition and potential biological effects. Conkright et al. found that an acute heavy resistance back squat exercise changed the surface EV protein density, such as CD63 and vesicle-associated membrane protein, in both men and women subjects [21]. A short time of high-intensity interval training exercise undertaken on a programmable bicycle ergometer has been shown to alter the composition of proteins in cEVs that involve processes such as cellular oxidant detoxification, the regulation of stress, the regulation of exocytosis and vesicle-mediated transport, and response to stimulus in seventeen young men [22]. Aerobic and resistance exercises have been suggested to improve blood lipid profiles, but limited information is available regarding the effects of exercise on EVs' lipid profiles. Taken together, based on known findings, we speculated that exercise training might affect cEV levels and functions under hypertensive conditions.

In this study, we investigated the effects of moderate-intensity exercise on cEV levels in a hypertensive mouse model and studied whether exercise-intervened cEVs could exhibit favorable effects in protecting cerebral microvascular endothelial cells against hypertension plus hypoxia-induced injury. The combination of exercise and cEV enhancement is crucial to understand in the context of ischemic stroke because it may point to a potential preventative and therapeutic approach to stroke in hypertension.

2. Materials and Methods

2.1. Animals

Human renin hypertensive transgenic mice (129S/SvEv-Tg; Alb1-Ren; 2Unc/CofJ; the Jackson Laboratory) were used in this study. All experimental mice were inbred and housed in 12 h light/dark cycles at the Marshall University Animal Facility. All mice were given complete free access to normal chow and water. The experimental mice were euthanized at the age of 15–16 weeks old.

2.2. Treadmill Exercise Protocol

The Alb1-Ren mice (male and female; 7–8 weeks old) were randomly assigned to exercise (ET) or sedentary (nET) groups. Exercise protocols were defined in a previous study [14]. All ET mice were adapted to the treadmill (Columbus Instruments, Columbus, OH, USA), running for five days before the beginning of treatment. During day 1 of training, mice ran at 5 m/min for 30 min, and each following day of training, the speed was increased by 1 m/min and the time by 10 min. Following training, the ET mice group underwent 60 min of running at 10 m/min, 5 days/week for 8 weeks.

2.3. Cell Culture

The mouse brain microvascular endothelial cells (mBMECs) were purchased from Cell Biologics (Chicago, IL, USA) and cultured according to the manufacturer's instructions. In brief, mBMECs were cultured in mouse endothelial medium (M1168, Cell Biologics, Chicago, IL, USA) containing growth factor supplements and fetal bovine serum. Cells were washed with 1× phosphate-buffered saline (PBS) every two days and subcultured at 70–80% confluency.

2.4. cEV Isolation and Characterization

After an 8-week exercise or sedentary period, the experimental mice were sacrificed. Blood samples were collected from the hearts in syringes containing EDTA anti-coagulant. The samples were centrifuged at 3000× g for 20 min to remove platelets. The plasma was then ultracentrifuged at 170,000× g for 90 min to collect cEVs. The cEVs isolated from exercised mice were denoted as ET-cEVs, and from sedentary mice were denoted as nET-cEVs. The pellet was resuspended with 100 μL filtered 1× PBS, of which 5 μL was further diluted in 695 μL filtered 1× PBS. This 700 μL sample of diluted cEVs was used for nanoparticle tracking analysis (NTA). Three videos were acquired for the NTA [23]. The camera level was set at nine, and the detection threshold was five. All EV samples were resuspended and diluted in the same way. The formula for EV absolute number in 100 µL of resuspension was calculated as follows: EV (absolute numbers) = NTA concentration (number of particles/mL) × dilution factor (140) × 0.1 (resuspension volume). The formula for EV concentration in plasma was calculated as follows: EV (number of particles/mL) = {NTA concentration (number of particles/mL) × dilution factor (140) × 0.1}/plasma volume (mL). The formula for EV concentration in blood was calculated as follows: EV (number of particles/mL) = {NTA concentration (number of particles/mL) × dilution factor (140) × 0.1}/whole volume (mL). For Western blot analysis, cEV pellets were directly resuspended with 80 µL lysis buffer (Fisher Scientific, Waltham, MA, USA) supplemented with a complete mini protease inhibitor tablet (Roche, Basel, Switzerland).

2.5. Internalization Assay of cEVs into mBMECs

To detect the uptake efficiency, cEVs were labeled with PKH26 (Sigma-Aldrich, St. Louis, MO, USA). The labeling protocol was described previously [14]. In brief, following ultracentrifugation, cEV pellets were resuspended with 500 µL PBS, 1 µL PKH26 was added to the suspension, and then the mixture was incubated for 5 min in the dark at room temperature. Then, 500 µL 1% bovine serum albumin (BSA) in PBS was added to stop the reaction. The samples were then ultracentrifuged at 170,000× *g* for 90 min to pellet the cEVs. Then, mBMECs (70–80% confluency) were divided into two groups and incubated with a culture medium supplemented with nET-cEVs or ET-cEVs. The concentration of cEVs was 1×10^9 cEVs/mL, which was chosen based on our previous study [14]. After 24 h of co-incubation, the medium was removed, and cells were rinsed with PBS. The cell nucleus was counterstained with DAPI. The uptake of cEVs by mBMECs was visualized using an inverted fluorescence microscope (Olympus XP70); Boston Industries, Inc., Walpole, MA, USA) equipped with an ACCU-SCOPE Excelis MPX-20RC cooled color microscopy camera (20 Megapixels; NewYork Microscope Company, Hicksville, NY, USA). The images were taken using the same exposure time and light intensity. Four random microscopic images (×20 objectives) in each well represented a group. A blinded investigator analyzed the mean of fluorescence intensities using Image J 1.54f software (NIH, Bethesda, MD, USA). Data were normalized to the fluorescence signal of nET-cEV. The experiment was repeated four times.

2.6. cEV Uptake Pathway Determination

We conducted an uptake pathway analysis to determine the internalization pathway of ET-cEVs. In brief, mBMECs were pre-treated with LY294002 (5 µM; inhibitor of macropinocytosis), Filipin (10 µg/mL; inhibitor of lipid rafts-mediated endocytosis), and chlorpromazine (20 µM; inhibitor of clathrin-mediated endocytosis) for 30 min before co-culture experiments. All inhibitors were purchased from Sigma-Aldrich (St. Louis, MO, USA) and were dissolved in DMSO or distilled water according to the manufacturer's instructions. As DMSO was used as a solvent, the toxic effect of DMSO on cells was evaluated. DMSO did not induce toxicity at the concentrations used, as evidenced by cell viability detection. Then, inhibitors were diluted in a culture medium to achieve the intended work concentrations. The inhibitor concentration was chosen based on previous reports [24]. After 30 min of pre-treatment with the inhibitor, the medium was removed, and cells were washed with 1× PBS. Then, a fresh c µL ture medium (500 µL) supplemented with ET-cEVs (1×10^9 cEVs/mL) was added. A well of cells with no inhibitor treatment served as a control. After 24 h of co-incubation, the medium was removed, and cells were rinsed with PBS. The cell nucleus was counterstained with DAPI. The uptake of cEVs by mBMECs was imaged using an inverted fluorescence microscope (Olympus XP70; Boston Industries,

Inc., Walpole, MA, USA) equipped with an ACCU-SCOPE Excelis MPX-20RC cooled color microscopy camera (20 Megapixels; NewYork Microscope Company, Hicksville, NY, USA). The images were taken using the same exposure time and light intensity. Four random microscopic images (20× objective) in each well represented a group. A blinded investigator analyzed the mean of fluorescence intensities using Image J software (NIH, Bethesda, MD, USA). Data were normalized to the fluorescence signal of mBMECs in the control group. The experiment was repeated four times.

2.7. Co-Incubation of cEVs with mBMECs Challenged by Ang II Plus Hypoxia

To evaluate the functions of cEVs on hypertension and hypoxia-injured brain endothelial cells, we first challenged the mBMECs with Angiotensin II (Ang II) and hypoxia (1% O_2 in a Biospherix hypoxia chamber; Biospeherix; BioSpherix, Ltd., Parish, NY, USA) to mimic hypertension and hypoxia injury in ischemic stroke. In brief, before being treated by cEVs, the culture medium of mBMECs in 24-well plates or culture slides was replaced with 500 μL serum and glucose-free medium containing growth factors and 1 uM Ang II (Sigma-Aldrich, St. Louis, MO, USA). Then, the cells were placed in a hypoxia chamber (1% O_2, 5% CO_2, and 95% N_2) for 6 h, followed by 24 h reoxygenation in a standard CO_2 incubator. During the reoxygenation period, the cells were assigned into different treatment groups and were either untreated or treated with ET-cEVs or nET-cEVs. Cells grown in complete media in the standard incubator were controls. Cells were assayed using the following procedures.

2.8. Migration Assay of mBMECs After cEV Treatment

We conducted a scratch assay to determine whether cEVs could rescue the migration capability of mBMECs compromised by Ang II plus hypoxia injury. The mBMECs were exposed to Ang II and hypoxic injury as described and assigned into different treatment groups: no treatment or treated with nET-cEVs or ET-cEVs. Cells cultured with complete culture media in the standard incubator were used as controls. At 0 h, when the cEVs were added to mBMECs, a scratch was made in the middle of each well using a 200 μL pipette tip. Each well was imaged at 0 and 24 h to visualize mBMEC migration. Images were taken using an inverted microscope (Olympus XP70). Image J was used to measure and quantify the scratch area. Data were calculated as Area of changes (%) = (the scratch area in 0 h—the scratch area in 24 h)/the scratch area in 0 h × 100%. Three to four random microscopic images in one well represent a group in each experiment. The experiment was repeated three times. All data were normalized to the fold of the control group.

2.9. Reactive Oxygen Species Quantification in mBMECs After cEV Treatment

To determine whether cEVs could impact oxidative stress in mBMECs challenged by Ang II plus hypoxia, we performed Dihydroethidium (DHE, Sigma-Aldrich) staining. In general, mBMECs were exposed to Ang II and hypoxic injury as described and assigned into different treatment groups: no treatment or treated with nET-cEVs or ET-cEVs. Cells cultured with complete culture media in the standard incubator were used as controls. After 24 h of cEV co-culture, 10 uM DHE was added to each well, and the plate was incubated for 70 min. Then, the medium was removed, and cells were rinsed with PBS. The DHE fluorescence signal was imaged with a fluorescent microscope equipped with an ACCU-SCOPE Excelis MPX-20RC cooled color microscopy camera (20 Megapixels). The images were taken using the same exposure time and light intensity. Four random microscopic images (20× objective) in each well represented a group for each experiment.

The means of fluorescence intensities were analyzed using Image J 1.54f software (NIH, Bethesda, MD, USA) by a blinded investigator. The experiment was repeated three times.

2.10. Western Blot Analysis

Following cEV treatment, cells were collected from each well. The proteins were extracted using lysis buffer supplemented with a complete mini protease inhibitor tablet. A bicinchoninic acid (BCA) assay was performed to quantify protein concentrations of cells and cEVs. Protein lysates were electrophoresed through SDS-PAGE gel before being transferred onto polyvinylidene fluoride (PVDF) membranes, which were blocked with BSA buffer. Primary antibodies CD63 (1:200; Abcam; cat# ab216130), Tsg 101 (1: 200; Abcam; cat# ab30871), Nox2 (1:1000; Abcam; cat# 129068), Akt (1:1000; Cell Signaling Technology; cat# 4691), p-Akt (1:1000; Cell Signaling Technology; cat# 4060), and β-actin (1:4000; Sigma-Aldrich; cat# A5441) were incubated at 4 °C overnight. The next day, membranes were washed and incubated with horseradish peroxidase-conjugated anti-rabbit or anti-mouse IgG (1:40,000; Jackson Immuno Research Lab, West Grove, PA, USA) for two hours at room temperature. Blots were imaged using chemiluminescent solutions in a ChemiDoc imager (Bio-Rad, Hercules, CA, USA) and analyzed using ImageJ 1.54f.

2.11. Statistical Analysis

Data are expressed as the mean ± SD. Comparisons between groups were performed using ordinary one-way ANOVA tests and an unpaired *t*-test for cEV quantification. GraphPad Prism 9 was implemented for data analysis. For all measurements, $p < 0.05$ was considered statistically significant.

3. Results

3.1. Treadmill Exercise Intervention Stimulates cEV Release in Hypertensive Transgenic Mice and Increases the Internalization of cEVs by mBMECs

cEVs were isolated from the plasma of exercised and sedentary hypertensive transgenic mice using the ultracentrifugation method and characterized using NTA and Western blot. According to the NTA analysis of particle size and distribution, the mode size of nET-cEVs was ~80 nm, and ET-cEVs was ~72 nm with another peak of ~106 nm, as shown in a representative plot (Figure 1A). Meanwhile, our data showed that the cEV concentration was approximately 2.24-fold higher in exercised hypertensive mice (2.24×10^{10} cEVs/mL of plasma) than in sedentary ones (0.99×10^{10} cEVs/mL of plasma) (Figure 1B). According to the Western blot analysis, both groups of cEVs positively expressed EV markers CD63 and Tsg101 (Figure 1C). These findings indicate that treadmill exercise intervention stimulated cEV release in hypertensive transgenic mice.

We recently showed that treadmill exercise improved the internalization of endothelial progenitor cell-derived EVs from exercised hypertensive mice by neuronal cells, but whether such an exercise regimen affects the internalization of cEVs by brain endothelial cells has not been studied. To reveal this, we assessed the effects of exercise on cEV uptake efficiency by brain microvascular ECs. The data showed that more ET-cEVs were internalized into the cytoplasm of mBMECs than that of mBMECs co-cultured with nET-cEVs, as evidenced by a high mean fluorescence intensity in mBMECs treated with ET-cEVs (0.023 vs. 0.046 for nET-cEVs and ET-cEVs, respectively; Figure 1D,E).

3.2. ET-cEVs Incorporate into mBMECs Through Endocytosis and Macropinocytosis

Several mechanisms, including endocytosis and micropinocytosis, of EV internalization have been proposed. We tested three specific blocking agents to unravel their contribution to cEV internalization by mBMECs. Ly294002, an inhibitor of phosphoinositide 3-kinase, participates in the signaling cascade that stimulates membrane ruffling and closes the macropinosomes during macropinocytosis [25]. Chlorpromazine blocks clathrin-dependent endocytosis by interfering with the association between clathrin and the plasma membrane [26]. Filipin is known to sequestrate cholesterol from the plasma membrane and destabilize caveolae formation. As shown in Figure 2, Ly294002 decreased the internalization of ET-cEVs into mBMECs by 72%, as indicated by the reduced fluorescence intensity in the cytoplasm of mBMECs following 24 h ET-cEV treatment as compared to that in the control group (ET-cEV only) (0.013 vs. 0.046 for ET-cEVs + LY294002 and ET-cEVs, respectively). Chlorpromazine decreased EV uptake by 58% (0.019 vs. 0.046 for ET-cEVs + Chlorpromazine and ET-cEVs, respectively), and Filipin decreased EV uptake by 48% (0.024 vs. 0.046 for ET-cEVs + Filipin and ET-cEVs, respectively). Interestingly, none of the inhibitors can completely block the uptake of labeled vesicles, indicating a combined contribution from both endocytosis and macropinocytosis pathways for EV uptake. Taken together, under the above conditions, Ly294002 exerted the highest inhibitory effect, suggesting that the macropinocytosis pathway may be the main intracellular route for EV intake.

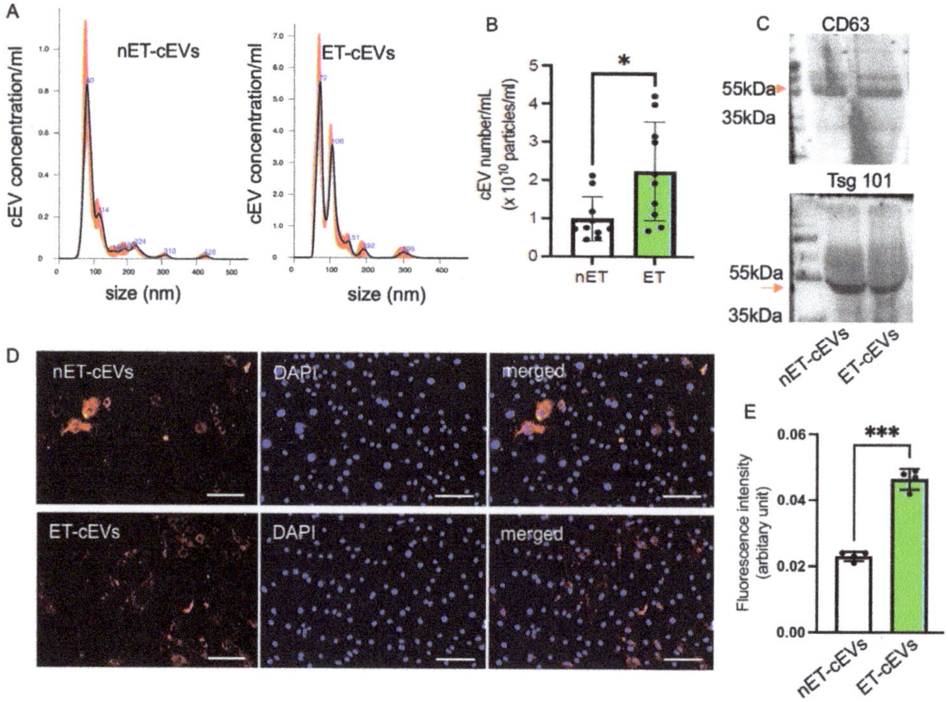

Figure 1. Exercise intervention stimulates cEV release and boosts the incorporation efficiency of cEVs into mBMECs. (**A**) Representative plots showing the size and distribution of nET-cEVs and ET-cEVs. (**B**) Summarized data on the level of the two groups of cEVs. Data are expressed as mean ± SD. * $p < 0.05$ vs. nET-cEV. n = 10/group. (**C**) Representative Western blot bands showing the expressions of EV-specific markers CD 63 and Tsg 101 (arrow). (**D**) Representative images showing the incorporation of cEVs with mBMECs after 24 h of co-culture. Blue: DAPI; red: PKH-26-labeled cEVs. Scale bar: 100 µm. 200× magnification. (**E**) Summary data of the uptake study. Data are expressed as mean ± SD. *** $p < 0.01$ vs. nET-cEV. n = 4/group.

3.3. Both nET-cEVs and ET-cEVs Improve the Migration Capability of mBMECs Compromised by Ang II Plus Hypoxia Injury

A scratch assay was conducted to assess the effects of cEVs on the migration ability of mBMECs. We calculated the area of the scratch in each image of interest. The larger the percentage change from baselines indicates a stronger migration capability of the cells. As expected, the Ang II plus hypoxia challenge significantly impaired the migration ability of mBMECs, as reflected by the smallest percentage change from baseline among all groups, suggesting the successful induction of the cell injury model. As shown in Figure 3, both nET-cEVs and ET-cEVs remarkably improved the migration capacity of mBMECs following Ang II plus hypoxia damage, indicated by a higher percentage change from baseline (at 0 h) compared to the cells without any treatment. Interestingly, there is no significant difference in the migration ability of mBMECs treated by nET-cEVs or ET-cEVs.

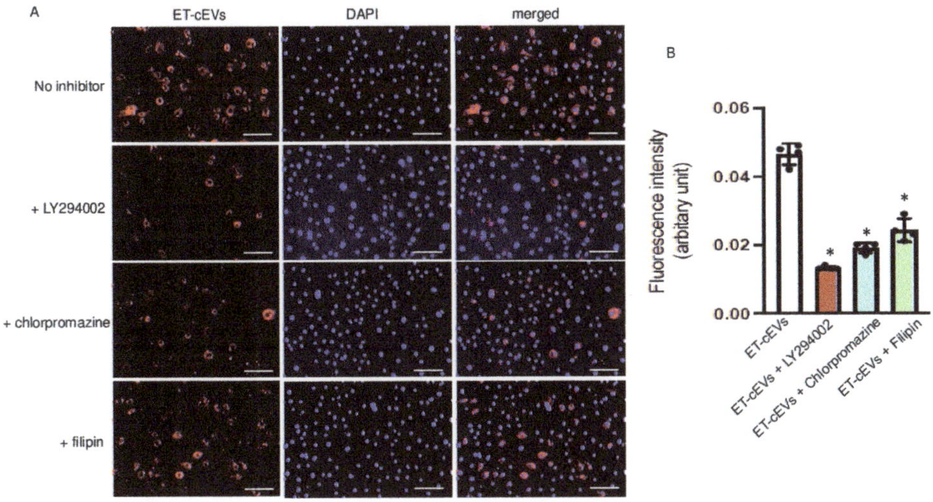

Figure 2. Macropinocytosis and endocytosis modulate the uptake of ET-cEVs into mBMECs. (**A**) Representative image showing the incorporation of ET-cEVs into the cytoplasm of mBMECs pre-treated with or without pathway inhibitors. Blue: DAPI; red: PKH-26-labeled cEVs. Scale bar: 100 μm. 200× magnification. (**B**) Summary data of the uptake mechanism study. Data are expressed as mean ± SD. * $p < 0.05$ vs. ET-cEV only (no inhibitor pre-treatment). n = 4/group.

3.4. ET-cEVs Exhibit Anti-Oxidative Effects in mBMECs Challenged by Ang II Plus Hypoxia

DHE staining was conducted to assess ROS overproduction of mBMECs. As shown in Figure 4, compared to the cells cultured in normal conditions, the Ang II plus hypoxia challenge remarkably raised the production of ROS, as revealed by a higher red fluorescence intensity in the cells. The data showed that nET-cEV co-culture alleviated ROS overproduction, but there was no significant difference as compared to that in the non-treated cells. Notably, ET-cEVs significantly decreased ROS overproduction as compared to those treated by nET-cEVs.

3.5. ET-cEVs Increase p-Akt/Akt and Decrease Nox2 Expressions in mBMECs Post-Ang II Plus Hypoxia Injury

Akt, also known as protein kinase B, is expressed in different cell types and plays a central role in various processes, such as migration and proliferation [27,28]. The cellular responses to Akt phosphorylation are executed via signal transduction pathways initiated by the phosphorylation of various Akt substrates [28]. Our data (Figure 5(A1,A2)) revealed that the total Akt expression was unchanged in mBMECs either challenged by Ang II plus hypoxia injury or post-treatment of cEVs. Ang II plus hypoxia challenge significantly decreased Akt activity in mBMECs, as reflected by a decreased ratio of p-Akt/Akt. However, both nET-cEV and ET-cEV treatments robustly restored the activity of Akt, as evidenced by a raised expression of p-Akt/Akt.

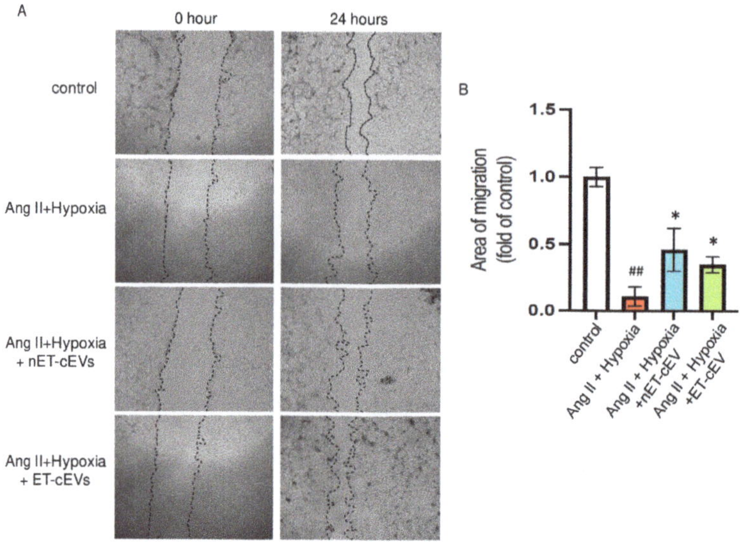

Figure 3. Migration assay of Ang II plus hypoxia-challenged mBMECs treated with cEVs. (**A**) Representative images of mBMEC migration at the baseline (0 h) and 24 h after the cEV treatment; 40× magnification. (**B**) Summary data depict the effects of cEVs on mBMEC migration following Ang II plus hypoxia injury. Data are shown as mean ± SD. ## $p < 0.01$ vs. control; * $p < 0.05$ vs. Ang II + hypoxia. n = 3/group.

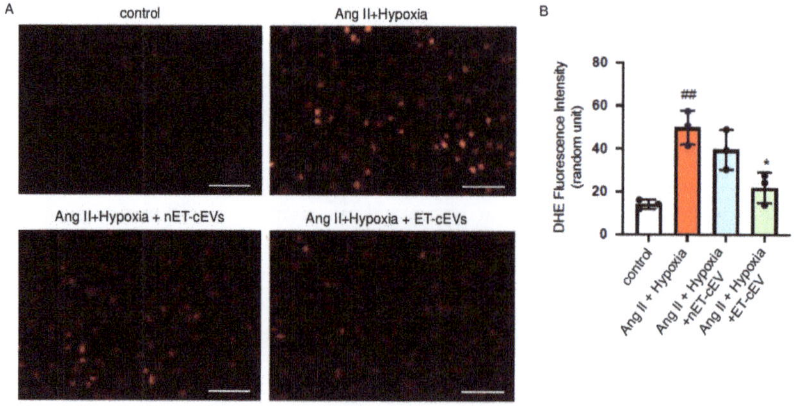

Figure 4. DHE overexpression in Ang II plus hypoxia-challenged mBMECs treated with cEVs. (**A**) Representative image showing DHE expression in hypoxia plus Ang II-injured mBMECs. Scale bar: 100 µm. 200× magnification. (**B**) Summary data of the DHE fluorescence intensity of mBMECs. Data are shown as mean ± SD. ## $p < 0.01$ vs. control; * $p < 0.05$ vs. Ang II + hypoxia. n = 3/group.

It is known that hypoxia is a major source of oxidative stress in hypertension and a potent activator of NADPH oxidases, including Nox2. Therefore, we analyzed the Nox2 level in mBMECs. As shown in Figure 5(B1,B2), Nox2 expression was significantly increased in Ang II and hypoxia-injured mBMECs. The nET-cEV treatment did not remarkably change Nox2 expression, but ET-cEVs significantly decreased Nox2 levels in mBMECs.

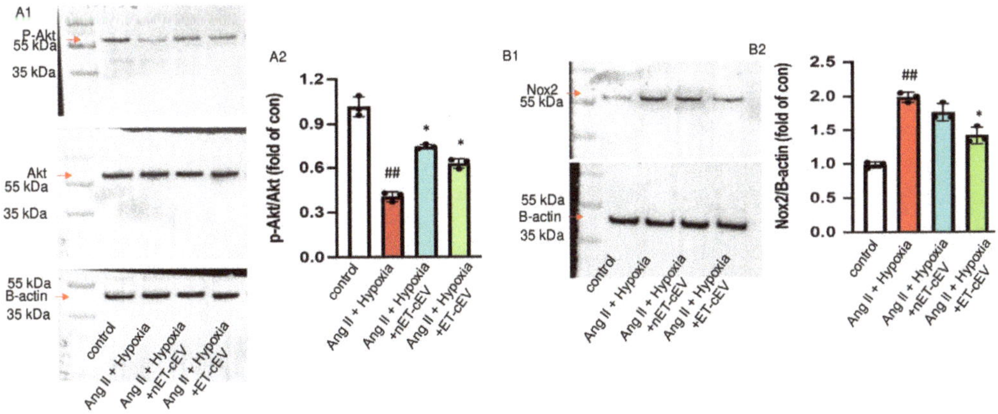

Figure 5. Akt phosphorylation and Nox2 expression in Ang II plus hypoxia-challenged mBMECs treated with cEVs. (**A1**,**A2**) Representative bands and summary data showing the ratio of p-Akt/Akt in mBMECs. (**B1**,**B2**) Representative bands and summary data showing the expression of Nox2 in mBMECs. Data are shown as mean ± SD. ## $p < 0.01$ vs. control; * $p < 0.05$ vs. Ang II + hypoxia. n = 3/group.

4. Discussion

In this study, we investigated the effects of exercise intervention on modulating cEV level and function under hypertensive conditions. Our key findings suggest that exercise intervention increased the production of cEVs from hypertensive mice and promoted the uptake of cEVs by mBMECs. The cEVs improved the migration capability of mBMECs, and cEVs from exercised mice further reduced ROS overproduction in Ang II plus hypoxia-challenged mBMECs. The potential mechanism is elucidated by the changes in proteins p-Akt/Akt and Nox2 in mBMECs.

Hypertension impairs endothelial function, which can lead to cerebral supply issues and make the outcomes of ischemic stroke more severe, as represented by increased mortality for hypertensive individuals who experienced an ischemic stroke [1,29]. Fortunately, exercise intervention has been shown to reduce these consequences, but the mechanisms by which this occurs are not clearly understood. Recent evidence indicates that EVs play a pivotal role in maintaining normal cardiovascular function and structure in healthy environments [30,31]. However, in disease conditions such as hypertensive conditions, EVs may decrease nitric oxide release while upregulating ROS production and cellular senescence, eventually leading to vascular lesions [32]. Previous studies showed that aerobic exercise stimulates the release of small EVs into circulation [33,34]. Indeed, exercise-induced EVs emerge as a novel class of exerkines that can exhibit systemic beneficial effects. Our group has previously demonstrated that moderate-intensity exercise stimulated the secretion of EVs from blood-derived stem cells [13]. In this study, we applied the same exercise regimen and studied its effects in hypertensive transgenic mice. Our data showed that moderate-intensity exercise can increase EV production in the blood circulation of hypertensive mice.

This trend supports the concept that exercise is an effective type of cellular stimulation regarding EV release. Meanwhile, we found multiple peaks in ET-cEVs according to the NTA analysis. Previous studies suggest that EV size varies depending on their cellular origin and specific cargoes. Yang and colleagues have demonstrated that urinary exosomes of different sizes originated from different types of cells and carry different lipid compositions [15]. The investigation of the specific molecular contents of these ET-cEVs is ongoing. Whether exercise intervention could alter the lipid composition of cEVs in hypertensive conditions and whether such alteration is responsible for the observed effects deserves further study. Additionally, our data showed that exercise intervention alters the uptake efficiency of cEVs. According to our co-culture study, exercise intervention upregulates the incorporation efficiency of cEVs by mBMECs challenged by Ang II and hypoxia, which mimics the injury of hypertension and ischemia in vitro. This finding might represent one of the potential mechanisms underlying the beneficial effects of exercise on ischemic stroke.

In the present study, we also elucidated the potential incorporation mechanism of cEVs by mBMECs. There are numerous mechanisms through which cells may internalize endocytic cargo. Generally, phagocytosis and pinocytosis are the two main subgroups of endocytosis. Phagocytosis involves the internalization of relatively large (>1 μm) particles and is typically restricted to specialized professional phagocytes, such as macrophages and dendritic cells. Pinocytosis is exhibited by all cells and is commonly classified into clathrin-dependent endocytosis, clathrin-independent endocytosis, and macropinocytosis. Several pathways, such as clathrin-mediated endocytosis [35,36] and micropinocytosis, have been reported to mediate EV internalization. Ajikumar and colleagues have demonstrated that endothelial cells take up materials from blood, including EVs, through macropinocytosis [37]. In the present study, we applied pharmaceutical inhibitors to unravel the uptake pathways involved in cEV incorporation. We found that macropinocytosis dominated the uptake pathways of cEVs by mBMECs. Of note, macropinocytosis is not the only pathway by which cEVs enter mBMECs. Endocytosis, to a lesser extent, also contributed to the internalization of cEVs to mBMECs. Future studies will further focus on the molecular mechanisms contributing to the observed internalization process. For instance, lipid compositions that are related to the size of EVs and subsequently influence EV-cell fusion and internalization mechanisms will be studied.

As we know, in an environment devoid of endothelial progenitor cells, endothelial regeneration relies on migration and proliferation, which are critical for cerebral ischemic recovery [38]. Wound scratch and Boyden chamber assays are commonly used to evaluate endothelial cell migration in vitro. In the present study, we conducted the wound scratch assay. We found that cEVs from both exercised and sedentary hypertensive mice substantially restored the migration capability of cerebral microvascular endothelial cells following ischemic hypertensive injury. Notably, the enhanced proliferation capability of cells might also affect their migration ability. Whether the EV cargoes such as miRs, mRNAs, or even DNA fragments could influence the proliferation of the cells has not been studied yet. In the current study, to further understand the corresponding molecular mechanisms of cEVs, we analyzed the expressions of Akt and its phosphorylation in the recipient cells. Akt, the serine-threonine kinase, is present in cells and tissues in both inactive and active (phosphorylated at T308 and S473) states. It is a key molecule in the PI3K/Akt pathway and plays an important role in modulating endothelial function [28]. Akt executes its role through phosphorylation rather than regulating its protein expression. Indeed, accumulating evidence has suggested that the expression level of p-Akt (Ser473) could be upregulated temporarily at the onset of focal cerebral ischemia and downregulated at 24 h after reperfusion, but the expression of Akt was not significantly changed [39]. In the present study, we found that the total expression of Akt was not disturbed by either ischemic hypertensive challenge or cEV treatment; however, the ratio of p-Akt/Akt was significantly decreased in mBMECs challenged by Ang II and hypoxia. Intriguingly, both nET-cEVs and ET-cEVs increased the ratio of p-Akt/Akt. These data are in line with the improved migration capability of mBMECs and are also supported by previous reports showing the positive effects of the Akt pathway in ischemic stroke [27,40]. Such overarching positive effects of cEVs on endothelial injury continue to point to the promise of utilizing cEVs in therapeutic settings for cerebrovascular injury. Previous reports have demonstrated that activation of the Akt pathway might alter the expression of hypoxia-inducible factor 1, which is a downstream target of Akt in cells such as breast cancer cells [41] and mesenchymal stem cells [42]. Whether cEV treatment could modulate the hypoxia-inducible factor 1 level in mBMECs and its potential roles will be investigated in our further studies.

Oxidative stress is a common feature of hypertension and hypoxia conditions. Experimental studies suggest that oxidants are mainly from NOXs in hypertension [43]. Growing evidence indicates that exercise prevents oxidative damage by reducing oxidative stress, an important factor in inflammation and hypertension [44]. However, what remains unclear is exactly how exercise modulates redox status and how it influences proinflammatory processes. In this study, we aimed to clarify this knowledge gap. We speculated that cEVs might be one of the mediators of exercise in decreasing ROS overproduction. Yao et al. have demonstrated that EVs from human mesenchymal stem cells can mitigate oxidative stress in the liver or on umbilical vein endothelial cells [45]. Nie and colleagues reported that skeletal muscle-derived exosomes can regulate the endothelial cell functions of angiogenesis [46]. Our group showed that exercise can regulate the functions of bone marrow endothelial progenitor cell-derived EVs [14]. Endothelial EVs have also been shown to promote the production of endothelial nitric oxide synthase and reduce the effects of oxidative stress [47]. Furthermore, as previously indicated, pathological states such as hypertension can cause cEVs to promote ROS production [32]. In the present study, we found the inability of cEVs from sedentary hypertensive mice to reduce ROS overproduction following hypertensive hypoxia injury, which supports previous findings. Meanwhile, it was abundantly clear to us that cEVs from exercised hypertensive mice can dramatically reduce ROS overproduction in mBMECs following ischemic hypertensive injury, indicating that exercise intervention can regulate cEV function in hypertensive conditions. Our data also revealed that ET-cEVs treatment significantly decreased Nox2 expression, while nET-cEVs did not in mBMECs challenged by Ang II and hypoxia. This is in line with the data showing that ET-cEV treatment reduced ROS overexpression. It is also supported by a recent study demonstrating that exercise-intervened endothelial progenitor cell-derived exosomes can protect neurons by improving mitochondrial function [48]. Knowing that cEVs from exercised conditions are more effective in reducing ROS, which suggests that their contents may change in response to aerobic activity, we strove to understand the mechanism behind the effects of cEVs on the endothelium at a deeper level. We will further analyze the contents of cEVs, such as miRs, and lipid compositions, and illustrate the underlying mechanism. Skeletal muscle is one of the major tissues that release EVs under exercise intervention. Whether skeletal muscle-derived EVs play a role in the effects elicited by ET-cEVs is unknown and will also be studied.

There are some limitations in this study: (1) We only investigated the effects of exercise intervention in cEVs in hypertensive transgenic mice. Whether this exercise regimen could affect the levels and functions of cEVs from normotensive mice needs to be investigated in future studies. (2) Subpopulations of cEVs, such as skeletal muscle-derived EVs, brain endothelial cell-derived EVs, bone marrow-stem cell-derived EVs, etc., that might play major roles in the observed effects require further investigation.

5. Conclusions

In conclusion, our data show that moderate-intensity exercise can stimulate cEV release in hypertensive conditions, and cEVs, specifically those from exercised mice, can protect mBMECs against hypertensive and hypoxia injury. The underlying mechanisms are ascribed to the anti-oxidative and pro-angiogenic effects of cEVs. Combining our findings regarding how ET-EVs can modulate oxidative stress pathways along with previous research showing that size-dependent EV lipid compositions [15] and oxidized lipids significantly contribute to endothelial dysfunction and atherosclerosis [46] provides important insight into how exercise might protect against cerebrovascular diseases such as stroke in the context of hypertension through EV-mediated mechanisms. Our findings solidify the importance of exercise intervention in maximizing the beneficial contributions of cEVs to alleviate the damage in cerebrovascular vessels caused by hypertension and hypoxia and have suggested that exercise-intervened cEVs might be a new therapeutic target for ischemic stroke in the context of hypertension.

Author Contributions: Conceptualization, J.W.; methodology, S.S., S.C., G.U. and J.W.; software, S.S., S.C. and J.W.; validation, S.S., S.C., G.U. and J.W.; Formal analysis, S.S., S.C. and J.W.; Investigation, S.S., S.C., G.U. and J.W.; resources, J.W.; Data curation, S.S., S.C., G.U. and J.W.; Writing—original draft, S.S.; Writing—review & editing, G.U. and J.W.; Supervision, J.W.; Project administration, J.W.; Funding acquisition, S.S. and J.W. All authors have read and agreed to the published version of the manuscript.

Funding: This work was partially supported by the NASA West Virginia Space Grant Consortium (80NSSC20M0055; SS), the American Heart Association (AHA) Career Development Award (935826; J.W.), the Pilot grant (J.W.) of the National Institute of General Medical Sciences (U54GM104942), and the AHA Transformational Project Award (24TPA1291189; J.W.).

Institutional Review Board Statement: The animal study protocol was approved by the Institutional Review Board Marshall University (protocol code 762 7 April 2021).

Informed Consent Statement: Not applicable.

Data Availability Statement: The datasets generated during the current study are available from the corresponding author upon reasonable request.

Acknowledgments: All authors thank Kaden Shaffer, Brandon Yu, and Annie Chen for proofreading the manuscript.

Conflicts of Interest: The authors declare no conflict of interest.

References

1. Boehme, A.K.; Esenwa, C.; Elkind, M.S. Stroke Risk Factors, Genetics, and Prevention. *Circ. Res.* **2017**, *120*, 472–495. [CrossRef] [PubMed]
2. Lin, Q.; Ye, T.; Ye, P.; Borghi, C.; Cro, S.; Damasceno, A.; Khan, N.; Nilsson, P.M.; Prabhakaran, D.; Ramirez, A.; et al. Hypertension in stroke survivors and associations with national premature stroke mortality: Data for 2.5 million participants from multinational screening campaigns. *Lancet Glob. Health* **2022**, *10*, e1141–e1149. [CrossRef] [PubMed]
3. Tsao, C.W.; Aday, A.W.; Almarzooq, Z.I.; Anderson, C.A.; Arora, P.; Avery, C.L.; Baker-Smith, C.M.; Beaton, A.Z.; Boehme, A.K.; Buxton, A.E.; et al. Heart Disease and Stroke Statistics-2023 Update: A Report From the American Heart Association. *Circulation* **2023**, *147*, e93–e621. [PubMed]
4. Dorans, K.S.; Mills, K.T.; Liu, Y.; He, J. Trends in Prevalence and Control of Hypertension According to the 2017 American College of Cardiology/American Heart Association (ACC/AHA) Guideline. *J. Am. Heart Assoc.* **2018**, *7*, e008888. [CrossRef]

5. Santisteban, M.M.; Iadecola, C. Hypertension, dietary salt and cognitive impairment. *J. Cereb. Blood Flow Metab.* **2018**, *38*, 2112–2128. [CrossRef]
6. Pires, P.W.; Dams Ramos, C.M.; Matin, N.; Dorrance, A.M. The effects of hypertension on the cerebral circulation. *Am. J. Physiol. Heart Circ. Physiol.* **2013**, *304*, H1598–H1614. [CrossRef]
7. Di Chiara, T.; Del Cuore, A.; Daidone, M.; Scaglione, S.; Norrito, R.L.; Puleo, M.G.; Scaglione, R.; Pinto, A.; Tuttolomondo, A. Pathogenetic Mechanisms of Hypertension-Brain-Induced Complications: Focus on Molecular Mediators. *Int. J. Mol. Sci.* **2022**, *23*, 2445. [CrossRef]
8. Andjelkovic, A.V.; Xiang, J.; Stamatovic, S.M.; Hua, Y.; Xi, G.; Wang, M.M.; Keep, R.F. Endothelial Targets in Stroke: Translating Animal Models to Human. *Arter. Thromb. Vasc. Biol.* **2019**, *39*, 2240–2247. [CrossRef]
9. Hou, L.; Li, M.; Wang, J.; Li, Y.; Zheng, Q.; Zhang, L.; Yao, Q.; Zhang, J.; Dong, S.; Zhou, M.; et al. Association between physical exercise and stroke recurrence among first-ever ischemic stroke survivors. *Sci. Rep.* **2021**, *11*, 13372. [CrossRef]
10. Howard, V.J.; McDonnell, M.N. Physical activity in primary stroke prevention: Just do it! *Stroke* **2015**, *46*, 1735–1739. [CrossRef]
11. Edward, J.A.; Cornwell III, W.K. Impact of Exercise on Cerebrovascular Physiology and Risk of Stroke. *Stroke* **2022**, *53*, 2404–2410. [CrossRef] [PubMed]
12. Higashi, Y. Exercise is a double-edged sword for endothelial function. *Hypertens. Res.* **2016**, *39*, 61–63. [CrossRef] [PubMed]
13. Ma, C.; Wang, J.; Liu, H.; Chen, Y.; Ma, X.; Chen, S.; Chen, Y.; Bihl, J.; Yang, Y. Moderate Exercise Enhances Endothelial Progenitor Cell Exosomes Release and Function. *Med. Sci. Sports Exerc.* **2018**, *50*, 2024–2032. [CrossRef] [PubMed]
14. Wang, J.; Liu, H.; Chen, S.; Zhang, W.; Chen, Y.; Yang, Y. Moderate exercise has beneficial effects on mouse ischemic stroke by enhancing the functions of circulating endothelial progenitor cell-derived exosomes. *Exp. Neurol.* **2020**, *330*, 113325. [CrossRef]
15. Yang, J.S.; Lee, J.C.; Byeon, S.K.; Rha, K.H.; Moon, M.H. Size Dependent Lipidomic Analysis of Urinary Exosomes from Patients with Prostate Cancer by Flow Field-Flow Fractionation and Nanoflow Liquid Chromatography-Tandem Mass Spectrometry. *Anal. Chem.* **2017**, *89*, 2488–2496. [CrossRef]
16. Sigdel, S.; Swenson, S.; Wang, J. Extracellular Vesicles in Neurodegenerative Diseases: An Update. *Int. J. Mol. Sci.* **2023**, *24*, 13161. [CrossRef]
17. Nopp, S.; van der Bent, M.L.; Kraemmer, D.; Königsbrügge, O.; Wojta, J.; Pabinger, I.; Ay, C.; Nossent, A.Y. Circulatory miR-411-5p as a Novel Prognostic Biomarker for Major Adverse Cardiovascular Events in Patients with Atrial Fibrillation. *Int. J. Mol. Sci.* **2023**, *24*, 3861. [CrossRef]
18. Bei, Y.; Xu, T.; Lv, D.; Yu, P.; Xu, J.; Che, L.; Das, A.; Tigges, J.; Toxavidis, V.; Ghiran, I.; et al. Exercise-induced circulating extracellular vesicles protect against cardiac ischemia-reperfusion injury. *Basic Res. Cardiol.* **2017**, *112*, 38. [CrossRef]
19. Hou, Z.; Qin, X.; Hu, Y.; Zhang, X.; Li, G.; Wu, J.; Li, J.; Sha, J.; Chen, J.; Xia, J.; et al. Longterm Exercise-Derived Exosomal miR-342-5p: A Novel Exerkine for Cardioprotection. *Circ. Res.* **2019**, *124*, 1386–1400. [CrossRef]
20. Chaturvedi, P.; Kalani, A.; Medina, I.; Familtseva, A.; Tyagi, S.C. Cardiosome mediated regulation of MMP9 in diabetic heart: Role of mir29b and mir455 in exercise. *J. Cell Mol. Med.* **2015**, *19*, 2153–2161. [CrossRef]
21. Conkright, W.R.; Beckner, M.E.; Sterczala, A.J.; Mi, Q.; Lovalekar, M.; Sahu, A.; Krajewski, K.T.; Martin, B.J.; Flanagan, S.D.; Greeves, J.P.; et al. Resistance exercise differentially alters extracellular vesicle size and subpopulation characteristics in healthy men and women: An observational cohort study. *Physiol. Genom.* **2022**, *54*, 350–359. [CrossRef] [PubMed]
22. Kobayashi, Y.; Eguchi, A.; Tamai, Y.; Fukuda, S.; Tempaku, M.; Izuoka, K.; Iwasa, M.; Takei, Y.; Togashi, K. Protein Composition of Circulating Extracellular Vesicles Immediately Changed by Particular Short Time of High-Intensity Interval Training Exercise. *Front. Physiol.* **2021**, *12*, 693007. [CrossRef] [PubMed]
23. Wang, J.; Guo, R.; Yang, Y.; Jacobs, B.; Chen, S.; Iwuchukwu, I.; Gaines, K.J.; Chen, Y.; Simman, R.; Lv, G.; et al. The Novel Methods for Analysis of Exosomes Released from Endothelial Cells and Endothelial Progenitor Cells. *Stem. Cells Int.* **2016**, *2016*, 2639728. [CrossRef] [PubMed]
24. Kwok, Z.H.; Wang, C.; Jin, Y. Extracellular Vesicle Transportation and Uptake by Recipient Cells: A Critical Process to Regulate Human Diseases. *Processes* **2021**, *9*, 273. [CrossRef]
25. Swanson, J.A.; Watts, C. Macropinocytosis. *Trends Cell Biol.* **1995**, *5*, 424–428. [CrossRef]
26. Wang, L.H.; Rothberg, K.G.; Anderson, R.G. Mis-assembly of clathrin lattices on endosomes reveals a regulatory switch for coated pit formation. *J. Cell Biol.* **1993**, *123*, 1107–1117. [CrossRef]
27. Shiojima, I.; Walsh, K. Role of Akt signaling in vascular homeostasis and angiogenesis. *Circ. Res.* **2002**, *90*, 1243–1250. [CrossRef]
28. Morales-Ruiz, M.; Fulton, D.; Sowa, G.; Languino, L.R.; Fujio, Y.; Walsh, K.; Sessa, W.C. Vascular endothelial growth factor-stimulated actin reorganization and migration of endothelial cells is regulated via the serine/threonine kinase Akt. *Circ. Res.* **2000**, *86*, 892–896. [CrossRef]

29. Satoh, M.; Ohkubo, T.; Asayama, K.; Murakami, Y.; Sugiyama, D.; Yamada, M.; Saitoh, S.; Sakata, K.; Irie, F.; Sairenchi, T.; et al. Lifetime Risk of Stroke and Coronary Heart Disease Deaths According to Blood Pressure Level: EPOCH-JAPAN (Evidence for Cardiovascular Prevention From Observational Cohorts in Japan). *Hypertension* **2019**, *73*, 52–59. [CrossRef]
30. Kumar, M.A.; Baba, S.K.; Sadida, H.Q.; Marzooqi, S.A.; Jerobin, J.; Altemani, F.H.; Algehainy, N.; Alanazi, M.A.; Abou-Samra, A.-B.; Kumar, R.; et al. Extracellular vesicles as tools and targets in therapy for diseases. *Signal Transduct. Target. Ther.* **2024**, *9*, 27.
31. Fu, S.; Zhang, Y.; Li, Y.; Luo, L.; Zhao, Y.; Yao, Y. Extracellular vesicles in cardiovascular diseases. *Cell Death Discov.* **2020**, *6*, 68. [CrossRef] [PubMed]
32. Buffolo, F.; Monticone, S.; Camussi, G.; Aikawa, E. Role of Extracellular Vesicles in the Pathogenesis of Vascular Damage. *Hypertension* **2022**, *79*, 863–873. [CrossRef] [PubMed]
33. Fruhbeis, C.; Helmig, S.; Tug, S.; Simon, P.; Kramer-Albers, E.M. Physical exercise induces rapid release of small extracellular vesicles into the circulation. *J. Extracell. Vesicles* **2015**, *4*, 28239. [CrossRef]
34. Whitham, M.; Parker, B.L.; Friedrichsen, M.; Hingst, J.R.; Hjorth, M.; Hughes, W.E.; Egan, C.L.; Cron, L.; Watt, K.I.; Kuchel, R.P.; et al. Extracellular Vesicles Provide a Means for Tissue Crosstalk during Exercise. *Cell Metab.* **2018**, *27*, 237–251e4. [CrossRef]
35. Escrevente, C.; Keller, S.; Altevogt, P.; Costa, J. Interaction and uptake of exosomes by ovarian cancer cells. *BMC Cancer* **2011**, *11*, 108. [CrossRef]
36. Nanbo, A.; Kawanishi, E.; Yoshida, R.; Yoshiyama, H. Exosomes derived from Epstein-Barr virus-infected cells are internalized via caveola-dependent endocytosis and promote phenotypic modulation in target cells. *J. Virol.* **2013**, *87*, 10334–10347. [CrossRef]
37. Ajikumar, A.; Long, M.B.; Heath, P.R.; Wharton, S.B.; Ince, P.G.; Ridger, V.C.; Simpson, J.E. Neutrophil-Derived Microvesicle Induced Dysfunction of Brain Microvascular Endothelial Cells In Vitro. *Int. J. Mol. Sci.* **2019**, *20*, 5227. [CrossRef]
38. Evans, C.E.; Iruela-Arispe, M.L.; Zhao, Y.Y. Mechanisms of Endothelial Regeneration and Vascular Repair and Their Application to Regenerative Medicine. *Am. J. Pathol.* **2021**, *191*, 52–65. [CrossRef]
39. Zhao, H.; Sapolsky, R.M.; Steinberg, G.K. Phosphoinositide-3-kinase/akt survival signal pathways are implicated in neuronal survival after stroke. *Mol. Neurobiol.* **2006**, *34*, 249–270. [CrossRef]
40. Wang, J.; Chen, Y.; Yang, Y.; Xiao, X.; Chen, S.; Zhang, C.; Jacobs, B.; Bin Zhao, B.; Bihl, J.; Chen, Y. Endothelial progenitor cells and neural progenitor cells synergistically protect cerebral endothelial cells from Hypoxia/reoxygenation-induced injury via activating the PI3K/Akt pathway. *Mol. Brain* **2016**, *9*, 12. [CrossRef]
41. Tian, Y.; Zhao, L.; Gui, Z.; Liu, S.; Liu, C.; Yu, T.; Zhang, L. PI3K/AKT signaling activates HIF1alpha to modulate the biological effects of invasive breast cancer with microcalcification. *NPJ Breast Cancer* **2023**, *9*, 93. [CrossRef] [PubMed]
42. Yun, S.P.; Lee, M.Y.; Ryu, J.M.; Song, C.H.; Han, H.J. Role of HIF-1alpha and VEGF in human mesenchymal stem cell proliferation by 17beta-estradiol: Involvement of PKC, PI3K/Akt, and MAPKs. *Am. J. Physiol. Cell Physiol.* **2009**, *296*, C317–C326. [CrossRef] [PubMed]
43. Montezano, A.C.; Touyz, R.M. Reactive oxygen species, vascular Noxs, and hypertension: Focus on translational and clinical research. *Antioxid. Redox Signal.* **2014**, *20*, 164–182. [CrossRef] [PubMed]
44. Schiffrin, E.L.; Touyz, R.M. From bedside to bench to bedside: Role of renin-angiotensin-aldosterone system in remodeling of resistance arteries in hypertension. *Am. J. Physiol. Heart Circ. Physiol.* **2004**, *287*, H435–H446. [CrossRef]
45. Yao, J.; Zheng, J.; Cai, J.; Zeng, K.; Zhou, C.; Zhang, J.; Li, S.; Li, H.; Chen, L.; He, L.; et al. Extracellular vesicles derived from human umbilical cord mesenchymal stem cells alleviate rat hepatic ischemia-reperfusion injury by suppressing oxidative stress and neutrophil inflammatory response. *FASEB J.* **2019**, *33*, 1695–1710. [CrossRef]
46. Nie, Y.; Sato, Y.; Garner, R.T.; Kargl, C.; Wang, C.; Kuang, S.; Gilpin, C.J.; Gavin, T.P. Skeletal muscle-derived exosomes regulate endothelial cell functions via reactive oxygen species-activated nuclear factor-kappaB signalling. *Exp. Physiol.* **2019**, *104*, 1262–1273. [CrossRef]
47. Kisielewska, M.; Rakoczy, K.; Skowron, I.; Górczyńska, J.; Kacer, J.; Bocheńska, A.; Choromańska, A. Utilizing Extracellular Vesicles for Eliminating 'Unwanted Molecules': Harnessing Nature's Structures in Modern Therapeutic Strategies. *Molecules* **2024**, *29*, 948. [CrossRef]
48. Chen, S.; Sigdel, S.; Sawant, H.; Bihl, J.; Wang, J. Exercise-Intervened Endothelial Progenitor Cell Exosomes Protect N2a Cells by Improving Mitochondrial Function. *Int. J. Mol. Sci.* **2024**, *25*, 1148. [CrossRef]

antioxidants

MDPI

Article

Restoration of Sestrin 3 Expression Mitigates Cardiac Oxidative Damage in Ischemia–Reperfusion Injury Model

Mina Park, Sunghye Cho and Dongtak Jeong *

Department of Medicinal & Life Science, College of Science and Convergence Technology, Hanyang University—ERICA, Ansan 15588, Republic of Korea; lampicka7119@hanyang.ac.kr (M.P.); josunghye88@gmail.com (S.C.)

* Correspondence: cooljdt@hanyang.ac.kr; Tel.: +82-31-400-5515

Abstract: Cardiac ischemia–reperfusion injury (IRI) occurs when blood flow is restored to the myocardium after a period of ischemia, leading to oxidative stress and subsequent myocardial cell damage, primarily due to the accumulation of reactive oxygen species (ROS). In our previous research, we identified that miR-25 is significantly overexpressed in pressure overload-induced heart failure, and its inhibition improves cardiac function by restoring the expression of SERCA2a, a key protein involved in calcium regulation. In this study, we aimed to investigate the role of miR-25 in the context of ischemia–reperfusion injury. We found that miR-25 was markedly upregulated under hypoxic conditions in both in vitro and in vivo models. Through in silico analysis, we identified Sestrin3 (SESN3), an antioxidant protein known for its protective effects against oxidative stress, as a novel target of miR-25. Based on these findings, we hypothesized that inhibiting miR-25 would restore Sestrin3 expression, thereby reducing ROS-induced myocardial cell damage and improving cardiac function. To test this hypothesis, we employed two model systems: a hypoxia/reoxygenation (H/R) stress model using H9c2 myoblasts and a surgically induced ischemia–reperfusion injury mouse model. Our results demonstrated that the use of miR-25 inhibitors significantly improved cardiac function and reduced myocardial damage in both models through the restoration of SESN3 expression. In conclusion, our findings suggest that targeting miR-25 may serve as a novel therapeutic modality to alleviate oxidative damage in the heart.

Keywords: ischemia–reperfusion injury; sestrin; miR-25; ROS; oxidative damage; apoptosis; cardiac dysfunction; hypoxia/reoxygenation; antioxidant

1. Introduction

Ischemic heart disease progresses to heart failure through myocardial infarction, resulting in negative outcomes [1–3]. A significant contributor to these results is oxidative stress, which arises from the sudden increase in oxygen supply when blood flow is restored to the ischemic area. This reperfusion injury is a common cause of damage in many patients [4–7]. Myocardial damage and myocardial cell death due to oxidative stress lead to a decline in cardiac function [8–10]. Representative changes include decreased contractility, decreased cardiac output, and structural changes such as cardiac remodeling [11–15]. Reducing oxidative stress in this pathological condition helps to minimize myocardial damage caused by ischemia–reperfusion injury (IRI) and offers cardioprotective benefits [16,17]. These benefits are mediated through various molecular mechanisms.

Recent studies have elucidated the role of antioxidant enzymes, such as superoxide dismutase and catalase, in mitigating oxidative stress-induced damage [18,19]. Furthermore, the activation of cellular survival pathways, including the PI3K/Akt and ERK1/2 signaling cascades [20–22], has been shown to confer cardioprotective effects against IRI. The modulation of mitochondrial function is another critical aspect of cardioprotection, as mitochondria are both sources and targets of reactive oxygen species during reperfusion [23–25]. Emerging research has also highlighted the potential of ischemic preconditioning and postconditioning strategies in reducing infarct size and preserving cardiac function. These approaches involve brief periods of ischemia and reperfusion applied either before or after the main ischemic insult, respectively, and have demonstrated promising results in experimental models and clinical trials. Additionally, pharmacological interventions targeting specific components of the oxidative stress pathway have shown potential in preclinical studies, although their translation to clinical practice requires further investigation [26,27].

The Sestrin family members also exhibit distinct regulatory mechanisms and tissue-specific expression patterns. SESN1 is ubiquitously expressed in human tissues, with the highest levels found in skeletal muscle, heart, liver, and brain. SESN2, initially identified as a hypoxia-inducible gene, is highly expressed in the kidneys, lungs, leukocytes, liver, gastrointestinal tract, and brain. SESN3, the least studied member, shows high expression in the brain, kidney, colon, small intestine, liver, and skeletal muscle [28–31]. Beyond their antioxidant functions, Sestrins play crucial roles in maintaining metabolic homeostasis. They regulate glucose homeostasis, insulin sensitivity, and lipid metabolism, primarily through their interaction with the AMPK/mTORC1 signaling pathway, where Sestrins activate AMPK and inhibit mTORC1, leading to improved metabolic outcomes. Additionally, Sestrins contribute to cellular stress responses by regulating autophagy, a critical process for cellular homeostasis. Through their interaction with the AMPK/mTOR signaling axis, Sestrins can promote autophagy induction, particularly under conditions of cellular stress or nutrient deprivation [32–36].

Noncoding RNAs, transcribed from DNA but not translated into proteins, are a type of functional RNA molecule. Among them, miRNAs act as post-transcriptional regulators of gene expression, and many studies have shown that changes in miRNA expression are related to various cardiovascular diseases [37–39]. In our previous study, we confirmed that upregulation of miR-25 suppresses the expression of SERCA2a, a master regulator of calcium signaling in cardiomyocytes [40]. This finding has significant implications for understanding the molecular mechanisms underlying cardiac dysfunction. SERCA2a plays a crucial role in maintaining calcium homeostasis in cardiomyocytes by facilitating the reuptake of calcium into the sarcoplasmic reticulum during diastole [41,42]. The reduced expression of SERCA2a has been associated with impaired cardiac contractility and relaxation, which are hallmarks of heart failure. The discovery that miR-25 regulates SERCA2a expression provides a potential therapeutic target for addressing calcium handling abnormalities in cardiovascular diseases.

Following these observations, this study also revealed a significant upregulation of miR-25 under hypoxic conditions, both in vitro and in vivo. Through a comprehensive in silico analysis utilizing three distinct miRNA target prediction algorithms, we identified SESN3, a member of the Sestrin family known for its antioxidant properties, as a potential target of miR-25.

Subsequently, we confirmed the inverse relationship between miR-25 and SESN3 expression under H/R stress conditions in vitro. Furthermore, the overexpression of SESN3 alone significantly reduced ROS-induced apoptosis. Based on these results, we delivered miR-25 TuD in vitro and in vivo models, successfully attenuating the expression of stress markers, including those associated with apoptosis and fibrosis. Notably, cardiac function was also substantially enhanced by miR-25 TuD, suggesting that its delivery may be a potential treatment for mitigating IRI-induced cardiac damage.

In summary, this study identifies SESN3 as a new target of miR-25 under oxidative stress conditions. Targeting miR-25 may serve as a promising strategy to alleviate IRI-induced cardiac dysfunction.

2. Materials and Methods

2.1. Cell Culture and Hypoxia/Reoxygenation In Vitro Model

H9c2 and HEK-293T cell lines were purchased from the American Type Culture Collection (ATCC, Manassas, VA, USA). Cells were cultured in 10 cm cell culture dishes in DMEM (CM002-050, GenDepot, Katy, TX, USA) supplemented with 10% fetal bovine serum (FBS; F0600-050, GenDepot, Katy, TX, USA) and 1% penicillin–streptomycin (CA005-010, GenDepot, Katy, TX, USA), at 37 °C with 5% CO_2 and 95% relative humidity. Cells were subcultured every 3 days to maintain subconfluence. H9c2 cells were starved in serum-free DMEM for 24 h after reaching 70–80% confluence, then exposed to either normoxia or hypoxia conditions for an additional 24 h in a hypoxia chamber (MIC-101, Billups-Rothenberg, Del Mar, CA, USA). For hypoxic conditions, the chamber was flushed with a hypoxia gas mixture containing 1% O_2, 5% CO_2, and 94% N_2, at 2 mmHg pressure for 3 min. The cells were then reoxygenated for an additional 2 h.

2.2. Predicted Gene Characteristics

The characteristics of the 148 predicted target genes of miR-25 were analyzed using the SRplot platform (www.bioinformatics.com (accessed on 15 November 2024)). The detailed results of this analysis are presented in Supplementary Table S1.

2.3. SESN3 3′-UTR Luciferase Assay

To verify that hsa-miR-25 directly binds to the SESN3 3′-UTR gene, we used a luciferase assay kit for analysis. HEK-293T cells were transfected with the plasmids described in Figure 1B using Lipofectamine 3000 (L3000015, Invitrogen, Waltham, MA, USA) transfection reagent. Measurements were made 24h after co-transfection with miRNA vectors, and luciferase (E1500, Promega, Madison, WI, USA) activity was measured using a luminescence microplate reader.

2.4. Measurement of Cellular ROS

ROS levels were analyzed using dichloro-dihydro-fluorescein diacetate (DCFH-DA, D6883, Sigma, Saint Louis, MO, USA) according to the manufacturer's instructions. Briefly, a final concentration of 10 μM of DCFH-DA was added to cells upon reoxygenation, and after 2 h, cells were washed with cold PBS, observed, and images were processed using a Leica microscope (DCF295, Leica, Berlin, Germany).

2.5. Immunofluorescence and TdT-Mediated dUTP Nick End-Labeling (TUNEL) Staining

Cells were plated on coverslips 24 h before transfection. After experimental treatment, cells were fixed for 30 min in 4% PFA (BYLABS, Hanam, Republic of Korea) and blocked with PBS-BT (1% BSA, 0.1% Triton X-100 in PBS) for 1 h. Cells were then incubated with primary antibodies overnight at 4 °C and incubated with Alexa Fluor 594-conjugated secondary antibodies (A-11012, Thermo Fisher Scientific, Waltham, MA, USA) for 1 h at room temperature. After staining with 4,6-diamidino-2-phenylindole (DAPI; D3571, Thermo Fisher Scientific, Waltham, MA, USA) for 5 min, cells were washed three times with

PBS and mounted on glass slides. TUNEL staining was performed to detect cell apoptosis in vitro according to the manufacturer's instructions using a commercially available kit (#64936, Cell Signaling, Danvers, MA, USA).

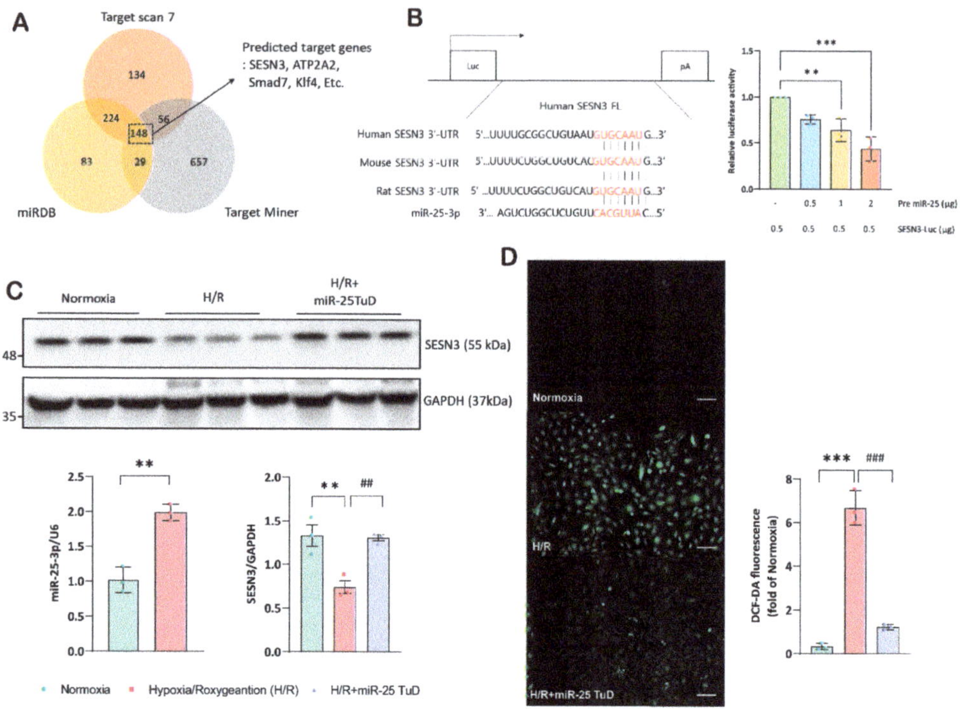

Figure 1. SESN3 is newly identified target of miR-25 as an ROS scavenger. (**A**) In silico identification of potential target genes for miR-25-3p. (**B**) The putative miR-25-3p binding site in the 3′-UTR region of the SESN3 mRNA was predicted using TargetScan. Pre-miR-25 and SESN3-Luc plasmids were transfected into HEK-293T cells. SESN3-Luciferase activity was subsequently analyzed in response to increasing pre-miR-25 transfection levels. (**C**) Protein expression of SESN3 was analyzed in H9c2 cells transfected with miR-25 TuD plasmids. (**D**) Representative fluorescence microscopy images of H9c2 cells stained with DCFDA to detect intracellular ROS levels. A scale bar indicates 50 μm respectively. (** $p < 0.01$, *** $p < 0.001$ vs. Normoxia, ## $p < 0.01$, ### $p < 0.001$ vs. H/R).

2.6. Animal Care

All animal experiments in this study were performed in accordance with the Animal Care and Use Committee of Hanyang University ERICA (Approval No. HY-IACUC-24-0058, HY-IACUC-24-0059, HY-IACUC-24-0074). Eight-week-old male C57BL/6 mice were purchased from Orient Bio (Seongnam, Republic of Korea). The animals were housed in a specific pathogen-free environment at a constant ambient temperature of 22 °C and 50% humidity with a 12 h light/dark cycle. Food and water were provided ad libitum.

2.7. Western Blot Analysis

Cells and tissues were lysed in RIPA buffer (R4100, GenDepot, Katy, TX, USA) supplemented with protease and phosphatase inhibitors (P3300, GenDepot, Katy, TX, USA). Lysates were centrifuged at 13,000 rpm for 10 min at 4 °C. Protein concentrations in lysates were quantified using BCA assay (23225, Thermo Fisher Scientific, Waltham, MA, USA) according to the manufacturer's instructions. Subsequently, they were transferred to nitrocellulose membranes (LC7033, GenDepot, Katy, TX, USA) via SDS-PAGE, and membranes were irradiated with primary and HRP-linked secondary antibodies and confirmed using the ECL detection system (K-12045-D50, Advansta, Menlo Park, CA, USA). Antibodies used for immunoblotting are listed in the Supplementary Table S2.

2.8. *Quantitative Real-Time PCR*

Total RNA and miRNA from cells and tissues were extracted using Hybrid R miRNA Isolation Kit (Geneall, Seoul, Republic of Korea), following the manufacturer's protocol. After elution, RNA purity was measured using a spectrophotometer (Multiskan SkyHigh, Thermo Fisher Scientific, Rockford, IL, USA), and only samples with a 260/280 nm ratio between 1.8 and 2.1 were used. Reverse transcription (RT) for miRNA was performed with 4 µg of total RNA in a total reaction volume of 20 µL using the Mir-X miRNA First-Strand Synthesis Kit (Takara Bio Inc., Shiga, Japan), and cDNA from total RNA was synthesized using the Tetro cDNA Synthesis Kit (BIO-65043, Bioline, Memphis, TN, USA) according to the manufacturer's protocol. mRNA expression was analyzed using Quantstudio 1 (Applied Biosystems, Waltham, CA, USA) and the $\Delta\Delta$CT method. The transcript abundance of miRNA was normalized to U6, and SESN1, SESN2, and SESN3 were normalized to 18S.

The reaction parameters were as follows for 40 cycles: 94 °C for 30 s, 60 °C for 30 s, with an initial cycle of 50 °C for 2 min followed by 95 °C for 10 min. The primers used for qRT-PCR are listed in Supplementary Table S3.

2.9. *Myocardial Ischemia–Reperfusion Injury (IRI) Model*

This was performed based on guidelines for experimental models of myocardial ischemia and infarction. Briefly, 8-week-old mice were anesthetized with ketamine (95 mg/kg) + xylazine (5 mg/kg) by intraperitoneal injection and then cannulated using a 22-gauge venous catheter. The mice received mechanical ventilation with medical oxygen. The surgery was performed on a 37 °C heating pad to prevent the body from cooling, and the left thoracotomy was performed after shaving the chest to prevent contamination during the surgery. A loose double knot was made with a suture under the left anterior descending artery, and polyethylene glycol tubing (20 gauge) was inserted and fixed, followed by ischemic injury for 30 min. After that, the knot was cut, the tube was removed, and the chest was closed in layers with sutures. In this study, 1E11vg of AAV9 was administered intravenously via tail vein.

2.10. *Evaluation of Heart Function by Echocardiography*

Functional assessment of I/R-injured hearts was performed using echocardiography. The mice were anesthetized with 2% isoflurane, and two-dimensional images and M-mode tracings were recorded in the short axis at the level of the left ventricular papillary muscles using a 14.0 MHz transducer to determine fractional shortening ratio and ventricular dimensions (Vivid S60N; GE HealthCare, Chicago, IL, USA). EF and FS, indices of LV systolic function, were calculated using the following equations, respectively:

$$\mathrm{EF}\ (\%) = 100 \times [(\mathrm{LVIDd}^2 - \mathrm{LVIDs}^2)/\mathrm{LVIDd}^2]$$

$$\mathrm{FS}\ (\%) = 100 \times [(\mathrm{LVIDd} - \mathrm{LVIDs})/\mathrm{LVIDd}]$$

2.11. Statistical Analysis

Statistical analyses for all experiments were performed using Prism version 9.5 (GraphPad Software, Inc., La Jolla, CA, USA). Data are representative of independent experiments and are expressed as the mean ± standard error of the mean (SEM). One-way ANOVA and Student's *t*-test were used to compare the groups, and * $p < 0.05$, ** $p < 0.01$, and *** $p < 0.001$ were considered statistically significant at different levels.

3. Results

3.1. SESN3 Is a Newly Identified Target of miR-25 as an ROS Scavenger

IRI induces severe oxidative stress in the heart [43–45], subsequently leading to myocardial cell damage and cardiac dysfunction. Recently, we observed a significant increase in the expression of miR-25 under hypoxia/reoxygenation (H/R) conditions, and pretreatment with miR-25 Tough Decoy (TuD) substantially reduced ROS generation. Therefore, we hypothesized that miR-25 may regulate potential antioxidant molecules. To identify novel targets of miR-25 involved in the regulation of oxidative damage, we conducted in silico analyses utilizing three databases: Target Miner (May 2012 version), TargetScan7 (TargetScanHuman 7.0), and miRDB (https://mirdb.org/ (accessed on 18 May 2022)). From a total of 148 candidate genes identified through these databases, we selected SESN3 for further investigation (Figure 1A, Supplementary Table S1) due to its antioxidant properties. Notably, the 3′-UTR of the SESN3 mRNA exhibited high conservation across species.

To verify the direct interaction between miR-25 and SESN3, we performed a luciferase reporter assay using a construct containing the SESN3 3′-UTR sequence. The results demonstrated a dose-dependent decrease in luciferase activity with increasing concentrations of pre-miR-25, suggesting that miR-25 directly targets the 3′-UTR region of SESN3 (Figure 1B). To validate these findings, we employed an in vitro hypoxia/reoxygenation (H/R) system using H9c2 myoblasts and evaluated the effect of inhibiting miR-25 on the SESN3 expression and ROS generation. Under H/R conditions, we first confirmed that miR-25 was highly expressed (Figure 1C). Importantly, pretreatment with the miR-25 TuD inhibitor under H/R conditions not only normalized the SESN3 expression (Figure 1C) but also significantly reduced ROS generation, as shown in Figure 1D. Collectively, these results provide compelling evidence that H/R-induced ROS generation is significantly reduced by the restoration of SESN3 expression through miR-25 inhibition.

3.2. SESN3 Overexpression Ameliorates ROS-Induced Apoptosis In Vitro

The SESN family consists of three isoforms: SESN1, SESN2, and SESN3. Most of the literature has focused on SESN1 and SESN2, likely due to their relatively higher expression levels [46–49]. In contrast, the antioxidant effects of SESN3, particularly in the heart, have not been fully elucidated. Therefore, we first characterized SESN3 activity to determine whether it can also scavenge ROS under hypoxia/reoxygenation (H/R) conditions. To this end, we evaluated the effect of SESN3 overexpression by measuring immunofluorescence against ROS and cell death under the H/R condition.

First, we observed that the apoptotic markers, cleaved PARP and cleaved caspase-9, significantly increased in the H/R group; however, these markers were substantially reduced with SESN3 overexpression (Figure 2A). These findings suggest that SESN3 effectively mitigates ROS-induced cell death (Figure 2B,C).

Based on these results, we further investigated the impact of miR-25 on SESN3 expression by treating cells with pre-miR-25 and performing immunofluorescence staining for SESN3. As shown in Supplementary Figure S1, the SESN3 expression was dramatically decreased in the pre-miR-25 transfected group. In summary, we confirmed that SESN3 alone fully mitigates ROS-induced apoptosis, and its expression can be negatively regulated by miR-25.

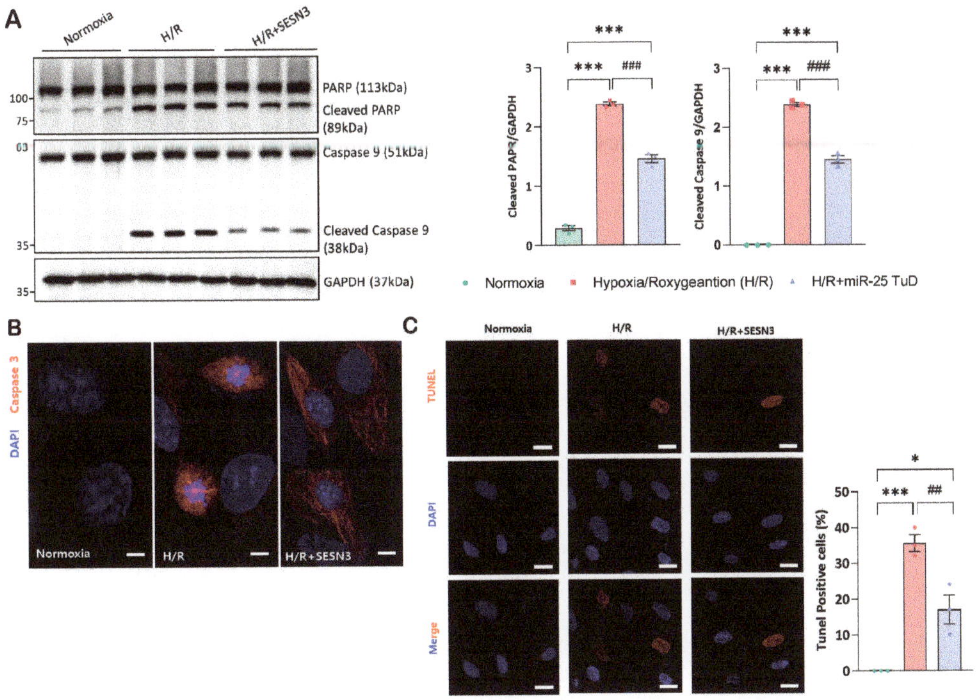

Figure 2. SESN3 overexpression ameliorates ROS-induced apoptosis in vitro. (**A**) Western blot analysis of SESN3, Caspase 9, and cleaved caspase 9 protein levels in myoblasts under Normoxia, HR, and HR+SESN3 overexpression conditions. GAPDH served as a loading control. Representative blots from three independent experiments are shown. (**B**) Representative fluorescence microscopy images of myoblasts stained for active caspase 3 (red). Nuclei were counterstained with DAPI (blue). The scale bar indicates 25 µm. (**C**) TUNEL assay for detection of apoptotic cells. Representative images showing TUNEL-positive nuclei (red) and total nuclei stained with DAPI (blue). The scale bar indicates 50 µm. (* $p < 0.05$, *** $p < 0.001$ vs. Normoxia, ## $p < 0.01$, ### $p < 0.001$ vs. H/R).

3.3. miR-25 TuD Delivery Attenuates Hypoxia/Reoxygenation-Induced Damage in H9c2 Cardiomyoblasts

Based on previous results, we next measured the expression of three forms of miR-25 (pri-, pre-, and mature forms) and three SESN isoforms following miR-25 TuD delivery to assess its specificity for SESN3. First, all three forms of miR-25 were substantially increased under H/R conditions, but miR-25 TuD delivery dramatically normalized their expression (Figure 3B). Under the same conditions, we examined the expression of all three SESN isoforms: SESN1, SESN2, and SESN3. SESN1 and SESN2 were significantly upregulated under H/R conditions, consistent with previous reports [49]. In contrast, the SESN3 expression was significantly decreased. To our surprise, miR-25 TuD delivery significantly increased the SESN3 expression while both SESN1 and SESN2 were downregulated (Figure 3C). These results suggest that normalizing SESN3 expression is sufficient to reduce ROS-induced damage, indicating that SESN1 and SESN2 levels could also normalize as a consequence.

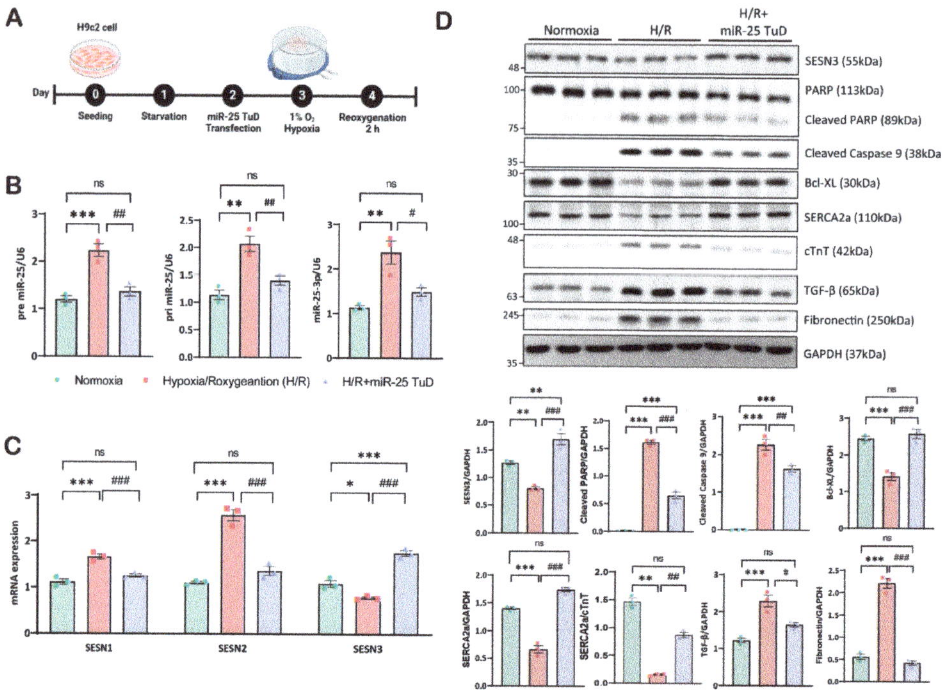

Figure 3. miR-25 TuD delivery attenuates hypoxia/reoxygenation-induced damage in H9c2 cardiomyoblasts. (**A**) Experimental design and procedures. (**B**,**C**) The expression levels of miR-25 (primary, precursor, and mature) and the expression levels of the SESN family were analyzed by qRT-PCR. (**D**) Immunoblotting analysis and quantification of protein levels in H9c2 cells subjected to hypoxia/reoxygenation (H/R) injury (* $p < 0.05$, ** $p < 0.01$, *** $p < 0.001$ vs. Normoxia, # $p < 0.05$, ## $p < 0.01$, ### $p < 0.001$ vs. H/R, ns: not significant).

Oxidative stress generally induces cell apoptosis, which, in many cases, exacerbates cardiac fibrosis [50]. Therefore, we further investigated the effect of miR-25 inhibition in both apoptosis and fibrosis. As shown in Figure 3D, the restoration of SESN3 expression through miR-25 TuD delivery remarkably decreased the levels of apoptotic markers, including cleaved PARP and cleaved caspase-9, while increasing the expression of the anti-apoptotic marker Bcl-XL. Furthermore, we observed a reduction in the expression of fibrosis markers, such as TGF-β and fibronectin (Figure 3D), and Collagen I/III (Supplementary Figure S4). Taken together, these results suggest that miR-25 inhibition via TuD delivery not only modulates the expression of the SESN family but also attenuates apoptosis and fibrosis through the regulation of oxidative stress.

3.4. miR-25 TuD Delivery Reduces ROS-Mediated Damage in a Cardiac IRI Model

Our results suggest that miR-25 inhibition successfully reduced ROS generation, apoptosis, and fibrosis through the restoration of SESN3 expression in vitro. To validate these findings and explore their clinical relevance, we extended our investigation to an in vivo mouse model of cardiac IRI, with or without miR-25 TuD delivery.

For this purpose, we utilized AAV9-EGFP (control) and AAV9-miR-25 TuD, administered via tail vein injection to 8-week-old mice, according to the experimental scheme (Figure 4A). Prior to evaluating cardiac function, we analyzed the biodistribution of AAV9-

GFP. The dissection of five major organs (brain, heart, lungs, liver, and kidneys) revealed that the heart exhibited the second highest level of expression (Supplementary Figure S2), indicating that AAV9 has significant adaptability for cardiac tissue [51–53]. We then confirmed that AAV9-miR-25 TuD delivery effectively reduced the levels of primary miR-25, precursor miR-25, and mature miR-25-3p in the mouse heart (Figure 4B). This reduction in miR-25 expression is crucial for the success of our subsequent experiments.

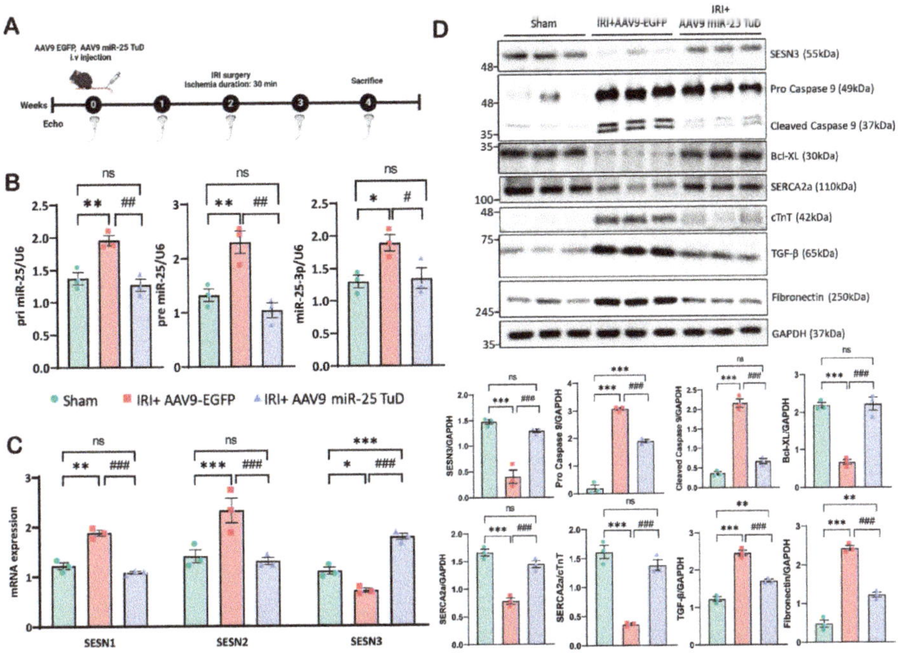

Figure 4. miR-25 TuD delivery reduces ROS-mediated damage in a cardiac IRI model. (**A**) Experimental scheme for the pretreatment of miR-25 TuD in the ischemia–reperfusion injury model. (**B**) The expression levels of different forms of endogenous miR-25 (primary, precursor, and mature) were evaluated to confirm the long-term effect of AAV9 miR-25 TuD. (**C**) SESNS family expression levels were analyzed using qRT-PCR. (**D**) Immunoblotting analysis and quantification of protein levels in the ischemia–reperfusion injury (IRI) mouse heart (* $p < 0.05$, ** $p < 0.01$, *** $p < 0.001$ vs. Sham, # $p < 0.05$, ## $p < 0.01$, ### $p < 0.001$ vs. IRI+AAV9-EGFP, ns: not significant).

We then examined the expression of the SESN isoforms, focusing particularly on SESN3, a novel target of miR-25. As shown in Figure 4C, SESN3 mRNA expression was restored following AAV9-miR-25 TuD delivery, while SESN1 and SESN2 were substantially reduced, consistent with our in vitro data. Next, we investigated the expression of key proteins related to apoptosis and fibrosis in the cardiac samples from these mice. As in in vitro conditions, the SESN3 expression was significantly increased. Additionally, cleaved caspase-9, a key mediator of apoptosis, was highly elevated but effectively mitigated by miR-25 TuD delivery (Figure 4D). In contrast, the anti-apoptotic marker Bcl-XL was substantially upregulated, indicating a shift towards cell survival and away from apoptotic pathways.

Furthermore, we observed a reduction in the TGF-β and fibronectin levels, both of which are associated with fibrotic processes, along with significant decreases in Collagen Type I and Type III (Figure 4D, Supplementary Figure S5). These findings indicate that miR-25 inhibition not only prevents cell apoptosis but also attenuates fibrotic remodeling in the injured myocardium.

In summary, our data demonstrate that miR-25 inhibition using miR-25 TuD is sufficient to alleviate oxidative stress in cardiac IRI. The restoration of SESN3 expression, along with the modulation of apoptotic and fibrotic markers, appears to be a key mechanism in preventing cell death and pathological remodeling.

3.5. miR-25 TuD Delivery Mitigates IRI-Induced Cardiac Dysfunction

To assess the impact of miR-25 TuD delivery on cardiac function, we performed weekly echocardiographic evaluations (Figure 5A). In the IRI model, the heart weight-to-body weight ratio was increased compared to that in the sham-operated mice, while the mice treated with AAV9 miR-25 TuD exhibited a ratio similar to that of the sham group (Figure 5B). Ventricular ejection fraction (EF) and fractional shortening (FS) were significantly higher in the AAV9 miR-25 TuD-treated group than in the IRI group (Figure 5C). The decreased IVSd and IVSs values observed in the IRI model suggest a loss of contractility due to ischemic injury. Notably, both values were preserved in the mice treated with AAV9 miR-25 TuD (Figure 5C).

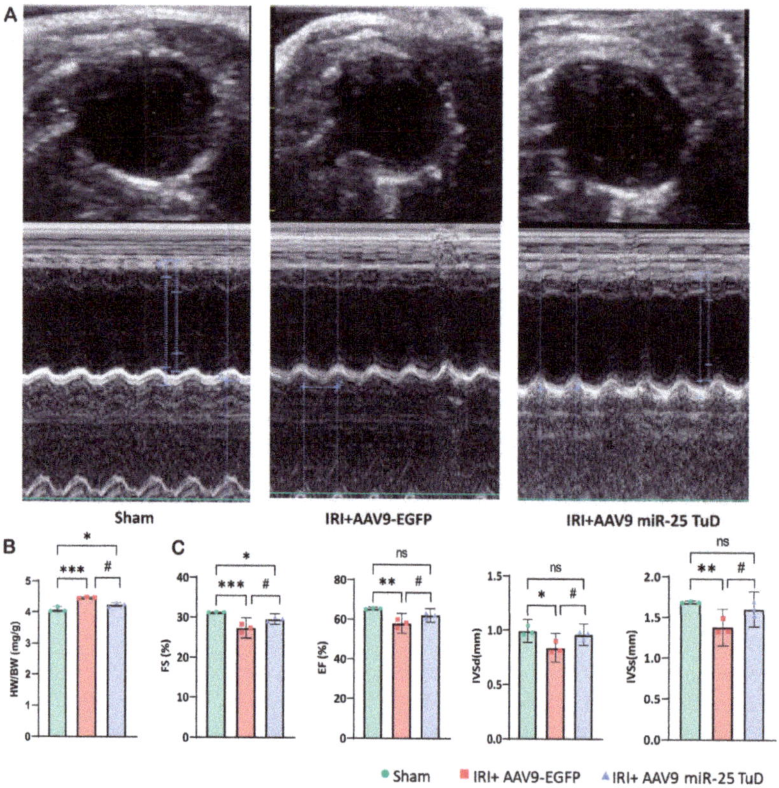

Figure 5. miR-25 TuD delivery mitigates IRI-induced cardiac dysfunction. (**A**) Representative left ventricular M-mode echocardiographic images of the sham, AAV9-EGFP, and AAV9 miR-25 TuD-transfected groups were obtained before sacrifice. (**B**) Quantitative results of heart weight/body weight (HW/BW) 2 weeks post-I/R surgery. (**C**) Left ventricular functional and remodeling parameters, including FS, EF, IVSd, and IVSs, are presented (* $p < 0.05$, ** $p < 0.01$, *** $p < 0.001$ vs. Sham, # $p < 0.05$ vs. IRI+AAV9-EGFP, ns: not significant).

Taken together, these results suggest that miR-25 inhibition using miR-25 TuD can effectively prevent ROS-induced cardiac dysfunction in vivo.

3.6. Knockdown of SESN3 Neutralizes the Effect of miR-25 TuD Delivery

Finally, we conducted additional experiments to verify whether the beneficial effects of miR-25 inhibition are mediated specifically through the regulation of SESN3 expression under H/R conditions. To this end, we used shSESN3 to knock down the SESN3 expression in combination with miR-25 TuD delivery. As shown in Figure 6A, the SESN3 expression was completely absent following SESN3 knockdown, even with miR-25 TuD treatment (Figure 6A, lanes 6–7). Furthermore, the beneficial effects of miR-25 TuD treatment were completely abrogated (Figure 6A). These findings were also substantiated at the mRNA level (Figure 6B), providing strong evidence that SESN3 is indeed a direct target of miR-25.

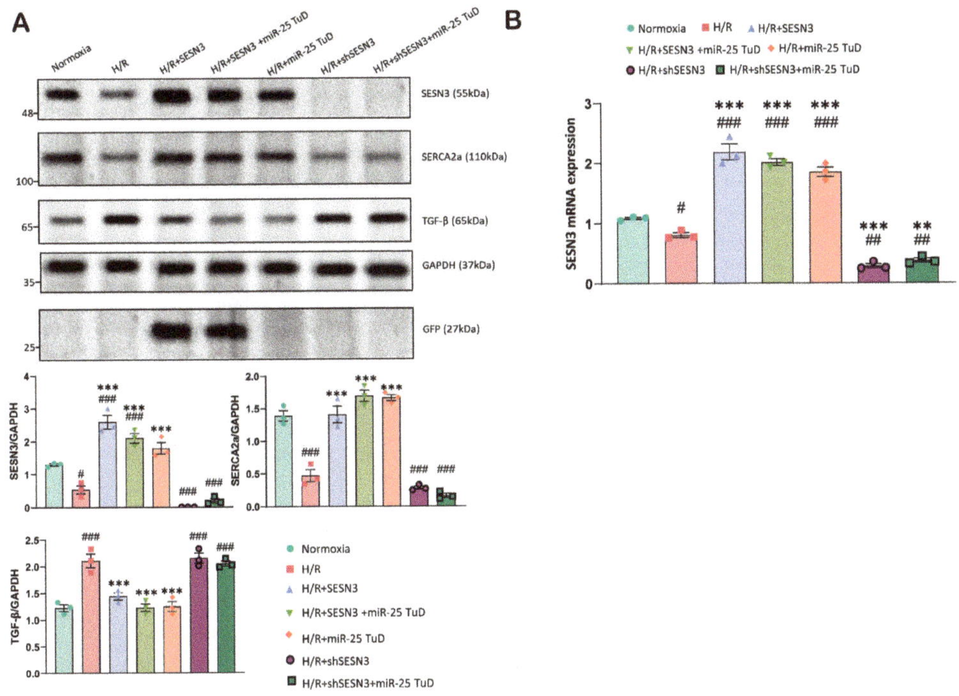

Figure 6. Knockdown of SESN3 neutralizes the effect of miR-25 TuD delivery. (**A**) SESN3 overexpression, miR-25 TuD treatments, and SESN3 knockdown were applied either individually or in various combinations in H9c2 cells under H/R conditions. Immunoblotting was then performed using anti-SERCA2a, TGF-β, and GFP antibodies. (**B**) SESN3 mRNA expression was measured in H9c2 cells under hypoxia/reoxygenation (H/R) conditions (** $p < 0.01$, *** $p < 0.001$ vs. Normoxia, # $p < 0.05$, ## $p < 0.01$, ### $p < 0.001$ vs. H/R).

Consequently, these results highlight the specificity of miR-25 in regulating SESN3 expression and demonstrate that the anti-apoptotic and anti-fibrotic effects of miR-25 TuD are mediated through SESN3 by reducing oxidative damage in the heart.

4. Discussion

The treatment of acute myocardial ischemia presents a paradoxical challenge in modern cardiology. While early and successful reperfusion remains the most effective strategy for salvaging ischemic myocardium, it can also exacerbate myocardial damage through a phenomenon known as ischemia–reperfusion injury (IRI) [4,5]. This injury manifests through various mechanisms, including endothelial dysfunction, myocardial cell necrosis, alterations in calcium handling, metabolic disturbances, and inflammation [54]. A significant contributor to IRI is the production of reactive oxygen species (ROS) and intracellular Ca^{2+} overload, both of which play central roles in myocardial damage.

Recent studies have shown that certain miRNAs play crucial roles in regulating oxidative stress responses in cardiovascular diseases. For instance, miR-15b, miR-29, and miR-222 have been shown to downregulate key antioxidant factors such as SIRT4, PGC-1α, and SOD, respectively, thereby disrupting cellular defenses against oxidative stress [55–57]. These findings underscore the potential of miRNAs as both biomarkers and therapeutic targets in cardiovascular pathologies. Interestingly, studies have shown contradictory roles for miR-25: while one study reported that increased miR-25 expression exacerbated ROS-induced cell damage [58], another study suggested that miR-25 upregulation protects cardiomyocytes from oxidative stress [59]. These opposing findings may be attributed to differences in experimental models, specific stressors, or the timing and duration of miR-25 modulation.

Our recent studies revealed that miR-25 is highly upregulated in the IRI model, and its overexpression exacerbates cardiac damage and impaired function. Thus, we hypothesized that miR-25 may have an additional target involved in regulating ROS generation. To explore this, we conducted in silico screening and identified SESN3 as a novel target of miR-25 in the context of ROS regulation.

The Sestrin family of proteins performs critical functions, such as protecting against oxidative stress [60], regulating mTORC1 signaling [61], and promoting autophagy [62]. Sestrin3, in particular, has gained attention for its diverse roles in various tissues. For example, in the liver, Sestrin3 has been shown to protect against metabolic stress and insulin resistance [31], while also modulating FOXO3-mediated ROS regulation [63]. However, its role is not universally protective across all tissues. In neurological diseases, Sestrin3 has been implicated in the promotion of epileptic seizures [64], and in a mouse model of colitis, increased Sestrin3 expression activated macrophages and promoted the production of inflammatory cytokines [65]. This highlights the context-dependent nature of Sestrin3 function and underscores the importance of carefully considering its therapeutic targeting.

The role of Sestrin3 in cardiovascular diseases, particularly in cardiac IRI, remains underexplored. While Sestrin2 has been shown to have protective roles in cardiac IRI, its interaction with Sestrin3 in this context has not been fully elucidated. Therefore, we performed experiments using an miR-25 TuD inhibitor to test our hypothesis. As expected, when the ROS levels increased under H/R conditions, the Sestrin3 expression was suppressed by pre-miR-25. However, miR-25 TuD delivery restored Sestrin3 expression (Figure 1C,D). Additionally, Sestrin3 overexpression alleviated ROS-induced apoptosis (Figure 2A,B). Further experiments confirmed that miR-25 TuD delivery reduced apoptosis and fibrosis (Figures 3D and 4C), consistent with previous findings that Sestrin3 inhibits TGF-β signaling to prevent fibrosis [66].

While this study provides strong evidence that miR-25 directly targets SESN3 and modulates oxidative stress-induced apoptosis and cardiac fibrosis, several areas require further investigation. First, the precise molecular mechanisms by which SESN3 overexpression mitigates ROS-induced apoptosis remain unclear. Elucidating these downstream signaling pathways could provide deeper insights into the protective effects of SESN3. Second, although we demonstrated that miR-25 regulates SESN3 expression in both H/R and IRI models, further research is needed to explore the regulation of other SESN isoforms under miR-25 TuD treatment. Lastly, while SESN3 is a confirmed target of miR-25, it is also important to investigate whether other miR-25 targets play significant roles in modulating oxidative stress and apoptosis.

Although this study demonstrates that miR-25 directly targets SESN3 and modulates oxidative stress-induced apoptosis and cardiac fibrosis, the timing of potential treatment strategies must be considered. Previous studies have shown that members of the miR-15 family confer cardioprotective effects when administered during ischemia–reperfusion injury [67]. Additionally, the inhibition of miR-192 and miR-128 prior to ischemic injury has been shown to significantly reduce infarct size, further highlighting their cardioprotective potential [68,69]. Moreover, reperfusion is most effective when performed within 90 min of ischemia onset [70,71]. Taken together, these findings suggest that therapeutic approaches targeting the miR-25/SESN3 axis would be most beneficial as a preventive measure in high-risk patients or as an immediate intervention following myocardial infarction. Future studies should focus on optimizing the timing and delivery of these treatments to maximize their cardioprotective potential.

5. Conclusions

Restoring blood flow is essential for treating acute myocardial ischemia, but reperfusion can paradoxically exacerbate myocardial damage through mechanisms such as ROS accumulation, calcium overload, and inflammation. In this study, we confirmed that miR-25 expression is upregulated in ischemia–reperfusion injury (IRI), and through in silico methods, we identified Sestrin3 (SESN3) as a novel target of miR-25. Additionally, we observed that using miR-25 Tough Decoy (TuD), a previously validated inhibitor of miR-25, restored SESN3 expression. This restoration of SESN3 expression resulted in reduced ROS-induced damage and improved cardiac function in both in vitro and in vivo models. In conclusion, these findings suggest that targeting the miR-25-SESN3 axis could be a promising therapeutic strategy for alleviating I/R injury.

Supplementary Materials: The following supporting information can be downloaded at https://www.mdpi.com/article/10.3390/antiox14010061/s1: Figure S1: SESN3 expression following Pre miR-25 transfection in H9c2 cells. H9c2 cardiac myoblast cells were either transfected with Scrambled control or Pre miR-25 for 24 h. Cells were then fixed, permeabilized, and stained for SESN3 (red) and nuclei (DAPI, blue); Figure S2: In vivo Expression of AAV9-EGFP in Various Organs. Two weeks after tail vein injection of AAV9-EGFP, five major organs (Brain, Heart, Lung, Liver and Kidney) were collected from mice receiving a single intravenous AAV9-EGFP administration. These tissues were subsequently subjected to Western blot analysis for GFP expression; Figure S3: miR-25 Expression Levels at 1 Week and 2 Weeks Post-Injury. Quantitative analysis of miR-25 expression in the heart following ischemia/reperfusion (I/R) injury. Mice were administered AAV9-miR-25 TuD via tail vein injection prior to I/R injury. Cardiac tissue was collected at 1 week and 2 weeks post-injury. miR-25 levels were assessed by qRT-PCR and normalized to U6. Data are presented as mean ± SEM ($n = 3$ per group). (* $p < 0.05$, ** $p < 0.01$, *** $p < 0.001$ vs. Sham); Figure S4: Expression of Collagen Type I and Type III in H9c2 cells under Normoxia and hypoxia/reoxygenation (H/R) conditions following miR-25 TuD treatment. H9c2 cardiac myoblast cells were subjected to normoxia, hypoxia/reoxygenation (H/R), and H/R with miR-25 TuD pretreatment. Collagen Type I and Type III expression levels were assessed by qRT-PCR and normalized to GAPDH. (* $p < 0.05$, ** $p < 0.01$, *** $p < 0.001$ vs. Normoxia, # $p < 0.05$, ## $p < 0.01$, ### $p < 0.001$ vs. H/R); Figure S5: Expression of Collagen Type I and Type III in Cardiac Tissue Following AAV9-miR-25 TuD delivery. Mice were subjected to sham surgery, ischemia/reperfusion (I/R) injury, and I/R with AAV9 miR-25 TuD pretreatment. The AAV9 miR-25 TuD was administered via tail vein injection prior to I/R injury. Collagen Type I and Type III expression levels were assessed by qRT-PCR and normalized to GAPDH. (* $p < 0.05$, ** $p < 0.01$, *** $p < 0.001$ vs. Sham, # $p < 0.05$, ## $p < 0.01$, ### $p < 0.001$ vs. IRI+AAV9-EGFP); Figure S6: SESN1, SESN2 mRNA expression in H9c2 cells under Normoxia and hypoxia/reoxygenation (H/R) conditions. SESN1 and 2 mRNA expression were measured in H9c2 cells subjected to various conditions using SESN3 overexpression, miR-25 TuD treatments, and SESN3 knockdown under normoxia and hypoxia/reoxygenation (H/R) conditions. (* $p < 0.05$, ** $p < 0.01$, *** $p < 0.001$ vs. Normoxia, # $p < 0.05$, ## $p < 0.01$, ### $p < 0.001$ vs. H/R); Table S1: Predicted miR-25 target genes and their characteristics; Table S2: Antibodies used for western blot; Table S3: Quantitative RT-PCR primer information.

Author Contributions: Conceptualization, D.J.; methodology, D.J.; validation, M.P., S.C. and D.J.; formal analysis, M.P. and S.C.; investigation, M.P. and S.C.; writing—original draft preparation, M.P. and D.J.; writing—review and editing, D.J.; supervision, D.J.; funding acquisition, D.J. All authors have read and agreed to the published version of the manuscript.

Funding: D.J. was supported by grants from the National Research Foundation of Korea (2021R1A2C1008058, 2021R1A4A5032463, and RS-2024-00440285) funded by the Korean Government (MSIP).

Institutional Review Board Statement: All experimental procedures were approved by the Institutional Animal Care and Use Committee of Hanyang University-ERICA. (Approval No. HY-IACUC-24-0058, approved on 30 July 2024; HY-IACUC-24-0059, approved on 31 July 2024; HY-IACUC-24-0074, approved on 22 September 2024).

Informed Consent Statement: Not applicable.

Data Availability Statement: Data is contained within the article or Supplementary Materials.

Conflicts of Interest: The authors have no relevant financial or non-financial interests to disclose.

References

1. Del Buono, M.G.; Moroni, F.; Montone, R.A.; Azzalini, L.; Sanna, T.; Abbate, A. Ischemic Cardiomyopathy and Heart Failure After Acute Myocardial Infarction. *Curr. Cardiol. Rep.* **2022**, *24*, 1505–1515. [CrossRef] [PubMed]
2. Panza, J.A.; Chrzanowski, L.; Bonow, R.O. Myocardial Viability Assessment Before Surgical Revascularization in Ischemic Cardiomyopathy: JACC Review Topic of the Week. *J. Am. Coll. Cardiol.* **2021**, *78*, 1068–1077. [CrossRef] [PubMed]
3. Cabac-Pogorevici, I.; Muk, B.; Rustamova, Y.; Kalogeropoulos, A.; Tzeis, S.; Vardas, P. Ischaemic cardiomyopathy. Pathophysiological insights, diagnostic management and the roles of revascularisation and device treatment. Gaps and dilemmas in the era of advanced technology. *Eur. J. Heart Fail.* **2020**, *22*, 789–799. [CrossRef] [PubMed]
4. Pizzino, G.; Irrera, N.; Cucinotta, M.; Pallio, G.; Mannino, F.; Arcoraci, V.; Squadrito, F.; Altavilla, D.; Bitto, A. Oxidative Stress: Harms and Benefits for Human Health. *Oxid. Med. Cell Longev.* **2017**, *2017*, 8416763. [CrossRef]
5. Li, T.; Zhang, X.; Jiang, K.; Liu, J.; Liu, Z. Dural effects of oxidative stress on cardiomyogenesis via Gata4 transcription and protein ubiquitination. *Cell Death Dis.* **2018**, *9*, 246. [CrossRef] [PubMed]
6. Munzel, T.; Camici, G.G.; Maack, C.; Bonetti, N.R.; Fuster, V.; Kovacic, J.C. Impact of Oxidative Stress on the Heart and Vasculature: Part 2 of a 3-Part Series. *J. Am. Coll. Cardiol.* **2017**, *70*, 212–229. [CrossRef]
7. Zhazykbayeva, S.; Hassoun, R.; Herwig, M.; Budde, H.; Kovacs, A.; Mannherz, H.G.; El-Battrawy, I.; Toth, A.; Schmidt, W.E.; Mugge, A.; et al. Oxidative stress and inflammation distinctly drive molecular mechanisms of diastolic dysfunction and remodeling in female and male heart failure with preserved ejection fraction rats. *Front. Cardiovasc. Med.* **2023**, *10*, 1157398. [CrossRef] [PubMed]
8. Duan, D.; Li, H.; Chai, S.; Zhang, L.; Fan, T.; Hu, Z.; Feng, Y. The relationship between cardiac oxidative stress, inflammatory cytokine response, cardiac pump function, and prognosis post-myocardial infarction. *Sci. Rep.* **2024**, *14*, 8985. [CrossRef]
9. Li, Q.; Ding, J.; Xia, B.; Liu, K.; Zheng, K.; Wu, J.; Huang, C.; Yuan, X.; You, Q. L-theanine alleviates myocardial ischemia/reperfusion injury by suppressing oxidative stress and apoptosis through activation of the JAK2/STAT3 pathway in mice. *Mol. Med.* **2024**, *30*, 98. [CrossRef]
10. Chen, Y.; Guo, X.; Zeng, Y.; Mo, X.; Hong, S.; He, H.; Li, J.; Fatima, S.; Liu, Q. Oxidative stress induces mitochondrial iron overload and ferroptotic cell death. *Sci. Rep.* **2023**, *13*, 15515. [CrossRef] [PubMed]

11. Cohn, J.N.; Ferrari, R.; Sharpe, N. Cardiac remodeling--concepts and clinical implications: A consensus paper from an international forum on cardiac remodeling. Behalf of an International Forum on Cardiac Remodeling. *J. Am. Coll. Cardiol.* **2000**, *35*, 569–582. [CrossRef]
12. Evans, S.; Weinheimer, C.J.; Kovacs, A.; Williams, J.W.; Randolph, G.J.; Jiang, W.; Barger, P.M.; Mann, D.L. Ischemia reperfusion injury provokes adverse left ventricular remodeling in dysferlin-deficient hearts through a pathway that involves TIRAP dependent signaling. *Sci. Rep.* **2020**, *10*, 14129. [CrossRef] [PubMed]
13. Hwang, J.-W.; Park, J.-H.; Park, B.-W.; Kim, H.; Kim, J.-J.; Sim, W.-S.; Mishchenko, N.P.; Fedoreyev, S.A.; Vasileva, E.A.; Ban, K.; et al. Histochrome Attenuates Myocardial Ischemia-Reperfusion Injury by Inhibiting Ferroptosis-Induced Cardiomyocyte Death. *Antioxidants* **2021**, *10*, 1624. [CrossRef]
14. Pluijmert, N.J.; Bart, C.I.; Bax, W.H.; Quax, P.H.A.; Atsma, D.E. Effects on cardiac function, remodeling and inflammation following myocardial ischemia-reperfusion injury or unreperfused myocardial infarction in hypercholesterolemic APOE*3-Leiden mice. *Sci. Rep.* **2020**, *10*, 16601. [CrossRef]
15. van der Bijl, P.; Abou, R.; Goedemans, L.; Gersh, B.J.; Holmes, D.R., Jr.; Marsan, N.A.; Delgado, V.; Bax, J.J. Left Ventricular Post-Infarct Remodeling: Implications for Systolic Function Improvement and Outcomes in the Modern Era. *JACC Heart Fail.* **2020**, *8*, 131–140. [CrossRef] [PubMed]
16. Ikeda, Y.; Young, L.H.; Scalia, R.; Ross, C.R.; Lefer, A.M. PR-39, a proline/arginine-rich antimicrobial peptide, exerts cardioprotective effects in myocardial ischemia-reperfusion. *Cardiovasc. Res.* **2001**, *49*, 69–77. [CrossRef] [PubMed]
17. Yang, J.; Wang, Z.; Chen, D.-L. Shikonin ameliorates isoproterenol (ISO)-induced myocardial damage through suppressing fibrosis, inflammation, apoptosis and ER stress. *Biomed. Pharmacother.* **2017**, *93*, 1343–1357. [CrossRef]
18. Glorieux, C.; Calderon, P.B. Catalase, a remarkable enzyme: Targeting the oldest antioxidant enzyme to find a new cancer treatment approach. *Biol. Chem.* **2017**, *398*, 1095–1108. [CrossRef]
19. Lai, L.; Yan, L.; Gao, S.; Hu, C.-L.; Ge, H.; Davidow, A.; Park, M.; Bravo, C.; Iwatsubo, K.; Ishikawa, Y.; et al. Type 5 adenylyl cyclase increases oxidative stress by transcriptional regulation of manganese superoxide dismutase via the SIRT1/FoxO3a pathway. *Circulation* **2013**, *127*, 1692–1701. [CrossRef]
20. Dudek, H.; Datta, S.R.; Franke, T.F.; Birnbaum, M.J.; Yao, R.; Cooper, G.M.; Segal, R.A.; Kaplan, D.R.; Greenberg, M.E. Regulation of neuronal survival by the serine-threonine protein kinase Akt. *Science* **1997**, *275*, 661–665. [CrossRef] [PubMed]
21. Kennedy, S.G.; Wagner, A.J.; Conzen, S.D.; Jordán, J.; Bellacosa, A.; Tsichlis, P.N.; Hay, N. The PI 3-kinase/Akt signaling pathway delivers an anti-apoptotic signal. *Genes Dev.* **1997**, *11*, 701–713. [CrossRef] [PubMed]
22. Widmann, C.; Gibson, S.; Jarpe, M.B.; Johnson, G.L. Mitogen-activated protein kinase: Conservation of a three-kinase module from yeast to human. *Physiol. Rev.* **1999**, *79*, 143–180. [CrossRef]
23. Nguyen, B.Y.; Ruiz-Velasco, A.; Bui, T.; Collins, L.; Wang, X.; Liu, W. Mitochondrial function in the heart: The insight into mechanisms and therapeutic potentials. *Br. J. Pharmacol.* **2019**, *176*, 4302–4318. [CrossRef] [PubMed]
24. Hollander, J.M.; Thapa, D.; Shepherd, D.L. Physiological and structural differences in spatially distinct subpopulations of cardiac mitochondria: Influence of cardiac pathologies. *Am. J. Physiol. Heart Circ. Physiol.* **2014**, *307*, H1-14. [CrossRef] [PubMed]
25. Ikeuchi, M.; Matsusaka, H.; Kang, D.; Matsushima, S.; Ide, T.; Kubota, T.; Fujiwara, T.; Hamasaki, N.; Takeshita, A.; Sunagawa, K.; et al. Overexpression of mitochondrial transcription factor a ameliorates mitochondrial deficiencies and cardiac failure after myocardial infarction. *Circulation* **2005**, *112*, 683–690. [CrossRef] [PubMed]
26. Forman, H.J.; Zhang, H. Targeting oxidative stress in disease: Promise and limitations of antioxidant therapy. *Nat. Rev. Drug Discov.* **2021**, *20*, 689–709. [CrossRef]
27. Rojo, A.I.; Salinas, M.; Martín, D.; Perona, R.; Cuadrado, A. Regulation of Cu/Zn-superoxide dismutase expression via the phosphatidylinositol 3 kinase/Akt pathway and nuclear factor-kappaB. *J. Neurosci.* **2004**, *24*, 7324–7334. [CrossRef] [PubMed]
28. Velasco-Miguel, S.; Buckbinder, L.; Jean, P.; Gelbert, L.; Talbott, R.; Laidlaw, J.; Seizinger, B.; Kley, N. PA26, a novel target of the p53 tumor suppressor and member of the GADD family of DNA damage and growth arrest inducible genes. *Oncogene* **1999**, *18*, 127–137. [CrossRef]
29. Peeters, H.; Debeer, P.; Bairoch, A.; Wilquet, V.; Huysmans, C.; Parthoens, E.; Fryns, J.P.; Gewillig, M.; Nakamura, Y.; Niikawa, N.; et al. PA26 is a candidate gene for heterotaxia in humans: Identification of a novel PA26-related gene family in human and mouse. *Hum. Genet.* **2003**, *112*, 573–580. [CrossRef] [PubMed]
30. Kumar, A.; Dhiman, D.; Shaha, C. Sestrins: Darkhorse in the regulation of mitochondrial health and metabolism. *Mol. Biol. Rep.* **2020**, *47*, 8049–8060. [CrossRef] [PubMed]
31. Tao, R.; Xiong, X.; Liangpunsakul, S.; Dong, X.C. Sestrin 3 protein enhances hepatic insulin sensitivity by direct activation of the mTORC2-Akt signaling. *Diabetes* **2015**, *64*, 1211–1223. [CrossRef] [PubMed]

32. Cordani, M.; Butera, G.; Dando, I.; Torrens-Mas, M.; Butturini, E.; Pacchiana, R.; Oppici, E.; Cavallini, C.; Gasperini, S.; Tamassia, N.; et al. Mutant p53 blocks SESN1/AMPK/PGC-1alpha/UCP2 axis increasing mitochondrial O_2^{-}. production in cancer cells. *Br. J. Cancer* **2018**, *119*, 994–1008. [CrossRef] [PubMed]
33. Deng, W.; Cha, J.; Yuan, J.; Haraguchi, H.; Bartos, A.; Leishman, E.; Viollet, B.; Bradshaw, H.B.; Hirota, Y.; Dey, S.K. p53 coordinates decidual sestrin 2/AMPK/mTORC1 signaling to govern parturition timing. *J. Clin. Investig.* **2016**, *126*, 2941–2954. [CrossRef]
34. Morsch, A.L.B.C.; Wisniewski, E.; Luciano, T.F.; Comin, V.H.; Silveira, G.d.B.; Marques, S.d.O.; Thirupathi, A.; Lock, P.C.S.; De Souza, C.T. Cigarette smoke exposure induces ROS-mediated autophagy by regulating sestrin, AMPK, and mTOR level in mice. *Redox Rep.* **2019**, *24*, 27–33. [CrossRef] [PubMed]
35. Xue, R.; Zeng, J.; Chen, Y.; Chen, C.; Tan, W.; Zhao, J.; Dong, B.; Sun, Y.; Dong, Y.; Liu, C. Sestrin 1 ameliorates cardiac hypertrophy via autophagy activation. *J. Cell Mol. Med.* **2017**, *21*, 1193–1205. [CrossRef]
36. Lear, T.B.; Lockwood, K.C.; Ouyang, Y.; Evankovich, J.W.; Larsen, M.B.; Lin, B.; Liu, Y.; Chen, B.B. The RING-type E3 ligase RNF186 ubiquitinates Sestrin-2 and thereby controls nutrient sensing. *J. Biol. Chem.* **2019**, *294*, 16527–16534. [CrossRef] [PubMed]
37. Ovchinnikova, E.S.; Schmitter, D.; Vegter, E.L.; ter Maaten, J.M.; Valente, M.A.; Liu, L.C.; van der Harst, P.; Pinto, Y.M.; de Boer, R.A.; Meyer, S.; et al. Signature of circulating microRNAs in patients with acute heart failure. *Eur. J. Heart Fail.* **2016**, *18*, 414–423. [CrossRef]
38. Sygitowicz, G.; Tomaniak, M.; Błaszczyk, O.; Kołtowski, Ł.; Filipiak, K.J.; Sitkiewicz, D. Circulating microribonucleic acids miR-1, miR-21 and miR-208a in patients with symptomatic heart failure: Preliminary results. *Arch. Cardiovasc. Dis.* **2015**, *108*, 634–642. [CrossRef] [PubMed]
39. Seronde, M.-F.; Vausort, M.; Gayat, E.; Goretti, E.; Ng, L.L.; Squire, I.B.; Vodovar, N.; Sadoune, M.; Samuel, J.-L.; Thum, T.; et al. Circulating microRNAs and Outcome in Patients with Acute Heart Failure. *PLoS ONE* **2015**, *10*, e0142237. [CrossRef] [PubMed]
40. Wahlquist, C.; Jeong, D.; Rojas-Muñoz, A.; Kho, C.; Lee, A.; Mitsuyama, S.; van Mil, A.; Park, W.J.; Sluijter, J.P.G.; Doevendans, P.A.F.; et al. Inhibition of miR-25 improves cardiac contractility in the failing heart. *Nature* **2014**, *508*, 531–535. [CrossRef] [PubMed]
41. Park, W.J.; Oh, J.G. SERCA2a: A prime target for modulation of cardiac contractility during heart failure. *BMB Rep.* **2013**, *46*, 237–243. [CrossRef] [PubMed]
42. del Monte, F.; Harding, S.E.; Schmidt, U.; Matsui, T.; Bin Kang, Z.; Dec, G.W.; Gwathmey, J.K.; Rosenzweig, A.; Hajjar, R.J. Restoration of contractile function in isolated cardiomyocytes from failing human hearts by gene transfer of SERCA2a. *Circulation* **1999**, *100*, 2308–2311. [CrossRef]
43. Zweier, J.L.; Flaherty, J.T.; Weisfeldt, M.L. Direct measurement of free radical generation following reperfusion of ischemic myocardium. *Proc. Natl. Acad. Sci. USA* **1987**, *84*, 1404–1407. [CrossRef] [PubMed]
44. Levraut, J.; Iwase, H.; Shao, Z.-H.; Hoek, T.L.V.; Schumacker, P.T. Cell death during ischemia: Relationship to mitochondrial depolarization and ROS generation. *Am. J. Physiol. Heart Circ. Physiol.* **2003**, *284*, H549–H558. [CrossRef]
45. Hoek, T.L.V.; Li, C.; Shao, Z.; Schumacker, P.T.; Becker, L.B. Significant levels of oxidants are generated by isolated cardiomyocytes during ischemia prior to reperfusion. *J. Mol. Cell Cardiol.* **1997**, *29*, 2571–2583. [CrossRef] [PubMed]
46. Kim, M.; Sujkowski, A.; Namkoong, S.; Gu, B.; Cobb, T.; Kim, B.; Kowalsky, A.H.; Cho, C.-S.; Semple, I.; Ro, S.-H.; et al. Sestrins are evolutionarily conserved mediators of exercise benefits. *Nat. Commun.* **2020**, *11*, 190. [CrossRef]
47. Tang, Y.; Zhang, J.; Wang(B), J.; Xiao, M.; Lu, G.; Li, J.; Liu, Q.; Guo, Y.; Gu, J. Cardiac SIRT1 ameliorates doxorubicin-induced cardiotoxicity by targeting sestrin 2. *Redox Biol.* **2022**, *52*, 102310. [CrossRef]
48. Haidurov, A.; Budanov, A.V. Sestrin family-the stem controlling healthy ageing. *Mech. Ageing Dev.* **2020**, *192*, 111379. [CrossRef] [PubMed]
49. Li, R.; Huang, Y.; Semple, I.; Kim, M.; Zhang, Z.; Lee, J.H. Cardioprotective roles of sestrin 1 and sestrin 2 against doxorubicin cardiotoxicity. *Am. J. Physiol. Heart Circ. Physiol.* **2019**, *317*, H39–H48. [CrossRef] [PubMed]
50. Moris, D.; Spartalis, M.; Spartalis, E.; Karachaliou, G.-S.; Karaolanis, G.I.; Tsourouflis, G.; Tsilimigras, D.I.; Tzatzaki, E.; Theocharis, S. The role of reactive oxygen species in the pathophysiology of cardiovascular diseases and the clinical significance of myocardial redox. *Ann. Transl. Med.* **2017**, *5*, 326. [CrossRef]
51. Guenther, C.M.; Brun, M.J.; Bennett, A.D.; Ho, M.L.; Chen, W.; Zhu, B.; Lam, M.; Yamagami, M.; Kwon, S.; Bhattacharya, N.; et al. Protease-Activatable Adeno-Associated Virus Vector for Gene Delivery to Damaged Heart Tissue. *Mol. Ther.* **2019**, *27*, 611–622. [CrossRef] [PubMed]
52. Wu, I.; Zeng, A.; Greer-Short, A.; Aycinena, J.A.; Tefera, A.E.; Shenwai, R.; Farshidfar, F.; Van Pell, M.; Xu, E.; Reid, C.; et al. AAV9:PKP2 improves heart function and survival in a Pkp2-deficient mouse model of arrhythmogenic right ventricular cardiomyopathy. *Commun. Med.* **2024**, *4*, 38. [CrossRef] [PubMed]
53. Li, J.; Richmond, B.; Cluntun, A.A.; Bia, R.; Walsh, M.A.; Shaw, K.; Symons, J.D.; Franklin, S.; Rutter, J.; Funai, K.; et al. Cardiac gene therapy treats diabetic cardiomyopathy and lowers blood glucose. *JCI Insight* **2023**, *8*, e166713. [CrossRef] [PubMed]

54. Verma, S.; Fedak, P.W.; Weisel, R.D.; Butany, J.; Rao, V.; Maitland, A.; Li, R.-K.; Dhillon, B.; Yau, T.M. Fundamentals of reperfusion injury for the clinical cardiologist. *Circulation* **2002**, *105*, 2332–2336. [CrossRef]
55. Lang, A.; Grether-Beck, S.; Singh, M.; Kuck, F.; Jakob, S.; Kefalas, A.; Altinoluk-Hambüchen, S.; Graffmann, N.; Schneider, M.; Lindecke, A.; et al. MicroRNA-15b regulates mitochondrial ROS production and the senescence-associated secretory phenotype through sirtuin 4/SIRT4. *Aging* **2016**, *8*, 484–505. [CrossRef] [PubMed]
56. Caravia, X.M.; Fanjul, V.; Oliver, E.; Roiz-Valle, D.; Morán-Álvarez, A.; Desdín-Micó, G.; Mittelbrunn, M.; Cabo, R.; Vega, J.A.; Rodríguez, F.; et al. The microRNA-29/PGC1alpha regulatory axis is critical for metabolic control of cardiac function. *PLoS Biol.* **2018**, *16*, e2006247. [CrossRef] [PubMed]
57. Dubois-Deruy, E.; Cuvelliez, M.; Fiedler, J.; Charrier, H.; Mulder, P.; Hebbar, E.; Pfanne, A.; Beseme, O.; Chwastyniak, M.; Amouyel, P.; et al. MicroRNAs regulating superoxide dismutase 2 are new circulating biomarkers of heart failure. *Sci. Rep.* **2017**, *7*, 14747. [CrossRef] [PubMed]
58. Li, Z.; Li, H.; Liu, B.; Luo, J.; Qin, X.; Gong, M.; Shi, B.; Wei, Y. Inhibition of miR-25 attenuates doxorubicin-induced apoptosis, reactive oxygen species production and DNA damage by targeting PTEN. *Int. J. Med. Sci.* **2020**, *17*, 1415–1427. [CrossRef]
59. Liu, Q.; Wang, Y.; Yang, T.; Wei, W. Protective effects of miR-25 against hypoxia/reoxygenation-induced fibrosis and apoptosis of H9c2 cells. *Int. J. Mol. Med.* **2016**, *38*, 1225–1234. [CrossRef] [PubMed]
60. Chen, C.-C.; Jeon, S.-M.; Bhaskar, P.T.; Nogueira, V.; Sundararajan, D.; Tonic, I.; Park, Y.; Hay, N. FoxOs inhibit mTORC1 and activate Akt by inducing the expression of Sestrin3 and Rictor. *Dev. Cell* **2010**, *18*, 592–604. [CrossRef] [PubMed]
61. Budanov, A.V.; Karin, M. p53 target genes sestrin1 and sestrin2 connect genotoxic stress and mTOR signaling. *Cell* **2008**, *134*, 451–460. [CrossRef] [PubMed]
62. Liu, X.; Niu, Y.; Yuan, H.; Huang, J.; Fu, L. AMPK binds to Sestrins and mediates the effect of exercise to increase insulin-sensitivity through autophagy. *Metabolism* **2015**, *64*, 658–665. [CrossRef] [PubMed]
63. Hagenbuchner, J.; Kuznetsov, A.; Hermann, M.; Hausott, B.; Obexer, P.; Ausserlechner, M.J. FOXO3-induced reactive oxygen species are regulated by BCL2L11 (Bim) and SESN3. *J. Cell Sci.* **2012**, *125*, 1191–1203. [CrossRef]
64. Johnson, M.R.; Behmoaras, J.; Bottolo, L.; Krishnan, M.L.; Pernhorst, K.; Santoscoy, P.L.M.; Rossetti, T.; Speed, D.; Srivastava, P.K.; Chadeau-Hyam, M.; et al. Systems genetics identifies Sestrin 3 as a regulator of a proconvulsant gene network in human epileptic hippocampus. *Nat. Commun.* **2015**, *6*, 6031. [CrossRef] [PubMed]
65. Ge, L.; Xu, M.; Brant, S.R.; Liu, S.; Zhu, C.; Shang, J.; Zhao, Q.; Zhou, F. Sestrin3 enhances macrophage-mediated generation of T helper 1 and T helper 17 cells in a mouse colitis model. *Int. Immunol.* **2020**, *32*, 421–432. [CrossRef]
66. Huang, M.; Kim, H.G.; Zhong, X.; Dong, C.; Zhang, B.; Fang, Z.; Zhang, Y.; Lu, X.; Saxena, R.; Liu, Y.; et al. Sestrin 3 Protects Against Diet-Induced Nonalcoholic Steatohepatitis in Mice Through Suppression of Transforming Growth Factor beta Signal Transduction. *Hepatology* **2020**, *71*, 76–92. [CrossRef] [PubMed]
67. Liu, L.F.; Liang, Z.; Lv, Z.R.; Liu, X.H.; Bai, J.; Chen, J.; Chen, C.; Wang, Y. MicroRNA-15a/b are up-regulated in response to myocardial ischemia/reperfusion injury. *J. Geriatr. Cardiol.* **2012**, *9*, 28–32. [CrossRef] [PubMed]
68. Varga, Z.V.; Zvara, Á.; Faragó, N.; Kocsis, G.F.; Pipicz, M.; Gaspar, R.; Bencsik, P.; Görbe, A.; Csonka, C.; Puskás, L.G.; et al. MicroRNAs associated with ischemia-reperfusion injury and cardioprotection by ischemic pre- and postconditioning: ProtectomiRs. *Am. J. Physiol. Heart Circ. Physiol.* **2014**, *307*, H216–H227. [CrossRef] [PubMed]
69. Zeng, X.C.; Li, L.; Wen, H.; Bi, Q. MicroRNA-128 inhibition attenuates myocardial ischemia/reperfusion injury-induced cardiomyocyte apoptosis by the targeted activation of peroxisome proliferator-activated receptor gamma. *Mol. Med. Rep.* **2016**, *14*, 129–136. [CrossRef]
70. Menees, D.S.; Peterson, E.D.; Wang, Y.; Curtis, J.P.; Messenger, J.C.; Rumsfeld, J.S.; Gurm, H.S. Door-to-balloon time and mortality among patients undergoing primary PCI. *N. Engl. J. Med.* **2013**, *369*, 901–909. [CrossRef] [PubMed]
71. Larsen, A.I.; Løland, K.H.; Hovland, S.; Bleie, Ø.; Eek, C.; Fossum, E.; Trovik, T.; Juliebø, V.; Hegbom, K.; Moer, R.; et al. Guideline-Recommended Time Less Than 90 Minutes from ECG to Primary Percutaneous Coronary Intervention for ST-Segment-Elevation Myocardial Infarction Is Associated with Major Survival Benefits, Especially in Octogenarians: A Contemporary Report in 11 226 Patients from NORIC. *J. Am. Heart Assoc.* **2022**, *11*, e024849. [CrossRef] [PubMed]

antioxidants

MDPI

Review

Lung Ischemia–Reperfusion Injury in Lung Transplant Surgery: Where Do We Stand?

Lawek Berzenji [1,2,*], Jeroen M. H. Hendriks [1,2], Stijn E. Verleden [1,2], Suresh Krishan Yogeswaran [1,2], Wen Wen [1,2], Patrick Lauwers [1,2], Geert Verleden [3], Rudi De Paep [4], Pieter Mertens [5], Inez Rodrigus [6], Dirk Adriaensen [7] and Paul Van Schil [1,2]

1 Department of Thoracic and Vascular Surgery, Antwerp University Hospital, Drie Eikenstraat 655, 2650 Edegem, Belgium; jeroen.hendriks@uza.be (J.M.H.H.); stijn.verleden@uantwerpen.be (S.E.V.); sureshkrishan.yogeswaran@uza.be (S.K.Y.); wen.wen@uza.be (W.W.); patrick.lauwers@uza.be (P.L.); paul.vanschil@uza.be (P.V.S.)
2 Antwerp Surgical Training, Anatomy and Research Centre, University of Antwerp, 2000 Antwerpen, Belgium
3 Department of Pulmonology, Antwerp University Hospital, 2650 Edegem, Belgium; geert.verleden@uza.be
4 Intensive Care Unit, Antwerp University Hospital, 2650 Edegem, Belgium; rudi.depaep@uza.be
5 Department of Anesthesiology, Antwerp University Hospital, 2650 Edegem, Belgium; pieter.mertens@uza.be
6 Department of Cardiac Surgery, Antwerp University Hospital, 2650 Edegem, Belgium; inez.rodrigus@uza.be
7 Laboratory of Cell Biology and Histology, University of Antwerp, 2000 Antwerpen, Belgium; dirk.adriaensen@uantwerpen.be
* Correspondence: lawek.berzenji@uza.be; Tel.: +32-(0)-821-43-61

Abstract

Lung ischemia–reperfusion injury (LIRI) remains a major contributor to perioperative morbidity and mortality in thoracic surgery, especially for lung transplantations, where it is one of the principal drivers of primary graft dysfunction (PGD). Although substantial advances have been made in surgical technique, donor management, and perioperative care, LIRI continues to pose a significant clinical challenge. Mechanistically, LIRI reflects a combined pathology of oxidative stress, endothelial and glycocalyx disruption, innate immune activation, mitochondrial dysfunction, and regulated cell death, resulting in loss of alveolar–capillary barrier integrity and gas exchange failure. Current management is phase-specific and multimodal, spanning donor care and preservation, controlled reperfusion and lung-protective ventilation, and pharmacological treatments. Treatment candidates that target oxidative stress and inflammatory cascades (e.g., antioxidants, complement and adenosine pathways, mesenchymal stromal cell products, and dipeptidyl-peptidase-4 inhibition) show promise, yet translation into a clinical scenario remains difficult. Increasing evidence supports endothelial-preserving and mitochondria-sparing strategies, rigorous perioperative bundles, and biomarker-guided trials to move from pathophysiology to practice. Ultimately, addressing LIRI requires an integrated, multidisciplinary approach that spans surgical, anesthetic, and pharmacologic domains, with the goal of improving both early outcomes and long-term graft survival in lung transplant patients.

Keywords: lung ischemia–reperfusion injury; thoracic surgery; lung transplantation; primary graft dysfunction

1. Introduction

Ischemia–reperfusion injury (IRI) refers to the detrimental effects on cellular function and homeostasis that occur when blood flow is restored to previously ischemic tissues [1].

Counterintuitively, the return of perfusion can sometimes cause greater tissue damage than the preceding ischemic episode itself, particularly during the reperfusion phase [1,2]. IRI involves a cascade of processes, such as sterile inflammation, increased oxidative stress, endothelial dysfunction, and activation of programmed cell death pathways (apoptosis) [3]. These events can provoke a widespread systemic response, even leading to remote organ injury and multiple organ failure (MOF) as it progresses [4].

Lungs are particularly susceptible to IRI and lung ischemia–reperfusion injury (LIRI) can arise in a variety of clinical settings, including pulmonary transplantation, oncological lung resections, cardiopulmonary bypass (CPB) during cardiac surgery, and even with the use of tourniquets during orthopedic procedures [1,2,5–9]. The key pathophysiological result is the breakdown of the pulmonary endothelial and epithelial barriers, resulting in pulmonary edema, subsequent impaired gas exchange, and an increase in pulmonary vascular resistance, which can result in pulmonary hypertension [10].

The clinical manifestations of LIRI are diverse and often severe. LIRI may present as acute lung injury (ALI) or acute respiratory distress syndrome (ARDS) following major lung resections, or as primary graft dysfunction (PGD) after lung transplantation, all of which are associated with higher morbidity and mortality rates [11,12]. In lung transplantation procedures, the donor lungs are kept in an ischemic state until placement on ex vivo lung perfusion (EVLP) or implantation, at which point reperfusion in the recipient can trigger LIRI and PGD, frequently resulting in prolonged mechanical ventilation and a longer hospital length of stay [10,12,13]. Furthermore, IRI is the most predominant risk factor for late graft failure in lung transplant procedures, including the development of chronic lung allograft dysfunction (CLAD) [10,14]. Due to the profound impact of LIRI on post-surgical and post-transplant results, significant research has focused on its prevention and management [15,16].

A variety of experimental and preclinical studies have explored pharmacological and non-pharmacological interventions aimed at limiting LIRI. These include the use of specialized organ preservation solutions, optimizing storage temperatures, EVLP, lung-protective ventilation strategies, antioxidants, anti-inflammatory drugs, and stem cell therapies [17–21]. More recently, scientific attention has shifted toward molecular targets, such as the endothelial glycocalyx, mitochondrial processes, and the regulation of autophagy [22–25]. Among the pharmacological approaches, dipeptidyl peptidase 4 inhibitors (DPP-4i) have emerged as promising agents due to their antioxidant, anti-inflammatory, and anti-apoptotic effects, and their potential to mitigate both acute IRI and chronic allograft injury in experimental models [26,27].

Nevertheless, the complex nature of LIRI pathogenesis and treatment remains a significant challenge. Many proposed interventions remain in the early stages of research or have not yet demonstrated clear benefit in clinical trials. Continued investigation is necessary to unravel the underlying mechanisms of LIRI and to identify and develop effective interventions to improve surgical and transplant outcomes.

In this review, we summarize the most recent advances in the understanding and management of LIRI and highlight novel therapeutic avenues within the broader context of oxidative stress and antioxidant defense.

2. Pathophysiology of LIRI

The pathophysiology of LIRI is multifactorial and initiated during an ischemic event or period (e.g., the ischemic storage of donor lungs), when cessation of blood flow leads to rapid depletion of adenosine triphosphate (ATP) and a shift to anaerobic metabolism. This aerobic energy depletion and shift is accompanied by intracellular acidosis, lactate accumulation, and the buildup of purine metabolites such as hypoxanthine, which serve as precursors for the subsequent generation of reactive oxygen species (ROS) by endothelial cells, macrophages, and other immune cells upon reperfusion [4,10,17,28].

Following the depletion of ATP, pulmonary cellular ion homeostasis is rapidly disrupted as ATP-dependent pumps such as the Na^+/K^+-ATPase fail, resulting in cellular edema and calcium overload. These changes activate phospholipases and proteases, and initiate the breakdown of cellular and mitochondrial membranes [2,29]. When alveolar oxygen is limited (e.g., during cold storage without ventilation), mitochondrial electron transport slows and succinate accumulates via reversal of succinate dehydrogenase; upon reperfusion, rapid succinate oxidation drives reverse electron transport at complex I, generating a burst of mitochondrial superoxide and amplifying tissue injury. In parallel, and importantly in lungs even when parenchymal oxygenation is preserved, ischemia alters endothelial shear sensing: stop-of-flow is detected by a caveolae-resident "mechanosome" (PECAM-1/VEGFR2/VE-cadherin), leading to KATP-channel closure, endothelial depolarization, opening of T-type Ca^{2+} channels and eNOS activation, and phosphoinositide 3-kinase (PI3K)–Akt–dependent assembly of NOX2 with ROS generation; the abrupt change in shear on reperfusion can further activate NOX2. Notably, because lung parenchyma can remain oxygenated during ischemia if ventilated, NOX2-driven mechanosignaling provides a hypoxia-independent route to ROS in lung IRI, whereas hypoxic storage adds the succinate-mediated mitochondrial ROS burst on reperfusion [3,10,30–32].

Reperfusion, although necessary to restore oxygen delivery and limit irreversible tissue loss due to ischemia, paradoxically triggers a dramatic burst of ROS generation [2,4]. This process is driven by both the metabolism of accumulated hypoxanthine by xanthine oxidase and activation of nicotinamide adenine dinucleotide phosphate (NADPH) oxidase isoforms in pulmonary endothelial cells, alveolar macrophages, and infiltrating leukocytes [33,34]. The resultant oxidative stress overwhelms the lung's endogenous antioxidant defenses, causing the peroxidation of membrane lipids, carbonylation and nitration of proteins, and deoxyribonucleic acid (DNA) strand breaks [35]. This primary oxidative injury is amplified by downstream effects on intracellular signaling pathways that further compromise cellular survival and function [28].

In addition to direct tissue damage, ROS can also serve as potent pro-inflammatory mediators, rapidly activating resident alveolar macrophages and endothelial cells. These cells release a broad array of cytokines and chemokines, including tumor necrosis factor-alpha (TNF-α), interleukin (IL)-1β, CXCL-8, and CXCL2, which initiate a cascade that recruits and activates neutrophils and other innate immune effectors. Neutrophil and macrophage infiltration are prominent features of LIRI and are associated with the release of additional ROS, proteases, elastases, and the formation of neutrophil extracellular traps (NETs), all of which contribute to the destruction of lung parenchyma and the microvascular barrier [3,28,36].

The pulmonary endothelium is a principal target of this injury. Oxidative and inflammatory damage cause cytoskeletal remodeling and disruption of intercellular junctions, resulting in increased vascular permeability and the leakage of protein-rich fluid into the interstitial and alveolar spaces [37,38]. This process is further exacerbated by the activation of the complement and coagulation cascades. Ischemia and early reperfusion trigger all three complement pathways in the lung: natural IgM/neoepitope binding (classical), mannose-binding lectin (MBL) sensing ischemia-induced glycan changes (lectin), and amplification via the alternative pathway. This culminates in generation of C3a/C5a (potent chemoattractants that up-regulate endothelial adhesion, prime neutrophils, and increase permeability) and assembly of the terminal complement complex (C5b-9) that directly injures endothelium and worsens microvascular leak and thrombosis. Clinically, local complement activation in the allograft within 24 h after transplant, i.e., elevated sC4d and sC5b-9 in bronchoalveolar lavage (BAL) and higher levels of C1q/C2/C4 (classical/lectin) and Ba (alternative), is associated with PGD, with MBL and ficolin-3 strongly correlating with terminal complement activity in BAL [39,40]. Systemically, rising plasma C5a between 6–24 h post-reperfusion correlates with both PGD and mortality, supporting a role for an early complement surge [40]. Early C3d/C4d deposition in lung allografts has likewise been observed after transplantation [41]. Together, these data support complement as a key amplifier of LIRI that links oxidative/endothelial injury to neutrophil recruitment, coagulation crosstalk, and early edema.

In addition, vasoactive mediators such as thromboxane A2 and platelet-activating factor further promote pulmonary edema formation [10]. The alveolar epithelium is also highly vulnerable, particularly its type II pneumocytes; injury to these cells impairs lung surfactant synthesis and turnover, contributing to alveolar instability and collapse, resulting in worsening gas exchange [42]. Figure 1 shows a schematic overview of the pathophysiology of LIRI.

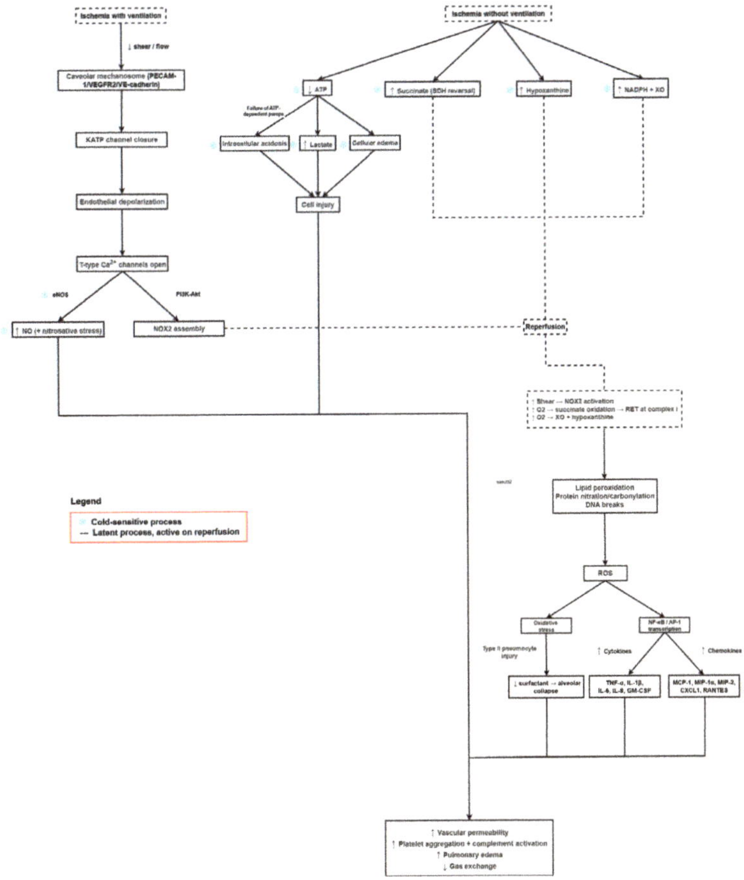

Figure 1. Schematic overview of lung ischemia–reperfusion injury. Ischemia with ventilation (left; mechanotransduction) and without ventilation (middle; oxygen debt) are shown with their respective pathways and links to reperfusion (right). Dashed boxes/lines indicate latent processes expressed on

reperfusion; ❄ marks cold-sensitive processes. Reperfusion combines start-of-flow–induced NOX2 activation with O_2-dependent bursts from succinate oxidation/reverse electron transport (RET) at complex I and from xanthine oxidase (XO). Reactive oxygen species (ROS) drive lipid peroxidation, protein nitration/carbonylation, and DNA breaks and activate NF-κB/AP-1, leading to cytokine/chemokine release, type II pneumocyte injury with ↓surfactant and alveolar collapse, increased vascular permeability, platelet/complement activation, pulmonary edema, and impaired gas exchange. AP-1, Activator Protein-1; ATP, adenosine triphosphate; CXCL1, CXC ligand 1; eNOS, endothelial nitric oxide synthase, GM-CSF, Granulocyte-macrophage colony-stimulating factor; IL, interleukin; KATP, ATP-sensitive potassium channel; MCP-1, Monocyte chemoattractant protein-1; MIP, Macrophage inflammatory protein; NADPH, nicotinamide adenine dinucleotide phosphate; NF-κB, nuclear factor kappa-B; NO, nitric oxide; NOX2, NADPH oxidase-2; PECAM-1, platelet endothelial cell adhesion molecule-1; PI3K–Akt, Phosphoinositide 3-kinase → Akt pathway; RANTES, "Regulated on Activation, Normal T-cell Expressed and Secreted"; ROS, reactive oxygen species; SDH, succinate dehydrogenase; TNF, tumor necrosis factor; VE-cadherin, vascular endothelial cadherin; VEGFR2, vascular endothelial growth factor receptor-2; XO, xanthine oxidase.

A growing body of evidence has identified the endothelial glycocalyx as a critical modulator of vascular homeostasis in the process of IRI [24,43]. In blood vessels, the endothelial glycocalyx is a glycoprotein- and proteoglycan-rich layer projecting into the vascular lumen that regulates vascular permeability, mechanotransduction, and inflammatory responses [44,45]. Ischemia and ROS-mediated degradation of the glycocalyx enhances leukocyte adhesion, disrupts vascular barrier integrity, and amplifies edema and inflammation [10]. In parallel, mitochondrial dysfunction, driven by calcium overload and sustained oxidative stress, triggers the opening of mitochondrial permeability transition pores and the release of pro-apoptotic factors, resulting in both apoptotic and necrotic cell death [46]. The subsequent release of damage-associated molecular patterns (DAMPs) into the extracellular space perpetuates the cycle of sterile inflammation and tissue injury [28].

While LIRI is initiated within the transplanted lung, the consequences are often systemic. The spillover of cytokines, DAMPs, and activated immune cells into the circulation can precipitate remote organ dysfunction and even failure. Notably, unilateral LIRI can elicit contralateral lung injury [10,28]. Despite advances in lung transplant surgery such as donor management, graft preservation, and surgical technique, these complex, destructive processes remain a significant challenge, and underscore the urgent need for targeted interventions. Novel therapeutic approaches focused on antioxidant administration, immune modulation, and preservation of endothelial integrity hold promise for attenuating LIRI and improving clinical outcomes in major lung surgery and transplantation [25,47].

3. Clinical Impact of LIRI–Lung Transplantation

The primary effect of LIRI is the breakdown of the alveolar–capillary barrier, leading to non-cardiogenic pulmonary edema and impaired ventilation-perfusion (V/Q) matching. This disruption causes pulmonary edema, impaired gas exchange, reduced static and dynamic lung compliance, and raises the alveolar-arterial oxygen gradient [(A-a)DO_2] [1,24]. Reperfusion also triggers precapillary vasoconstriction, which can triple pulmonary vascular resistance, often resulting in pulmonary hypertension and worsening hydrostatic edema. Clinically, severe LIRI presents as ALI or ARDS, with bilateral pulmonary edema and refractory hypoxemia that are indistinguishable from other causes of ARDS [4,48]. There are no specific diagnostic markers, making LIRI essentially a diagnosis of exclusion once cardiogenic edema and other etiologies are ruled out.

3.1. Lung Transplantation and PGD

In the context of lung transplantation, LIRI manifests as PGD, an ALI syndrome and the leading cause of early post-transplant morbidity and mortality [3]. It is associated with a 30-day mortality rate that is approximately sevenfold higher than that in patients without PGD [49]. PGD is characterized by hypoxemia (low PaO_2/FiO_2 ratio) and diffuse pulmonary infiltrates on chest X-ray without other identifiable causes [50]. Multiple risk factors have been identified; including donor, recipient, and procedural variables. Notable variables include donor smoking and alcohol history, donor age, pulmonary embolism, size mismatch, recipient disease etiology, recipient body mass index (BMI), use of extracorporeal life support perioperatively, ischemic times, polytransfusion, and timing of transplants [15,51]. Many of these risk factors influence the development of PGD through mechanisms that converge on IRI, the central pathophysiologic process underlying early allograft dysfunction. Donor exposures such as smoking and alcohol use are associated with endothelial dysfunction, oxidative stress, and impaired alveolar fluid clearance, which prime the graft for exaggerated inflammatory and oxidative responses upon reperfusion [52,53]. Older donor age similarly heightens susceptibility to IRI owing to reduced cellular stress-response capacity and augmented baseline inflammation [54]. Hemodynamic and mechanical stressors, such as pulmonary hypertension, size mismatch, and obesity, exacerbate microvascular shear and capillary leak during reperfusion, further amplifying IRI-related endothelial injury [55–58]. Procedural factors including prolonged ischemic times, the use of extracorporeal life support, and excessive transfusion burden can each potentiate the release of DAMPs, complement activation, and neutrophil recruitment, thereby intensifying the inflammatory cascade characteristic of IRI and PGD [10,59–61]. These variables likely act in concert rather than isolation, with cumulative "hits" to the donor lung and recipient environment synergistically amplifying the IR response and translating into higher grades of PGD [24].

Histologically, PGD corresponds to diffuse alveolar damage (similar to ARDS) caused largely by IRI to the transplanted lung. LIRI-induced sterile inflammation and damage to transplanted lungs results in diffuse alveolar damage with flooding of alveoli, loss of ventilating surface, and severe gas exchange impairment. Clinically, this manifests as PGD grades 1–3 (with grade 3 being $PaO_2/FiO_2 < 200$ and bilateral infiltrates) in the hours after transplant [15,50]. Severe PGD is not only a leading cause of early post-transplant morbidity and mortality, but is also associated with worse long-term outcomes, including a higher risk of developing CLAD [12]. Despite advances in surgical technique and preservation, LIRI-induced PGD still occurs in up to 30% of lung transplant recipients, underscoring the need to understand its pathophysiology and develop targeted interventions [12,62,63].

The primary approach of PGD prevention lies in identifying and minimizing modifiable risk factors in both donors and recipients, which highlights the necessity of a thorough risk-factor assessment before transplantation [64,65]. Contemporary efforts also focus on optimizing reperfusion and ventilation strategies, along with improving lung preservation techniques, including EVLP, to mitigate LIRI [63]. Extended ischemic (cold storage) time has been consistently recognized as a strong procedure-related risk factor for PGD, underscoring the importance of reducing ischemic duration through careful surgical and anesthetic planning [66]. Preventive strategies therefore include optimizing donor lung storage temperatures, adopting controlled reperfusion protocols, using lung-protective ventilation, and applying targeted pharmacologic interventions to modulate the inflammatory and oxidative pathways that drive LIRI [10,21].

3.2. Risk Factors and Selection of Donor/Recipient

Due to the fact that PGD is mainly a clinical expression of LIRI, donor and recipient risk factors are best understood by how they prime the endothelium/epithelium for reperfusion or increase the IRI "dose." Donor lungs subjected to pre-procurement hypoxemia or hypotension frequently accompany brain death-related catecholamine surges and inflammatory activation, which injure the alveolar–capillary barrier and glycocalyx and lower the threshold for edema and hypoxemia upon reperfusion [10,24,62,67]. Previous studies have shown that these donor lungs with prolonged hypoxemia or hypotension prior to organ retrieval also have higher PGD rates [12,62]. Brain death itself triggers a systemic cascade of cytokines and complement with neutrophil recruitment in the lung; this "first hit" potentiates IRI during implantation, thus priming the lung for PGD after transplant [62,63,67–69].

Donor demographics (e.g., increased age) can further heighten IRI susceptibility through reduced stress-response capacity and "inflammaging," although results vary across cohorts [10,62,67]. Donor smoking and chronic alcohol abuse are consistently associated with higher PGD risk and mortality, possibly via baseline endothelial dysfunction, oxidant burden, impaired surfactant and alveolar fluid clearance, all of which amplify IRI signaling at reperfusion [52,53]. Donor smoking history has been identified as one of the strongest predictors of PGD [52]. Other donor injuries (aspiration, chest trauma) and prolonged mechanical ventilation add inflammatory and ventilator-induced stresses that sensitize the graft to IRI; conversely, donor lung-protective ventilation and careful fluid/hemodynamic management can mitigate these effects [12,50,62,70].

On the recipient side, factors that raise mechanical/hemodynamic stress at first reperfusion or increase baseline inflammatory tone intensify IRI and PGD risk. Higher BMI is associated with a dose–response increase in PGD, likely reflecting systemic low-grade inflammation, impaired respiratory mechanics, and higher peri-operative transfusion/support needs that magnify IRI [71]. Overweight and obese lung transplant recipients have a significantly higher incidence of PGD with an estimated risk increase of 6% for BMI 25–30 and 11% for BMI > 30 [12,55]. Pre-existing pulmonary hypertension in the recipient is another known risk factor, as high pulmonary artery pressures (PAPs) can exacerbate reperfusion injury in the new lung by increasing shear and transvascular hydrostatic load across a vulnerable endothelial barrier during reperfusion [56,72]. Certain diagnoses leading to transplant, such as idiopathic pulmonary fibrosis or sarcoidosis, have been associated with higher PGD rates, possibly due to the severe lung fibrosis/vascular remodeling and inflammation present in those diseases, which can lead to prolonged ischemic exposures and increase initial reperfusion pressures [12,50,56,57,62]. In addition, donor–recipient size matching is an important aspect in modulating LIRI and PGD [73]. Previous studies have shown that oversizing allografts have been linked to a reduced risk of postoperative PGD, particularly in patients without chronic obstructive pulmonary disease (COPD), possibly due to decreased shear upon reperfusion [74]. In summary, carefully optimizing the recipient's condition and selection of appropriate donor–recipient matches are important steps to reduce LIRI burden and PGD risk.

3.3. Donor Procedure and Preservation

The prevalence of IRI-induced PGD and donor shortage in lung transplantation surpasses that of all other organ transplants [10,75]. Therefore, the process of donor lung procurement and preservation needs to minimize ischemic injury and optimally prepare the organ for transplantation.

After flushing, donor lungs are transported in a cooled state to minimize metabolic activity leading to IRI and preserve tissue integrity. Traditional ice-on-cooler methods produce uneven, sometimes near-freezing temperatures around 0 °C, risking cold-induced cellular and endothelial injury and variable cooling across lobes; controlled hypothermia avoids this pitfall [21,76]. However, emerging clinical and translational evidence now supports controlled hypothermic storage at approximately 10 °C as optimal for lung preservation [77,78]. This slightly warmer temperature better maintains mitochondrial function and cellular metabolism, thereby attenuating the metabolic drivers of IRI while avoiding the risks of uneven or excessively cold exposure seen with traditional ice storage [21,77,79–83]. Mechanistically, holding lungs at ~10 °C maintains a low but viable metabolic state that limits ATP collapse and DAMP release, curbs mitochondrial priming (e.g., succinate-driven ROS burst) and protects the endothelium/glycocalyx, all of which translate into a smaller reperfusion inflammatory surge [10,24,81–85]. In a prospective, multicenter, nonrandomized trial, prolonged preservation at 10 °C resulted in low rates of PGD grade 3 and similar outcomes to lungs transplanted using conventional methods with shorter preservation times [86]. Although longer cold storage would ordinarily be expected to increase the ischemic dose, controlled hypothermia at ~10 °C slows metabolism while preserving mitochondrial homeostasis and limiting ischemic succinate build-up, the key driver of the early reperfusion ROS burst, thereby attenuating IRI at reperfusion [21,77,81,86,87]. Consistent with this mechanism, a multicenter clinical series reported safe preservation approaching 24 h without excess PGD [77]. Currently, there is an ongoing randomized, controlled trial investigating whether lung preservation at 10 °C is non-inferior to standard cooling temperatures.

Additionally, the lungs are not completely collapsed during storage; they are partially inflated to about 50% of total lung capacity using a low volume of air or oxygen. This strategy preserves surfactant function and maintains alveolar recruitment, improving compliance and reducing atelectatic injury during the ischemic period [12,88]. Furthermore, maintaining partial inflation during cold storage may limit atelectrauma and necrosis that drive sterile DAMP release, particularly high mobility group box 1 protein (HMGB1), which is implicated in early ischemia–reperfusion lung injury and primary graft dysfunction [89]. The combination of precise hypothermia and controlled partial inflation has been shown to enhance cell viability and membrane integrity, supporting better early graft function following implantation [78].

Both cold and warm ischemia durations are kept as short as possible to prevent LIRI. Prolonged total ischemic time (from donor cross-clamp to reperfusion in the recipient) is a well-established risk factor for IRI-induced PGD [12,90]. In practice, teams coordinate logistics (donor timing, transport, operating room readiness) and increasingly use controlled hypothermia at ~10 °C (with or without EVLP when indicated) to shorten warm phases and buffer the cold phase metabolically, thereby dampening the reperfusion inflammatory cascade and lowering PGD incidence [20,21,77,80,91–93].

3.4. Lung Implantation Procedure

The intraoperative and immediate postoperative management of a lung transplant are crucial in modulating the severity of LIRI. Perioperatively, the unclamping of the pulmonary artery is generally performed in a stepwise manner, allowing a controlled reperfusion and thus preventing an onslaught of full cardiac output to the cold ischemic lung [94]. By partially unclamping the pulmonary artery or using a brief, low-pressure, low-flow reintroduction of blood (over ~2–5 min, with normoxic FiO_2), the initial surge in shear stress and oxygen delivery is blunted, allowing endothelial Ca^{2+} handling, nitric-oxide–mediated vasodilation, and glycocalyx recovery, thereby limiting capillary leak and the early mitochondrial ROS burst that drives lung IRI [10,24,84,85,87,88]. This graded reperfusion/postconditioning approach is mechanistically aligned with lung IRI biology: a sudden full-flow, hyperoxic reperfusion increases endothelial shear, glycocalyx shedding, Ca^{2+} overload, and reverse-electron transport (RET)–mediated ROS at complex I fueled by ischemic succinate accumulation. Slowing the first minutes of reperfusion reduces these triggers [10,24,84,85,87]. In lung transplantation, clinical "modified/controlled reperfusion" strategies have been associated with lower severe PGD and better early physiology, and preclinical/EVLP models show that lower initial flow reduces edema and inflammatory cytokines [50,62,95]. Avoiding hyperoxia at first reperfusion (using lower FiO_2) further attenuates oxidative injury and has been linked to a lower risk of severe PGD [96]. Cross-organ data support the same principle: in the liver, end-ischemic hypothermic oxygenated perfusion (HOPE), often followed by controlled oxygenated rewarming (COR) and then warm normothermic machine perfusion (NMP), metabolizes ischemic succinate and replenishes ATP under low metabolic demand, thereby dampening the subsequent reperfusion burst. Randomized trials in DCD livers show reduced biliary complications with (dual) HOPE versus static cold storage [97–101]. In the heart, stepwise/controlled reflow and ischemic postconditioning reduce infarct size and endothelial dysfunction, reinforcing the value of gradual re-reperfusion to mitigate IRI [102]. Together, these data justify stepwise, normoxic, low-pressure reperfusion of the lung allograft as a practical, mechanism-based countermeasure to LIRI.

Another approach is modified reperfusion, where a catheter is placed in the pulmonary artery in order to administer leukocyte-depleted blood mixed with vasodilators before full circulation is restored. In a series of 100 patients managed with this technique, the incidence of severe PGD was remarkably low (around 2%) and early outcomes were excellent [50,103]. The rationale is that flushing out activated donor leukocytes and providing a vasodilated, controlled flow reduces the "trigger" for endothelial injury at first contact with recipient blood. While not all centers use specialized reperfusion circuits, the general principle is to avoid an immediate high-pressure, high-oxygen surge to the graft [94]. Additionally, reperfusion is ideally done with the lung already being gently ventilated with oxygen to avoid blood flowing into a completely collapsed and hypoxic lung. Some protocols also recommend keeping the FiO_2 moderate during the first few minutes of reperfusion [62,104]. In fact, use of very high FiO_2 (>0.4) during initial reperfusion has been associated with higher rates of PGD, likely because excessive oxygen tension exacerbates ROS generation in the newly perfused lung [12,105]. Therefore, many centers will start reperfusion on 40–50% oxygen rather than 100% oxygen, increasing it later as needed [10,16].

Post-implantation, the donor lung is extremely vulnerable to ventilator-induced injury. Mechanical ventilation itself can cause shear stress and inflammatory injury, especially in an acutely injured lung. To avoid compounding the reperfusion injury, a lung-protective ventilation strategy is used from the time of reperfusion onward [96]. This includes low tidal volumes (typically 6–8 mL/kg or less of predicted body weight) and adequate positive end-expiratory pressure (PEEP) to prevent alveolar collapse, similar to ARDS ventilation protocols [12,106]. Studies have shown that tidal volumes > 8–10 mL/kg in the early postoperative period can induce PGD, whereas limiting volumes can decrease neutrophil infiltration and cytokine release in the graft [12]. It is also important to avoid excessive driving pressures; keeping plateau pressures in a safe range (<30 cm H_2O) and using gentle recruitment maneuvers if needed [96,106]. If a size mismatch occurs (e.g., smaller donor lungs in a larger recipient), special care must be taken to avoid over-ventilating the graft as size mismatches can lead to inadvertent delivery of too large a volume per lung volume [107]. In fact, donor–recipient lung size mismatch is recognized as a modifiable risk factor for PGD, precisely because of the ventilation implications [12,70]. Early extubation can be considered if the patient is stable, as this allows the patient to breathe spontaneously and may reduce ventilator-associated injury; however, this must be balanced against the need for adequate support if the lung is still recovering [108,109].

Transplanted lungs should be protected from acute hydrostatic pressure overload. Reperfusion injury can be worsened by high pulmonary capillary pressures, leading to stress edema [110]. Thus, transplant teams often aim to keep the patient "dry" and limit intravenous (IV) fluids in the intraoperative and immediate postoperative phase [111,112]. In practice, a low central venous pressure (CVP) or PAP is maintained to reduce the burden on the fragile pulmonary capillaries. Inotropic support and vasodilators may be used to optimize the right heart function and pulmonary circulation without volume loading [110]. Some centers avoid CPB for lung transplant when possible, opting for off-pump or ECMO support if needed, as CPB is associated with greater inflammatory response and capillary leak, which can elevate PGD risk [12,62]. If CPB or ECMO is used perioperatively, for example, in cases of hemodynamic instability or double-lung transplant in very sick patients, meticulous management of anticoagulation and perfusion flows is required to minimize inflammatory activation [113–115].

ECMO has become an important rescue strategy in severe PGD. If a patient develops life-threatening PGD, veno-venous ECMO allows the patient's blood to be oxygenated externally, "resting" the transplanted lung [12]. ECMO support for a few days can allow the reperfusion injury to abate while avoiding additional ventilator-induced injury [116,117]. Clinical series have reported successful recovery of graft function in many PGD patients bridged through the acute phase on ECMO [118]. Thus, in an expert center, early deployment of ECMO for refractory PGD is considered a protective measure to prevent multi-organ failure. Overall, a combination of gradual reperfusion, protective ventilation, careful circulatory management, and timely supportive interventions form the cornerstone of PGD prevention and management in the perioperative setting [119,120].

3.5. LIRI in Donation After Circulatory Death

Donation after circulatory death (DCD) presents a distinct scenario for lung transplantation, with unique implications for IRI compared to donation after brain death (DBD) [121]. In controlled DCD, the agonal phase is the interval after withdrawal of life-sustaining therapy (WLST) until circulatory arrest (followed by a 2–5 min "no-touch" period before declaration of death) [122]. During this time, donors commonly exhibit intense spontaneous respiratory efforts/gasping with progressive hypoxemia and hypercapnic acidosis. These conditions drive patient self-inflicted lung injury (P-SILI), large negative intrathoracic pressure swings, "pendelluft", and cyclic recruitment/derecruitment that promote edema and epithelial injury, thereby sensitizing the alveolar–capillary barrier to reperfusion [123–125]. Furthermore, they trigger hypoxic pulmonary vasoconstriction and acidosis-augmented increases in pulmonary vascular resistance, raising microvascular shear at first reflow [126,127]. In parallel, warm low-flow/no-flow metabolism accelerates ATP depletion and succinate accumulation, so that reperfusion rapidly generates mitochondrial ROS via reverse-electron transport at complex I, amplifying the endothelial injury that characterizes LIRI [24,87,128]. Hypoxia and hypercapnia also impair alveolar fluid clearance by down-regulating ENaC/Na, K-ATPase, further predisposing to reperfusion edema once circulation resumes [129–131]. These agonal-phase stresses explain why real-world tolerance is often shorter than the experimental "~60 min if oxygenated" benchmark, and why many programs target strict limits on functional warm ischemic time (e.g., from SBP < 50 mmHg or SpO_2 < 70% to cold flush) rather than WLST-to-flush alone [132,133].

In controlled DCD (Maastricht category III, where withdrawal of life support is planned in a hospital setting), the agonal time can be anticipated and kept short. Indeed, it is a guiding principle that the agonal phase be <1 h to prevent irreversible lung injury [134]. By contrast, uncontrolled DCD (unexpected arrest) is more challenging due to indeterminate down-time; lungs from uncontrolled DCD (uDCD) donors are far less commonly used, or they may require ex vivo assessment before use [135]. Earlier data suggested that uncontrolled DCD lungs may be more prone to developing PGD; however, more recent data suggest that, when appropriately implemented, uDCD lung transplantation is feasible and safe [136].

Conversely, while DCD lungs suffer warm ischemic stress, they may avoid some of the injury associated with brain death. In DBD, a significant catecholamine storm often occurs at the time of brain herniation, causing severe hemodynamic swings and neurogenic pulmonary edema [137]. Additionally, brain death triggers systemic inflammatory responses that can prime donor organs with elevated cytokines and immune activation [68]. Studies have shown that some inflammatory markers are actually lower in DCD donor lungs compared to DBD [138]. Transcriptomic analyses similarly show that DBD lungs have upregulation of inflammatory pathways, due to a catecholamine surge and systemic "cytokine storm," which primes the lung endothelium and leukocyte trafficking, thereby pre-activating inflammatory arms of IRI even before cold storage. DCD lungs, by contrast, show more activation of hypoxia and cell-death pathways due to the warm ischemia insult, on reperfusion, this state favors a mitochondrial ROS burst and sterile inflammation, rather than leukocyte-primed injury [63]. In practical terms, this means each donor type has a different profile of injury: DBD lungs are "pre-injured" by inflammation before ischemia, and DCD lungs are injured by lack of perfusion/oxygen during warm ischemia [138]. Both mechanisms can lead to PGD, via different routes. One notable difference is that inducible nitric oxide synthase (iNOS) signaling is more activated in marginal DBD lungs than in DCD lungs, suggesting that NO-related oxidative injury may be a feature of brain death-related lung damage [138]. Nevertheless, the key determinant in DCD lung outcomes is the duration of warm ischemia; longer durations correlate with more severe mitochondrial dysfunction and structural injury in donor organs [139–141]. Therefore, aggressive measures are taken to mitigate warm ischemia in DCD: as soon as the donor is pronounced dead, the transplant team will intubate/re-intubate and ventilate the donor, instill preservation solution into the lungs, and cool the organs as quickly as possible [68,134,142]. In some centers, normothermic regional perfusion (NRP) is used for DCD donors, using ECMO within the donor's body to perfuse the organs with oxygenated blood before procurement [143]. NRP has been explored as a way to shorten the effective warm ischemic time and possibly recondition DCD lungs in situ, and there is evidence that it may reduce PGD, although data are still emerging [144,145]. Additionally, EVLP is playing a pivotal role in DCD lung transplantation. In a growing number of centers, lungs from both DBD and DCD donors are assessed on EVLP after procurement to ensure they meet functional criteria before implantation [146,147]. EVLP can also be used to treat donor lungs by removing excess fluid and delivering antioxidants or anti-inflammatory agents prior to transplant, thus acting as a bridge to improve DCD lung quality [20].

PGD remains a concern in DCD lung transplants, but recent data show that while DCD recipients may experience slightly higher rates of early PGD, the difference levels out within 72 h. Kashem et al. noted in their multicenter analysis of lung transplantation after DCD vs. DBD that at 1 h post-transplant the DCD group had more frequent severe PGD than the DBD group, but by 48–72 h there was no significant difference in PGD incidence between the two groups [148]. It appears that any initial damage in DCD lungs can often be overcome with supportive care, and the lung recovers similarly to a DBD lung. Importantly, when DCD protocols are properly followed (i.e., short agonal time, careful handling, use of EVLP when needed), the rates of successful transplantation are high [132,149,150].

4. Treatment Strategies

Due to the fact that LIRI involves a complex cascade with multiple overlapping pathways, a multi-faceted approach is necessary. Strategies include modifying surgical and perfusion techniques (to minimize ischemic time and reperfusion shocks), non-pharmacologic interventions (ventilatory strategies, extracorporeal support, positioning, conditioning), and pharmacologic or cellular therapies (antioxidants, anti-inflammatories, etc.). Below are some of the possible treatment strategies that have been proposed. The origin of the data regarding these treatment strategies vary from small-animal and large-animal models to EVLP studies using human donor lungs and clinical data (observational cohorts and randomized trials). Table 1 shows the mechanisms, evidence classes, net signals and translational status for each intervention category. Figure 2 shows a timeline overview of the different treatment modalities for LIRI, both established and experimental.

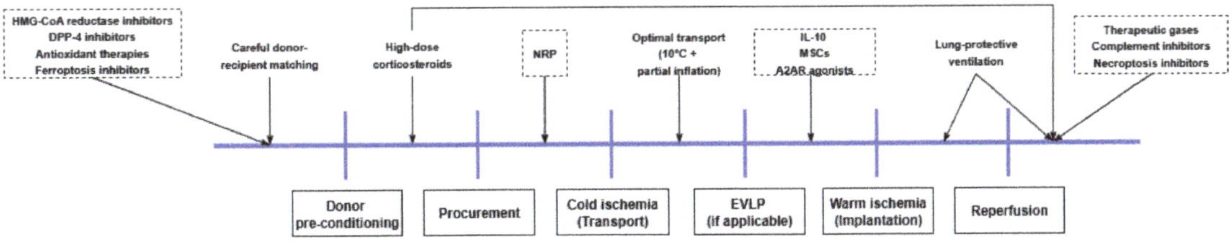

Figure 2. Overview of established and experimental treatment strategies within a lung transplant timeline. Each treatment strategy has been placed at its respective timing of (proposed) use. Dotted boxes indicate experimental/proposed strategies. A2AR, adenosine A_{2A} receptor; DPP-4, dipeptidyl peptidase 4; EVLP, ex vivo lung perfusion; HMG-CoA, 3-hydroxy-3-methylglutaryl coenzyme A; IL, interleukin; MSCs, mesenchymal stem cells; NRP, normothermic regional perfusion; NADPH, nicotinamide adenine dinucleotide phosphate; ROS, reactive oxygen species; TNF, tumor necrosis factor.

4.1. Lung-Protective Ventilation and Hypercapnia

Lung-protective ventilation is a key strategy in mitigating lung injury in the context of lung transplantation and other LIRI scenarios [106]. Mechanical ventilation can worsen pulmonary damage by inducing shear stress, volutrauma, and biotrauma, which in turn activate proinflammatory pathways such as nuclear factor kappa B (NF-κB) and mitogen-activated protein kinase, increase endothelial permeability, and promote cytokine release and neutrophil infiltration [96,106,151]. Evidence from ARDS literature and transplant cohorts supports the use of low tidal volumes (typically <6–8 mL/kg predicted body weight) combined with appropriate levels of PEEP to reduce these effects [12,106,152,153]. In a large retrospective study by Tague et al., donor-size–indexed low tidal volume ventilation after bilateral lung transplantation was associated with significantly lower rates of primary graft dysfunction (PGD) grade 3 and increased ventilator-free days [70]. Mechanistic insights from translational studies have shown that IRI activates sterile inflammation, damages the alveolar–capillary barrier, and leads to diffuse alveolar damage; hallmarks of PGD that can be attenuated through protective ventilator settings [15,154]. International survey data confirm that most transplant centers now routinely implement lung-protective ventilation strategies in the early post-reperfusion period, reflecting broad consensus on their clinical benefit [155]. These practices mirror findings from large ARDS trials, where limiting tidal volume and maintaining moderate PEEP consistently reduced inflammation, mechanical stress, and mortality [156–158]. Together, the preclinical rationale and clinical data make a compelling case for protective ventilation as a central component of supportive care during and after lung transplantation. Some experimental studies have suggested that a moderate hypercapnic acidosis (e.g., by reducing minute ventilation) can have protective effects. In isolated rat lungs, hypercapnic acidosis attenuated IRI, and in in vivo studies hypercapnia reduced lung injury by decreasing TNF-α levels, vascular leak, and apoptosis [159–162]. Hypercapnia appears to inhibit NF-κB activation and free radical generation, thereby blunting inflammation and cell death [12].

Table 1. Evidence map of interventions targeting lung ischemia–reperfusion injury (LIRI)/primary graft dysfunction (PGD) in lung transplantation.

Intervention	Proposed Mechanism(s)	Evidence Classes	Net Signal	Translational Status
LPV ± permissive hypercapnia	- ↓ Volutrauma/atelectrauma - Hypercapnia → ↓ NF-κB signaling and ROS injury	- Small animal ✓ - Human observational ✓	- LPV favorable - Hypercapnia preclinical favorable	- LPV standard of care - Hypercapnia investigational
Controlled/gradual reperfusion at implantation	Pressure/flow-limited reperfusion → ↓ endothelial shear/ROS burst	- Small animal ✓ - Large animal ✓ - Human observational ✓	Favorable	Standard of care
EVLP	- Normothermic assessment and reconditioning - Reduces ischemic time - Delivery vehicle for therapies	- Large animal ✓ - Human observational ✓ - RCT non-inferior vs. conventional preservation	Favorable	Established adjunct in many centers
iNO	- Selective pulmonary vasodilation - Improves V/Q matching - Theoretical anti-inflammatory effects	- Human RCT	- Neutral for PGD prevention - Useful as rescue/support	Supportive therapy
iCO	- Cytoprotective gas - Anti-inflammatory/anti-apoptotic via HO-1 and mito-signaling	- Small animal ✓ - Large animal ✓	Favorable (preclinical)	Investigational
iH_2	- Scavenges •OH/$ONOO^-$ - Activates Nrf2/HO-1 - Anti-apoptotic	- Large animal ✓ - EVLP (DCD) ✓	Favorable (preclinical/EVLP)	- Investigational - EVLP add-on candidate
Statins (pre-LTx exposure)	Pleiotropic anti-inflammatory and endothelial stabilizing	- Human observational ✓	Mixed/neutral	Not recommended specifically for PGD prevention
High-dose corticosteroids (peri-operative)	General anti-inflammatory part of standard immunosuppression	- Human observational ✓	Neutral for PGD prevention	Standard immunosuppression; not targeted PGD therapy
Mitochondria targeted agents	- Preserve mitochondrial integrity - Reduce mPTP opening - Reverse-electron-transport ROS	- Small animal ✓ - Large animal ✓ - EVLP model ✓	Favorable (preclinical)	Investigational
Metformin	- Activates AMPK - Dampens inflammation/oxidative stress - May limit necroptosis	- Small animal ✓	Favorable (preclinical)	Investigational (repurposing candidate)
DPP-4i	- Preserve VIP/chemokine tone - Anti-inflammatory/anti-apoptotic	- Small animal ✓ - Large animal ✓ - Human observational ✓	Favorable signal	Investigational (early clinical signal)

Table 1. *Cont.*

Intervention	Proposed Mechanism(s)	Evidence Classes	Net Signal	Translational Status
A_2A RA	- Immune-cell deactivation - Limits neutrophil-endothelium interactions	- Small animal ✓ - EVLP ✓ - RCT ✓	Biomarker signal; clinical efficacy unproven	Early-phase clinical; more trials needed
IL-10 therapy	- Potent anti-inflammatory cytokine - Shifts macrophage/T-cell responses	- Large animal ✓ - EVLP model ✓	Favorable (preclinical)	Investigational (EVLP delivery under refinement)
MSCs	- Paracrine immunomodulation - Antioxidant & endothelial protection	- Small animal ✓ - Large animal ✓ - EVLP model ✓	Favorable (preclinical); early human safety	Investigational/early clinical
"Classic" antioxidants	- Direct ROS scavenging - Glutathione repletion	- Small animal ✓ - EVLP model ✓	Inconsistent; no proven clinical benefit for PGD	Stalled—insufficient evidence for routine use
TLR pathway antagonists	Dampen innate immune activation to DAMPs	- Small animal ✓	Favorable (preclinical)	Investigational
Fibrinolytics	- Dissolve donor pulmonary thrombi - Improve perfusion/oxygenation	- EVLP model ✓	Favorable in selected EVLP cases	Selective EVLP tool; not PGD-directed therapy
Necroptosis inhibitors	- Block RIPK1/RIPK3/MLKL-mediated regulated necrosis	- Small animal ✓	Favorable (preclinical)	Investigational
Ferroptosis inhibitors	- Limit iron-dependent lipid peroxidation and cell death	- Small animal ✓	Favorable (preclinical)	Investigational

AMPK, AMP-activated protein kinase; A_2A RA, adenosine A_2A receptor agonist; DAMPs, damage-associated molecular patterns; DCD, donation after circulatory death; DPP-4i, dipeptidyl peptidase-4 inhibitor(s); EVLP, ex vivo lung perfusion; HO-1, heme oxygenase-1; iCO, inhaled carbon monoxide; iH2, inhaled hydrogen; IL-10, interleukin-10; iNO, inhaled nitric oxide; LIRI, lung ischemia–reperfusion injury; LPV, lung-protective ventilation; LTx, lung transplantation; MLKL, mixed lineage kinase domain-like protein; mPTP, mitochondrial permeability transition pore; MSCs, mesenchymal stromal cells; NF-κB, nuclear factor kappa-light-chain-enhancer of activated B cells; Nrf2, nuclear factor erythroid 2-related factor 2; ONOO-, peroxynitrite; PGD, primary graft dysfunction; RCT, randomized controlled trial; RIPK1, receptor-interacting serine/threonine-protein kinase 1; RIPK3, receptor-interacting serine/threonine-protein kinase 3; ROS, reactive oxygen species; TLR, Toll-like receptor; V/Q, ventilation/perfusion; VIP, vasoactive intestinal peptide; •OH, hydroxyl radical.

4.2. EVLP

In 2000, Steen et al. successfully performed the first lung transplantation using DCD lungs after evaluating the donor lungs using a novel technique called EVLP, which led to the development of the "Lund protocol" [163,164]. Subsequently, the Toronto group reported the results of a significant clinical trial using EVLP to evaluate the function of marginal donor lungs and DCD lungs, which laid the foundation for the "Toronto protocol" [20]. The group conducted 372 EVLP procedures between 2008 and 2017, increasing the annual lung transplantation rate by 70% during this period. EVLP has emerged in the last decade as a platform to rehabilitate and assess donor lungs before transplantation. Donor lungs are perfused and ventilated at normothermia in a specialized circuit for several hours. Clinically, EVLP allows marginal lungs to be evaluated and even treated prior to implantation [12]. Cypel et al. demonstrated that high-risk donor lungs treated with 4 h of EVLP had post-transplant outcomes comparable to standard lungs [165]. EVLP reduces the effective IRI burden by washing out DAMPs/cytokines linked to PGD, minimizing leukocyte/complement activation with acellular perfusate, and metabolically re-priming the graft under controlled flow/FiO_2. These effects diminish succinate-driven mitochondrial ROS at reperfusion and has been associated with less warm-ischemia-related damage and lower PGD3 after transplant [87,91,166–171]. In a retrospective, single-center study of 538 lungs from the Toronto Lung transplant Program database, lungs that received EVLP recovered significantly faster from PGD grade 3 compared to lungs that did not receive EVLP [172]. Similarly, in a recent United Network for Organ Sharing database analysis of 10,342 patients that underwent lung transplantation between 2015 and 2023, EVLP was associated with decreased PGD grade 3 development [171]. These promising results of EVLP have led to the development of the Organ Care System (OCS) Lung™ (TranMedic, Andover, MA, USA), a portable EVLP platform that enables normothermic perfusion with donor blood and ventilation of the donor lungs during storage and transportation. In contrast to standard EVLP, this mobile system could potentially recondition donor lungs as soon as they are procured and (almost) completely eliminate cold ischemia during transport [173,174]. Very recently, the results of the EXPAND trial were published, a prospective, single-arm multicenter trial that assessed long-term clinical outcomes after use of OCS before transplantation of extended criteria donor lungs. The outcomes were compared to control cohorts from the same centers. The results showed similar 5-year overall survival rates. Furthermore, no significant differences were found between the EXPAND and control cohorts for the development of any grade of bronchiolitis obliterans syndrome [59].

EVLP can also serves as a delivery platform for therapies: drugs, gene therapy vectors, or cells can be administered ex vivo without risking systemic effects [91,175,176]. For example, experimental studies have shown that adenoviral IL-10 gene therapy given during EVLP in damaged human lungs led to improved lung function and reduced inflammation, making previously unusable lungs fit for transplant [177,178]. Likewise, EVLP studies in animal models show that adding treatments such as mesenchymal stem cells (MSCs), A2A adenosine receptor agonists, beta-2 agonists, or perfusate filtration can act on core LIRI pathways, lowering perfusate DAMP/cytokine burden and leukocyte activation, preserving endothelial/mitochondrial homeostasis, and improving alveolar fluid clearance, thereby reducing the reperfusion ROS/inflammation surge and improving early graft physiology [12,166]. EVLP is now routine in many major centers and has expanded the donor pool while also acting as a research bridge between bench and bedside for LIRI interventions [12,179].

4.3. Therapeutic Gases–NO, Carbon Monoxide, and Hydrogen

NO is a pulmonary vasodilator that can improve oxygenation and reduce PAP [180]. It has theoretical benefits in LIRI by improving perfusion and possibly modulating inflammation through cGMP signaling. By terminating lipid peroxidation chain reactions and S-nitrosation of mitochondrial complex I at the onset of reperfusion, it can theoretically dampen RET–mediated ROS generation [180,181]. Conversely, when superoxide levels are high, NO rapidly forms peroxynitrite ($ONOO^-$), which amplifies oxidative/nitrative injury to lipids, proteins, and mitochondria; this helps explain why antioxidant benefits may not consistently translate at the bedside [182,183]. In practice, many transplant centers administer inhaled NO after reperfusion for severe PGD [10,12]. However, a double-blinded, placebo-controlled randomized trial in 84 lung transplant patients found no significant reduction in PGD incidence or outcomes with prophylactic inhaled NO [184]. Thus, inhaled NO is used as a supportive rescue therapy for hypoxemia, but evidence does not support it as a definitive preventive treatment for LIRI [185].

Low-dose CO exerts anti-inflammatory and anti-apoptotic effects via heme oxygenase-1 (HO-1) and stabilization of hypoxia-inducible factor (HIF-1α) [186,187]. In animal models of IRI, inhaling low concentrations of CO reduced IL-6 and TNF-α levels, decreased cell death, and improved oxygenation [188]. CO appears to induce a preconditioning-like state, upregulating cytoprotective pathways. A key mechanism is CO's ability to modulate macrophage activation toward an anti-inflammatory phenotype and to suppress NF-κB [189,190]. Some early clinical studies in other organ transplants hint at safety of low-dose CO inhalation [191,192].

Hydrogen gas is a reactive free radical scavenger that can neutralize hydroxyl radicals [193]. It also activates the Nrf2 antioxidant response [194]. In multiple other organ IRI models, inhaled H_2 or hydrogen-rich solutions reduced oxidative damage and improved outcomes [12]. In the lung, H_2 has been shown to attenuate inflammatory cytokines and cell death in LIRI by boosting endogenous antioxidants [195,196]. One murine study found that combining inhaled H_2 with NO provided additive protection against LIRI [196]. The main limitation is delivery: H_2 is flammable, thus giving it during organ transport or to patients poses logistic challenges. However, hydrogen-rich saline can be administered intravenously or used as an organ flush [197]. In rat and LIRI models, hydrogen-enriched preservation solutions significantly reduced reperfusion injury [10,196].

4.4. Pharmacological Therapies

Several pharmacological therapies have been proposed as possible treatments or preventive measures for LIRI. Activation of complement is a key event in reperfusion injury [40]. Complement system activation increases the inflammatory reaction by producing anaphylatoxins such as C3a and C5a, resulting in an increased vascular permeability. In a multicenter cohort study, patients with increased plasma C5a levels at 6 h and 24 h post lung transplant were more likely to develop severe PGD and had higher mortality rates [39,40]. Furthermore, patients with PGD had higher bronchoalveolar lavage levels of complement activation fragments 24 h after lung transplantation [39].

HMG-CoA (3-hydroxy-3-methylglutaryl coenzyme A) reductase inhibitors (statins) have anti-inflammatory and endothelial-stabilizing properties beyond cholesterol lowering [198]. Observational studies indicate that lung transplant recipients on statin therapy have lower rates of PGD [199,200]. In a retrospective analysis (1999–2014), PGD occurred in 34.8% of patients on perioperative statins vs. 57.9% of those not on statins [199]. After propensity adjustment, statin use was independently associated with reduced PGD risk

(OR 0.4). Some centers now consider continuing or starting statins in the peri-transplant period as an adjunct protective strategy [199,200].

High-dose corticosteroids are often given to the donor before organ procurement and to the recipient before reperfusion, primarily to attenuate immune activation and hyperacute rejection [201]. While not studied in randomized trials specifically for IRI prevention, steroids likely attenuate some early cytokine surges in LIRI (TNF, IL-1, etc.) [202]. Almost all lung transplant protocols include steroids (partly for anti-rejection), so their effect is entangled with standard care [203]. Experimental data in animals support that steroids reduce LIRI edema and inflammation, but careful timing and dosing are needed to balance risks such as infection and impaired healing [204,205].

Because mitochondrial ROS bursts, bioenergetic collapse, and defective mitophagy are central in LIRI, several mitochondria-directed strategies are being pursued. Mitochondria-targeted antioxidants and peptides, such as elamipretide (SS-31), which binds cardiolipin to stabilize cristae, and mitochondrial quinones like MitoQ, aim to reduce electron leak and limit mitochondrial ROS. Although most efficacy data come from heart and kidney IRI, the mechanisms are directly relevant to LIRI and EVLP may allow organ-specific delivery [206–208]. Complementary "metabolic re-wiring" at reperfusion seeks to blunt reverse electron transport–driven ROS by modulating succinate dehydrogenase activity (e.g., malonate or dimethyl-malonate prodrugs) [128,209]. Restoring mitophagy and mitochondrial quality control via Sirtuin1 (SIRT1)–PTEN-induced kinase 1 (PINK1)/Parkin signaling, illustrated by adiponectin-mediated rescue in diabetic lung-transplant models, can preserve mitochondrial integrity and reduce injury [210]. An orthogonal approach is mitochondrial transfer or transplantation, either through endogenous MSC-to-epithelium donation or exogenous delivery, which has improved lung mechanics, ATP content, and inflammation in preclinical lung-injury studies [46,211,212]. Collectively, these modalities are biologically compelling yet supported by limited lung-specific clinical data.

Metformin has emerged as a possible treatment candidate in LIRI. In a type-2 diabetic rat LTx model, metformin improved graft function and reduced necroptosis by activating adenosine monophosphate-activated protein kinase (AMPK); its benefits were reversed by an AMPK inhibitor, supporting on-target activity. Independent groups have replicated protection in LTx IRI models and extended benefits to CLAD in rats [213,214]. Mechanistically, metformin's complex-I modulation dampens mitochondrial ROS and engages AMPK-dependent cytoprotective pathways that intersect with mitophagy and endothelial barrier preservation, pathways already implicated in diabetic LIRI. A 2024–2025 cross-organ IRI literature synthesis positions metformin as a plausible peri-reperfusion adjunct, though no randomized human LTx trials have reported to date [215,216].

4.5. Anti-Inflammatory and Immunomodulatory Approaches

Activation of A2A receptors on immune cells has broad anti-inflammatory effects (increasing cAMP and inhibiting neutrophil/macrophage activation) [217,218]. In animal models of LIRI, selective A2A agonists given during EVLP improved lung compliance and reduced pro-inflammatory cytokines and neutrophil infiltration [219–221]. These promising results have led to a recent blinded multicenter randomized controlled trial of regadenoson, an A2A agonist, in lung transplant patients, recently showed a trend towards reducing IRI [222].

IL-10 is an anti-inflammatory cytokine that suppresses production of TNF-α, IL-1β, and other harmful mediators [223]. Gene therapy to overexpress IL-10 in donor lungs via EVLP has shown promising results [12]. In large animal models and human lungs deemed unsuitable for transplant, delivering IL-10 with an adenoviral vector during EVLP significantly attenuated subsequent reperfusion injury and even improved 30-day graft survival post-transplant [224,225]. IL-10 gene therapy effectively "preconditions" the lung by attenuating the inflammatory cascade upon reperfusion. To mitigate risks, the ex vivo delivery of the gene therapy confines it to the graft [179].

Dipeptidyl peptidase-4 (DPP-4/CD26) is a cell-surface serine protease highly expressed in the lung on capillary endothelium and alveolar cells [226,227]. It inactivates several cytoprotective peptides: GLP-1, vasoactive intestinal peptide (VIP), and stromal cell–derived factor-1α (SDF-1α) [17]. Pharmacologic DPP-4 inhibition preserves these substrates and exerts anti-inflammatory, antioxidant, and endothelial-protective effects [17,228–230]. Mechanistically, VIP limits NF-κB activation, reduces caspase activity, and suppresses pro-inflammatory cytokines while promoting broncho- and vasodilation; DPP-4 inhibition increases VIP-positive macrophages after reperfusion [17,231–234]. SDF-1α recruits bone-marrow progenitors and activates cell-survival signaling via CXCR4; DPP-4 inhibition raises intact SDF-1α and enhances progenitor homing [229,235]. GLP-1 receptor activation elevates cAMP, downregulates NADPH oxidase (reducing superoxide), and induces endogenous antioxidant enzymes; in endotoxemia models, DPP-4 inhibitors reduce vascular oxidative stress, NOX2 expression, inducible NOS, NF-κB activation, and inflammatory cytokine release while upregulating SOD, GPx, and thioredoxin [236–242].

Preclinical lung IRI and transplant studies corroborate these mechanisms. In ex vivo rat lung perfusion, irreversible DPP-4 inhibition improved oxygenation and lowered pulmonary artery pressures; in vivo, pretreatment improved compliance, reduced edema and neutrophil infiltration, and lessened histologic injury, with greater VIP staining [228]. In a mouse orthotopic transplant with 18 h cold ischemia, DPP-4 inhibition improved post-reperfusion function, reduced macrophage/neutrophil activation, and attenuated acute rejection. Donor-lung preconditioning with vildagliptin during cold storage decreased macrophage/neutrophil influx and ICAM-1 expression, improved oxygenation, and yielded better structure and function up to 14 days, accompanied by higher SDF-1α, more IL-10, and M2 macrophage polarization; CD26-knockout recipients showed similar protection, implicating DPP-4 activity directly [229].

Human data are limited to a retrospective diabetic-recipient cohort, where DPP-4 inhibitor use associated with higher 5-year survival and freedom from CLAD, and explanted tissues from non–DPP-4i patients showed higher CD26 expression [26]. While encouraging, these findings require confirmation in prospective trials to define dosing, timing (donor, EVLP, or recipient), and patient selection for preventing LIRI and possibly reducing downstream CLAD.

Bone marrow-derived MSCs possess immunomodulatory and pro-repair properties. They can release anti-inflammatory cytokines, growth factors, and microvesicles that reduce endothelial permeability and promote tissue repair [10]. In mouse lung transplant models, MSC infusion protected lungs from IRI, reducing inflammatory cell infiltration and apoptosis [10]. MSC-derived extracellular vesicles (EVs), nano-sized vesicles enriched in miRNAs, proteins and lipids, recapitulate much of the parent cells' immunomodulatory and reparative effects while avoiding concerns about persistence, embolism, or ectopic differentiation. These MSC-derived EVs have similarly shown potential to attenuate lung inflammation in IRI by reducing neutrophil influx and cytokine release, preserving alveolar–capillary barrier function, and improve oxygenation. Mechanisms include transfer of regulatory miRNAs (e.g., miR-21-5p, miR-146a) to alveolar macrophages and epithelial cells, promotion of epithelial repair programs, and enhancement of alveolar fluid clearance [195,197,243–245]. Several studies have indicated that MSC therapy protects the alveolar-epithelial barrier during ALI, likely due to improved permeability, alveolar fluid clearance, and oxygenation [12,246]. Safety of allogeneic MSCs has been shown in a Phase 2a trial for ARDS where no infusion-related toxicity was demonstrated [247]. Consequently, early-phase trials of MSC therapy for lung transplant patients (to prevent PGD or treat chronic rejection) are in development [246]. Two delivery avenues are especially promising for translation. First, EVLP provides a controllable window to administer EVs (or engineered EVs) directly to donor lungs before implantation. Contemporary reviews highlight EVLP as a practical bridge for EV/MSC products in LTx, with dosing and manufacturing standardization as the next hurdles [179,243,248]. Second, regional airway delivery is feasible: nebulized, miR-146a–engineered human umbilical cord MSC-EVs attenuated LIRI and improved graft oxygenation in an orthotopic rat LTx model by suppressing NLRP3 inflammasome signaling. Earlier work also showed anti-inflammatory activity of human MSC-EVs in reperfusion models [249].

During LIRI, endogenous danger signals like HMGB1 and extracellular ribonucleic acid (RNA) trigger toll-like receptors (TLRs) and inflammasomes. Experimental agents that neutralize HMGB1 or block TLR4 signaling (e.g., TLR4 antagonist eritoran) have shown reductions in LIRI in animal studies [10]. Similarly, inhibiting the NOD-like receptor family pyrin domain containing 3 (NLRP3) inflammasome or caspase-1 to reduce pyroptosis, a form of inflammatory cell death, is being explored. For instance, one study found that a glucagon-like peptide-1 (GLP-1) receptor agonist added during EVLP modulated pyroptosis pathways and improved lung graft function [236].

An often under-recognized contributor to LIRI is microthrombosis in the pulmonary microvasculature. Donor lungs, especially from DCD cases, can contain fibrin clots that impede reperfusion and prolong ischemia in parts of the lung [250]. Fibrinolytics like tissue plasminogen activator (tPA) or plasmin given to the donor lung have been tested to dissolve these clots [251,252]. Notably, administering plasmin during EVLP effectively cleared microthrombi and led to improved post-transplant lung function in recent studies [10]. Some EVLP protocols routinely include fibrinolytic treatment, particularly for DCD lungs where intravascular coagulation is a concern [10,253].

Another possible therapy includes inhibiting necroptosis, a programmed necrosis driven by receptor-interacting serine/threonine-protein kinases 1 and 3 (RIPK1/RIPK3) and mixed lineage kinase domain like pseudokinase (MLKL), contributing to endothelial and epithelial death in IRI [254]. Necrostatin-1 (Nec-1), a RIPK1 inhibitor, has shown efficacy in a mouse hilar clamp model of LIRI [255]. Nec-1 treatment significantly reduced lung injury scores, lowered pro-inflammatory cytokines, and decreased necroptotic markers in lung tissue. In vitro, Nec-1 also protected pulmonary cells from cold hypoxia-reoxygenation injury by preventing necrosome (RIPK1/RIPK3 complex) formation. Interestingly, Nec-1 not only blocked necroptosis but also reduced caspase-dependent apoptosis of epithelial cells, and it promoted apoptosis of neutrophils, thereby accelerating resolution of inflammation. By inhibiting both necroptosis and apoptosis, and encouraging clearance of neutrophils, Nec-1 provided multi-faceted protection. The authors concluded Nec-1 could be a promising therapy to prevent PGD [255]. Similarly, necrosulfonamide (an MLKL inhibitor) has shown protective effects in a rat LIRI model by blocking necroptosis of airway cells [256]. These findings underscore the therapeutic potential of targeting regulated necrosis in LIRI.

4.6. Antioxidant Therapies

Classic antioxidants like N-acetylcysteine (NAC), vitamin C, and superoxide dismutase mimetics have been studied in various IRI models [257–259]. NAC, a glutathione precursor, has been shown in some animal studies to reduce LIRI edema and malondialdehyde (lipid peroxidation) levels, although high doses are needed [259,260]. While antioxidants are intuitively beneficial, human data are limited.

Beyond inhaled NO as a vasodilator, strategies to enhance endogenous NO signaling are considered cytoprotective. For example, nitrite (NO_2^-) can be enzymatically reduced to NO during ischemia, acting as an oxygen-independent NO donor. In some organ IRI models, nitrite infusion before reperfusion improved microvascular flow and reduced ROS due to the fact that NO can outcompete superoxide to form peroxynitrite instead of hydroxyl radical formation [261,262]. Soluble guanylate cyclase activators, which amplify NO signaling, are another avenue; however, their role in LIRI is speculative [263]. Balancing NO is complex because excess inducible NOS during reperfusion can be harmful [10]. Antioxidant cocktails have not yet conclusively improved clinical outcomes in lung transplant or ARDS, possibly because timing and delivery to cells are challenging [264]. Nevertheless, managing oxidative stress remains a cornerstone concept, and these agents could be part of a multimodal regimen in the future.

Another possible avenue is targeting ferroptosis, iron-dependent lipid peroxidation-driven cell death [10]. Injured lungs often show signs of ferroptosis: iron accumulation, depleted glutathione, lipid peroxides, and several methods of targeting this pathway have been proposed in recent years [265]. Maresin-1 (MaR1), an endogenous pro-resolving lipid mediator, was recently shown to protect mouse lung transplants by inhibiting ferroptosis [10]. In a 2025 study, MaR1 given to mice undergoing lung transplantation preserved glutathione levels, prevented lipid peroxidation, and reduced ultrastructural mitochondrial damage in grafts [266]. Mechanistically, MaR1 activated Protein Kinase A and the Hippo-YAP pathway, which in turn reduced ferroptosis signaling. The authors concluded that MaR1 effectively attenuated LIRI and suggested it as a basis for organ-protective therapy. Beyond MaR1, classical iron chelators like deferoxamine or lipophilic antioxidants such as liproxstatin-1 could theoretically be applied to donor lungs to curb ferroptotic injury [267]. This area is still emerging, but targeting ferroptosis is promising given its central role in IR-induced cell death [10].

5. Conclusions

LIRI remains an important cause of morbidity and mortality in thoracic surgery, particularly in the context of lung transplantation, where it is the principal driver of PGD and a major contributor to the development of CLAD. Despite advances in surgical technique, organ preservation, and perioperative care, the incidence and impact of LIRI remain substantial, particularly with increasing reliance on extended-criteria donors and DCD lungs.

Over the past decade, considerable progress has been made in deciphering the complex pathobiology of LIRI, including the central roles of oxidative stress, endothelial dysfunction, inflammatory cell recruitment, and disruption of the alveolar–capillary barrier. Experimental models have further elucidated mechanisms such as endothelial glycocalyx degradation, mitochondrial injury, and regulated cell death pathways, all of which converge to exacerbate pulmonary edema, gas exchange impairment, and long-term allograft dysfunction.

Clinically, the evolution of lung-protective ventilation strategies, controlled reperfusion protocols, and the application of EVLP has improved early postoperative outcomes and expanded the donor pool. These advances reflect the growing recognition that a multimodal and phase-specific approach to LIRI prevention, beginning with donor management and extending through procurement, implantation, and postoperative care, is essential.

While different pharmacologic interventions have been proposed, including antioxidants, complement inhibitors, vasodilators, and immunomodulatory agents, few have translated successfully into routine clinical use. However, the growing understanding of cellular and molecular targets continues to inform the development of novel therapies. These include strategies to preserve the endothelial barrier, modulate innate immune activation, and inhibit key inflammatory mediators. Emerging approaches such as mesenchymal stem cell therapies, cytokine modulation, and inhibition of regulated necrosis (e.g., necroptosis, ferroptosis) hold particular promise but require further clinical validation.

LIRI spans heterogeneous donor and recipient states (DBD vs. DCD, ischemic times, size mismatch, pulmonary hypertension, ECMO use), making effect sizes small and context-dependent. Timing and route of delivery (intra-donor, EVLP, intra-op reperfusion, early post-op) are critical yet inconsistently standardized. Surrogate endpoints vary (e.g., PGD grade vs. biomarker panels), and negative or neutral trials of intuitive therapies (e.g., prophylactic inhaled NO) highlight the need for biomarker-guided enrichment and platform trials. Manufacturing and regulatory issues also slow cellular/EV products. We outline these issues to guide realistic translation of promising preclinical findings.

The future management of LIRI will depend on the integration of mechanistic insights with real-time biomarkers for injury prediction, early detection, and therapeutic monitoring. Translational and clinical research need to bridge the gap between bench and bedside, ideally through multicenter trials and standardized outcome measures.

Author Contributions: Conceptualization, L.B. and P.V.S.; writing—original draft preparation, L.B., J.M.H.H., S.E.V., S.K.Y., W.W., P.L., G.V., R.D.P., P.M., I.R., D.A., and P.V.S.; writing—review and editing, L.B., J.M.H.H., S.E.V., S.K.Y., W.W., P.L., G.V., R.D.P., P.M., I.R., D.A., and P.V.S.; visualization, L.B.; supervision, J.M.H.H., S.E.V., S.K.Y., W.W., P.L., G.V., R.D.P., P.M., I.R., D.A., and P.V.S.; final approval—L.B., J.M.H.H., S.E.V., S.K.Y., W.W., P.L., G.V., R.D.P., P.M., I.R., D.A., and P.V.S. All authors have read and agreed to the published version of the manuscript.

Funding: This research received no external funding.

Institutional Review Board Statement: Not applicable.

Data Availability Statement: No new data were created or analyzed in this study. Data sharing is not applicable to this article.

Conflicts of Interest: The authors declare no conflicts of interest.

Abbreviations

The following abbreviations are used in this manuscript:

ALI	Acute Lung Injury
ARDS	Acute Respiratory Distress Syndrome
ATP	Adenosine Triphosphate
BAL	Bronchoalveolar lavage
BMI	Body Mass Index
cAMP	Cyclic Adenosine Monophosphate
CD26	Cluster of Differentiation 26
cGMP	Cyclic Guanosine Monophosphate
CLAD	Chronic Lung Allograft Dysfunction
CO	Carbon Monoxide
COPD	Chronic Obstructive Pulmonary Disease
COR	Controlled Oxygenated Rewarming
CPB	Cardiopulmonary Bypass
CVP	Central Venous Pressure
CXCL	C-X-C Ligand
DAMP	Damage-associated Molecular Patterns

DBD	Donation after Brain Death
DCD	Donation after Circulatory Death
DNA	Deoxyribonucleic Acid
DPP-4	Dipeptidyl Peptidase-4
ECMO	Extracorporeal Membrane Oxygenation
EV	Extracellular Vesicles
EVLP	Ex Vivo Lung Perfusion
FiO_2	Fraction of Inspired Oxygen
GLP	Glucagon-like Peptide
GM-CSF	Granulocyte-Macrophage Colony-Stimulating Factor
HIF	Hypoxia-inducible Factor
HMG-CoA	3-Hydroxy-3-Methylglutaryl Coenzyme A
HMGB1	High Mobility Group Box 1
HOPE	Hypothermic Oxygenated Perfusion
ICU	Intensive Care Unit
IL	Interleukin
iNOS	Inducible Nitric Oxide Synthase
IR	Ischemia–Reperfusion
IRI	Ischemia–Reperfusion Injury
IV	Intravenous
KATP	ATP-Sensitive Potassium Channel
LIRI	Lung Ischemia–Reperfusion Injury
MaR1	Maresin-1
MLKL	Mixed Lineage Kinase Domain Like Pseudokinase
MOF	Multiple Organ Failure
MSC	Mesenchymal Stem Cell
NAC	N-acetylcysteine
NADPH	Nicotinamide Adenine Dinucleotide Phosphate
NET	Neutrophil Extracellular Traps
NF-κB	Nuclear Factor Kappa B
NLRP3	NOD-like Receptor Family Pyrin Domain Containing 3
NMP	Normothermic Machine Perfusion
NO	Nitric Oxide
NOS	Nitric Oxide Synthase
NOX	NADPH Oxidase 2
NRP	Normothermic Regional Perfusion
OCS	Organ Care System
OLV	One-lung Ventilation
PAP	Pulmonary Artery Pressure
PECAM-1	Platelet Endothelial Cell Adhesion Molecule
PEEP	Positive End-Expiratory Pressure
PGD	Primary Graft Dysfunction
PI3K-Akt	Phosphoinositide 3-Kinase–Akt pathway
PINK1	PTEN-induced kinase 1
RANTES	Regulated upon Activation, Normal T cell Expressed and Secreted
RIC	Remote Ischemic Conditioning
RIPK1/3	Receptor-interacting Serine/Threonine-Protein Kinases 1/3
RNA	Ribonucleic Acid
ROS	Reactive Oxygen Species
SDF	Stromal-cell Derived Factor
SIRT1	Sirtuin 1
TLR	Toll-like Receptor
TNF	Tumor Necrosis Factor

tPA	Tissue Plasminogen Activator
uDCD	Uncontrolled Donation after Circulatory Death
VEGFR2	Vascular Endothelial Growth Factor Receptor 2
VIP	Vasoactive Intestinal Peptide
V/Q	Ventilation/Perfusion
XO	Xanthine Oxidase

References

1. Vlastos, D.; Zeinah, M.; Ninkovic-Hall, G.; Vlachos, S.; Salem, A.; Asonitis, A.; Chavan, H.; Kalampalikis, L.; Al Shammari, A.; Alvarez Gallesio, J.M.; et al. The effects of ischaemic conditioning on lung ischaemia–reperfusion injury. *Respir. Res.* **2022**, *23*, 351. [CrossRef] [PubMed]
2. Den Hengst, W.A.; Gielis, J.F.; Lin, J.Y.; Van Schil, P.E.; De Windt, L.J.; Moens, A.L. Lung ischemia-reperfusion injury: A molecular and clinical view on a complex pathophysiological process. *Am. J. Physiol.-Heart Circ. Physiol.* **2010**, *299*, H1283–H1299. [CrossRef] [PubMed]
3. Laubach, V.E.; Sharma, A.K. Mechanisms of lung ischemia-reperfusion injury. *Curr. Opin. Organ. Transplant.* **2016**, *21*, 246–252. [CrossRef]
4. Ferrari, R.S.; Andrade, C.F. Oxidative Stress and Lung Ischemia-Reperfusion Injury. *Oxid. Med. Cell. Longev.* **2015**, *2015*, 590987. [CrossRef]
5. Rowe, C.J.; Walsh, S.A.; Dragon, A.H.; Rhodes, A.M.; Pak, O.L.; Ronzier, E.; Levi, B.; Potter, B.K.; Spreadborough, P.J.; Davis, T.A. Tourniquet-induced ischemia creates increased risk of organ dysfunction and mortality following delayed limb amputation. *Injury* **2023**, *54*, 1792–1803. [CrossRef]
6. Dulu, A.; Pastores, S.M.; Park, B.; Riedel, E.; Rusch, V.; Halpern, N.A. Prevalence and mortality of acute lung injury and ARDS after lung resection. *Chest* **2006**, *130*, 73–78. [CrossRef]
7. Li, C.; Li, Y.S.; Xu, M.; Wen, S.H.; Yao, X.; Wu, Y.; Huang, C.Y.; Huang, W.Q.; Liu, K.X. Limb remote ischemic preconditioning for intestinal and pulmonary protection during elective open infrarenal abdominal aortic aneurysm repair: A randomized controlled trial. *Anesthesiology* **2013**, *118*, 842–852. [CrossRef]
8. Hu, Q.; Luo, W.; Huang, L.; Huang, R.; Chen, R.; Gao, Y. Multiorgan protection of remote ischemic perconditioning in valve replacement surgery. *J. Surg. Res.* **2016**, *200*, 13–20. [CrossRef]
9. Suzuki, T. Additional lung-protective perfusion techniques during cardiopulmonary bypass. *Ann. Thorac. Cardiovasc. Surg.* **2010**, *16*, 150–155.
10. Chen-Yoshikawa, T.F. Ischemia-Reperfusion Injury in Lung Transplantation. *Cells* **2021**, *10*, 1333. [CrossRef] [PubMed]
11. Sayah, D.M.; Mallavia, B.; Liu, F.; Ortiz-Muñoz, G.; Caudrillier, A.; DerHovanessian, A.; Ross, D.J.; Lynch III, J.P.; Saggar, R.; Ardehali, A.; et al. Neutrophil Extracellular Traps Are Pathogenic in Primary Graft Dysfunction after Lung Transplantation. *Am. J. Respir. Crit. Care Med.* **2015**, *191*, 455–463. [CrossRef] [PubMed]
12. Talaie, T.; DiChiacchio, L.; Prasad, N.K.; Pasrija, C.; Julliard, W.; Kaczorowski, D.J.; Zhao, Y.; Lau, C.L. Ischemia-reperfusion Injury in the Transplanted Lung: A Literature Review. *Transplant. Direct* **2021**, *7*, e652. [CrossRef] [PubMed]
13. Carter, Y.M.; Gelman, A.E.; Kreisel, D. Pathogenesis, Management, and Consequences of Primary Graft Dysfunction. *Semin. Thorac. Cardiovasc. Surg.* **2008**, *20*, 165–172. [CrossRef] [PubMed]
14. Miller, C.L.; O, J.M.; Allan, J.S.; Madsen, J.C. Novel approaches for long-term lung transplant survival. *Front. Immunol.* **2022**, *13*, 931251. [CrossRef]
15. Van Slambrouck, J.; Van Raemdonck, D.; Vos, R.; Vanluyten, C.; Vanstapel, A.; Prisciandaro, E.; Willems, L.; Orlitová, M.; Kaes, J.; Jin, X.; et al. A Focused Review on Primary Graft Dysfunction after Clinical Lung Transplantation: A Multilevel Syndrome. *Cells* **2022**, *11*, 745. [CrossRef]
16. Forgie, K.A.; Fialka, N.; Freed, D.H.; Nagendran, J. Lung Transplantation, Pulmonary Endothelial Inflammation, and Ex-Situ Lung Perfusion: A Review. *Cells* **2021**, *10*, 1417. [CrossRef]
17. Beckers, P.A.J.; Gielis, J.F.; Van Schil, P.E.; Adriaensen, D. Lung ischemia reperfusion injury: The therapeutic role of dipeptidyl peptidase 4 inhibition. *Ann. Transl. Med.* **2017**, *5*, 129. [CrossRef]
18. De Sousa, S.G.; Nascimento da Silva, G.V.; Costa Rodrigues, A.M.; Meireles Fernandes da Silva, T.M.; Costa, F.C.; Freitas Teixeira da Silva, A.; Santana de Macedo, B.F.; Brito, M.V.H. Organ Preservation Solutions in Transplantation: A Literature Review. *Exp. Clin. Transplant.* **2021**, *19*, 511–521. [CrossRef]
19. Latchana, N.; Peck, J.R.; Whitson, B.; Black, S.M. Preservation solutions for cardiac and pulmonary donor grafts: A review of the current literature. *J. Thorac. Dis.* **2014**, *6*, 1143–1149. [CrossRef]

20. Ahmad, K.; Pluhacek, J.L.; Brown, A.W. Ex Vivo Lung Perfusion: A Review of Current and Future Application in Lung Transplantation. *Pulm. Ther.* **2022**, *8*, 149–165. [CrossRef]
21. Cenik, I.; Van Slambrouck, J.; Provoost, A.L.; Barbarossa, A.; Vanluyten, C.; Boelhouwer, C.; Vanaudenaerde, B.M.; Vos, R.; Pirenne, J.; Van Raemdonck, D.E.; et al. Controlled Hypothermic Storage for Lung Preservation: Leaving the Ice Age Behind. *Transpl. Int.* **2024**, *37*, 12601. [CrossRef]
22. Hofmann, J.; Pühringer, M.; Steinkellner, S.; Holl, A.-S.; Meszaros, A.T.; Schneeberger, S.; Troppmair, J.; Hautz, T. Novel, Innovative Models to Study Ischemia/Reperfusion-Related Redox Damage in Organ Transplantation. *Antioxidants* **2023**, *12*, 31. [CrossRef]
23. Mathis, S.; Putzer, G.; Schneeberger, S.; Martini, J. The Endothelial Glycocalyx and Organ Preservation-From Physiology to Possible Clinical Implications for Solid Organ Transplantation. *Int. J. Mol. Sci.* **2021**, *22*, 4019. [CrossRef] [PubMed]
24. Ta, H.Q.; Kuppusamy, M.; Sonkusare, S.K.; Roeser, M.E.; Laubach, V.E. The endothelium: Gatekeeper to lung ischemia-reperfusion injury. *Respir. Res.* **2024**, *25*, 172. [CrossRef] [PubMed]
25. Jungraithmayr, W. Novel Strategies for Endothelial Preservation in Lung Transplant Ischemia-Reperfusion Injury. *Front. Physiol.* **2020**, *11*, 581420. [CrossRef] [PubMed]
26. Yamada, Y.; Sato, T.; Oda, H.; Harada, N.; Yoshizawa, A.; Nishikawa, S.; Kayawake, H.; Tanaka, S.; Yutaka, Y.; Hamaji, M.; et al. Favorable effect of CD26/DPP-4 inhibitors on postoperative outcomes after lung transplantation: A propensity-weighted analysis. *J. Heart Lung Transplant.* **2024**, *43*, 66–76. [CrossRef]
27. Jang, J.-H.; Yamada, Y.; Janker, F.; De Meester, I.; Baerts, L.; Vliegen, G.; Inci, I.; Chatterjee, S.; Weder, W.; Jungraithmayr, W. Anti-inflammatory effects on ischemia/reperfusion-injured lung transplants by the cluster of differentiation 26/dipeptidylpeptidase 4 (CD26/DPP4) inhibitor vildagliptin. *J. Thorac. Cardiovasc. Surg.* **2017**, *153*, 713–724.e714. [CrossRef]
28. Pak, O.; Sydykov, A.; Kosanovic, D.; Schermuly, R.T.; Dietrich, A.; Schröder, K.; Brandes, R.P.; Gudermann, T.; Sommer, N.; Weissmann, N. Lung Ischaemia–Reperfusion Injury: The Role of Reactive Oxygen Species. In *Pulmonary Vasculature Redox Signaling in Health and Disease*; Wang, Y.-X., Ed.; Springer International Publishing: Cham, Switzerland, 2017; pp. 195–225.
29. Kalogeris, T.; Baines, C.P.; Krenz, M.; Korthuis, R.J. Cell biology of ischemia/reperfusion injury. *Int. Rev. Cell Mol. Biol.* **2012**, *298*, 229–317. [CrossRef]
30. Granger, D.N.; Kvietys, P.R. Reperfusion injury and reactive oxygen species: The evolution of a concept. *Redox Biol.* **2015**, *6*, 524–551. [CrossRef]
31. Xiang, M.; Lu, Y.; Xin, L.; Gao, J.; Shang, C.; Jiang, Z.; Lin, H.; Fang, X.; Qu, Y.; Wang, Y.; et al. Role of Oxidative Stress in Reperfusion following Myocardial Ischemia and Its Treatments. *Oxid. Med. Cell. Longev.* **2021**, *2021*, 6614009. [CrossRef]
32. Chatterjee, S.; Nieman, G.F.; Christie, J.D.; Fisher, A.B. Shear stress-related mechanosignaling with lung ischemia: Lessons from basic research can inform lung transplantation. *Am. J. Physiol.-Lung Cell. Mol. Physiol.* **2014**, *307*, L668–L680. [CrossRef]
33. Li, C.; Jackson, R.M. Reactive species mechanisms of cellular hypoxia-reoxygenation injury. *Am. J. Physiol.-Cell Physiol.* **2002**, *282*, C227–C241. [CrossRef]
34. Vishwakarma, V.K.; Upadhyay, P.K.; Gupta, J.K.; Yadav, H.N. Pathophysiologic role of ischemia reperfusion injury: A review. *J. Indian Coll. Cardiol.* **2017**, *7*, 97–104. [CrossRef]
35. Rogers, L.K.; Cismowski, M.J. Oxidative stress in the lung—The essential paradox. *Curr. Opin. Toxicol.* **2018**, *7*, 37–43. [CrossRef] [PubMed]
36. Mittal, M.; Siddiqui, M.R.; Tran, K.; Reddy, S.P.; Malik, A.B. Reactive oxygen species in inflammation and tissue injury. *Antioxid. Redox Signal* **2014**, *20*, 1126–1167. [CrossRef] [PubMed]
37. Qiao, X.; Yin, J.; Zheng, Z.; Li, L.; Feng, X. Endothelial cell dynamics in sepsis-induced acute lung injury and acute respiratory distress syndrome: Pathogenesis and therapeutic implications. *Cell Commun. Signal* **2024**, *22*, 241. [CrossRef]
38. Matthay, M.A.; Zemans, R.L.; Zimmerman, G.A.; Arabi, Y.M.; Beitler, J.R.; Mercat, A.; Herridge, M.; Randolph, A.G.; Calfee, C.S. Acute respiratory distress syndrome. *Nat. Rev. Dis. Primers* **2019**, *5*, 18. [CrossRef]
39. Kulkarni, H.S.; Ramphal, K.; Ma, L.; Brown, M.; Oyster, M.; Speckhart, K.N.; Takahashi, T.; Byers, D.E.; Porteous, M.K.; Kalman, L.; et al. Local complement activation is associated with primary graft dysfunction after lung transplantation. *JCI Insight* **2020**, *5*, e138358. [CrossRef]
40. Shah, R.J.; Emtiazjoo, A.M.; Diamond, J.M.; Smith, P.A.; Roe, D.W.; Wille, K.M.; Orens, J.B.; Ware, L.B.; Weinacker, A.; Lama, V.N.; et al. Plasma Complement Levels Are Associated with Primary Graft Dysfunction and Mortality after Lung Transplantation. *Am. J. Respir. Crit. Care Med.* **2014**, *189*, 1564–1567. [CrossRef]
41. Westall, G.P.; Snell, G.I.; McLean, C.; Kotsimbos, T.; Williams, T.; Magro, C. C3d and C4d deposition early after lung transplantation. *J. Heart Lung Transplant.* **2008**, *27*, 722–728. [CrossRef]

42. Ruaro, B.; Salton, F.; Braga, L.; Wade, B.; Confalonieri, P.; Volpe, M.C.; Baratella, E.; Maiocchi, S.; Confalonieri, M. The History and Mystery of Alveolar Epithelial Type II Cells: Focus on Their Physiologic and Pathologic Role in Lung. *Int. J. Mol. Sci.* **2021**, *22*, 2566. [CrossRef] [PubMed]
43. Duni, A.; Liakopoulos, V.; Koutlas, V.; Pappas, C.; Mitsis, M.; Dounousi, E. The Endothelial Glycocalyx as a Target of Ischemia and Reperfusion Injury in Kidney Transplantation—Where Have We Gone So Far? *Int. J. Mol. Sci.* **2021**, *22*, 2157. [CrossRef] [PubMed]
44. Foote, C.A.; Soares, R.N.; Ramirez-Perez, F.I.; Ghiarone, T.; Aroor, A.; Manrique-Acevedo, C.; Padilla, J.; Martinez-Lemus, L. Endothelial Glycocalyx. *Compr. Physiol.* **2022**, *12*, 3781–3811. [CrossRef] [PubMed]
45. Kimura, A.; Suehiro, K.; Yamada, T.; Shinta, Y.; Juri, T.; Fujimoto, Y.; Hirano, S.; Mori, T. Protective Effects of Hydrogen-Rich Saline Against Hemorrhagic Shock in Rats via an Endothelial Glycocalyx Pathway. *Biomedicines* **2025**, *13*, 833. [CrossRef]
46. Moskowitzova, K.; Orfany, A.; Liu, K.; Ramirez-Barbieri, G.; Thedsanamoorthy, J.K.; Yao, R.; Guariento, A.; Doulamis, I.P.; Blitzer, D.; Shin, B.; et al. Mitochondrial transplantation enhances murine lung viability and recovery after ischemia-reperfusion injury. *Am. J. Physiol.-Lung Cell. Mol. Physiol.* **2020**, *318*, L78–L88. [CrossRef]
47. Li, Q.; Nie, H. Advances in lung ischemia/reperfusion injury: Unraveling the role of innate immunity. *Inflamm. Res.* **2024**, *73*, 393–405. [CrossRef]
48. Fard, N.; Saffari, A.; Emami, G.; Hofer, S.; Kauczor, H.-U.; Mehrabi, A. Acute respiratory distress syndrome induction by pulmonary ischemia–reperfusion injury in large animal models. *J. Surg. Res.* **2014**, *189*, 274–284. [CrossRef]
49. Christie, J.D.; Kotloff, R.M.; Ahya, V.N.; Tino, G.; Pochettino, A.; Gaughan, C.; DeMissie, E.; Kimmel, S.E. The effect of primary graft dysfunction on survival after lung transplantation. *Am. J. Respir. Crit. Care Med.* **2005**, *171*, 1312–1316. [CrossRef]
50. Morrison, M.I.; Pither, T.L.; Fisher, A.J. Pathophysiology and classification of primary graft dysfunction after lung transplantation. *J. Thorac. Dis.* **2017**, *9*, 4084–4097. [CrossRef]
51. Avtaar Singh, S.S.; Das De, S.; Al-Adhami, A.; Singh, R.; Hopkins, P.M.; Curry, P.A. Primary graft dysfunction following lung transplantation: From pathogenesis to future frontiers. *World J. Transplant.* **2023**, *13*, 58–85. [CrossRef]
52. Diamond, J.M.; Cantu, E.; Calfee, C.S.; Anderson, M.R.; Clausen, E.S.; Shashaty, M.G.S.; Courtwright, A.M.; Kalman, L.; Oyster, M.; Crespo, M.M.; et al. The Impact of Donor Smoking on Primary Graft Dysfunction and Mortality after Lung Transplantation. *Am. J. Respir. Crit. Care Med.* **2024**, *209*, 91–100. [CrossRef]
53. Lowery, E.M.; Kuhlmann, E.A.; Mahoney, E.L.; Dilling, D.F.; Kliethermes, S.A.; Kovacs, E.J. Heavy alcohol use in lung donors increases the risk for primary graft dysfunction. *Alcohol Clin. Exp. Res.* **2014**, *38*, 2853–2861. [CrossRef]
54. Roesel, M.J.; Sharma, N.S.; Schroeter, A.; Matsunaga, T.; Xiao, Y.; Zhou, H.; Tullius, S.G. Primary Graft Dysfunction: The Role of Aging in Lung Ischemia-Reperfusion Injury. *Front. Immunol.* **2022**, *13*, 891564. [CrossRef]
55. Bennett, R.M.; Reilly, J.P.; Diamond, J.M.; Cantu, E.; Shashaty, M.; Benvenuto, L.; Singer, J.P.; Palmer, S.M.; Christie, J.D.; Anderson, M.R. Body mass index and mortality following primary graft dysfunction: A Lung Transplant Outcomes Group study. *JHLT Open* **2024**, *5*, 100107. [CrossRef] [PubMed]
56. Fang, A.; Studer, S.; Kawut, S.M.; Ahya, V.N.; Lee, J.; Wille, K.; Lama, V.; Ware, L.; Orens, J.; Weinacker, A.; et al. Elevated pulmonary artery pressure is a risk factor for primary graft dysfunction following lung transplantation for idiopathic pulmonary fibrosis. *Chest* **2011**, *139*, 782–787. [CrossRef] [PubMed]
57. Jenkins, J.A.; Verdiner, R.; Omar, A.; Farina, J.M.; Wilson, R.; D'Cunha, J.; Reck Dos Santos, P.A. Donor and recipient risk factors for the development of primary graft dysfunction following lung transplantation. *Front. Immunol.* **2024**, *15*, 1341675. [CrossRef] [PubMed]
58. Lederer, D.J.; Kawut, S.M.; Wickersham, N.; Winterbottom, C.; Bhorade, S.; Palmer, S.M.; Lee, J.; Diamond, J.M.; Wille, K.M.; Weinacker, A.; et al. Obesity and primary graft dysfunction after lung transplantation: The Lung Transplant Outcomes Group Obesity Study. *Am. J. Respir. Crit. Care Med.* **2011**, *184*, 1055–1061. [CrossRef]
59. Loor, G.; Warnecke, G.; Villavicencio, M.A.; Smith, M.A.; Zhou, X.; Kukreja, J.; Ardehali, A.; Hartwig, M.G.; Daneshmand, M.A.; Hertz, M.I.; et al. Long-term outcomes of the international EXPAND trial of Organ Care System (OCS) Lung preservation for lung transplantation. *eClinicalMedicine* **2025**, *85*, 103334. [CrossRef]
60. Seay, T.; Guinn, N.; Maisonave, Y.; Fuller, M.; Poisson, J.; Pollak, A.; Bryner, B.; Haney, J.; Klapper, J.; Hartwig, M.; et al. The Association of Increased FFP:RBC Transfusion Ratio to Primary Graft Dysfunction in Bleeding Lung Transplantation Patients. *J. Cardiothorac. Vasc. Anesth.* **2020**, *34*, 3024–3032. [CrossRef]
61. Vandervelde, C.M.; Vos, R.; Vanluyten, C.; Fieuws, S.; Verleden, S.E.; Van Slambrouck, J.; De Leyn, P.; Coosemans, W.; Nafteux, P.; Decaluwé, H.; et al. Impact of anastomosis time during lung transplantation on primary graft dysfunction. *Am. J. Transplant.* **2022**, *22*, 1418–1429. [CrossRef]
62. Hunt, M.L.; Cantu, E. Primary graft dysfunction after lung transplantation. *Curr. Opin. Organ. Transplant.* **2023**, *28*, 180–186. [CrossRef]

63. Jennekens, J.; Braithwaite, S.A.; Luijk, B.; van der Kaaij, N.P.; Vrisekoop, N.; de Jager, S.C.A.; de Heer, L.M. Primary Graft Dysfunction in Lung Transplantation: An Overview of the Molecular Mechanisms. *Int. J. Mol. Sci.* **2025**, *26*, 6776. [CrossRef]
64. Jin, Z.; Suen, K.C.; Wang, Z.; Ma, D. Review 2: Primary graft dysfunction after lung transplant-pathophysiology, clinical considerations and therapeutic targets. *J. Anesth.* **2020**, *34*, 729–740. [CrossRef]
65. Shaver, C.M.; Ware, L.B. Primary graft dysfunction: Pathophysiology to guide new preventive therapies. *Expert Rev. Respir. Med.* **2017**, *11*, 119–128. [CrossRef]
66. Wong, K.H.M.; Hsin, K.Y.M. Primary graft dysfunction in lung transplantation: Still a thorn in the side of lung transplant. *J. Thorac. Dis.* **2024**, *16*, 1–5. [CrossRef]
67. Snell, G.I.; Yusen, R.D.; Weill, D.; Strueber, M.; Garrity, E.; Reed, A.; Pelaez, A.; Whelan, T.P.; Perch, M.; Bag, R.; et al. Report of the ISHLT Working Group on Primary Lung Graft Dysfunction, part I: Definition and grading—A 2016 Consensus Group statement of the International Society for Heart and Lung Transplantation. *J. Heart Lung Transplant.* **2017**, *36*, 1097–1103. [CrossRef] [PubMed]
68. Hyun, S.; Haam, S. Donation after Circulatory Death in Lung Transplantation. *J. Chest Surg.* **2022**, *55*, 283–287. [CrossRef] [PubMed]
69. Avlonitis, V.S.; Wigfield, C.H.; Kirby, J.A.; Dark, J.H. The Hemodynamic Mechanisms of Lung Injury and Systemic Inflammatory Response Following Brain Death in the Transplant Donor. *Am. J. Transplant.* **2005**, *5*, 684–693. [CrossRef] [PubMed]
70. Tague, L.K.; Bedair, B.; Witt, C.; Byers, D.E.; Vazquez-Guillamet, R.; Kulkarni, H.; Alexander-Brett, J.; Nava, R.; Puri, V.; Kreisel, D.; et al. Lung protective ventilation based on donor size is associated with a lower risk of severe primary graft dysfunction after lung transplantation. *J. Heart Lung Transplant.* **2021**, *40*, 1212–1222. [CrossRef]
71. Upala, S.; Panichsillapakit, T.; Wijarnpreecha, K.; Jaruvongvanich, V.; Sanguankeo, A. Underweight and obesity increase the risk of mortality after lung transplantation: A systematic review and meta-analysis. *Transpl. Int.* **2016**, *29*, 285–296. [CrossRef]
72. Porteous, M.K.; Lee, J.C.; Lederer, D.J.; Palmer, S.M.; Cantu, E.; Shah, R.J.; Bellamy, S.L.; Lama, V.N.; Bhorade, S.M.; Crespo, M.M.; et al. Clinical Risk Factors and Prognostic Model for Primary Graft Dysfunction after Lung Transplantation in Patients with Pulmonary Hypertension. *Ann. Am. Thorac. Soc.* **2017**, *14*, 1514–1522. [CrossRef]
73. Catelli, C.; D'Alessandro, M.; Lloret Madrid, A.; Fossi, A.; Franchi, F.; Bennett, D.; Paladini, P.; Bargagli, E.; Luzzi, L. Donor-Recipient Mismatch in Lung Transplantation: The Role of Graft Sizing in Clinical Outcomes. *Transpl. Int.* **2025**, *38*, 14387. [CrossRef]
74. Eberlein, M.; Reed, R.M.; Bolukbas, S.; Diamond, J.M.; Wille, K.M.; Orens, J.B.; Brower, R.G.; Christie, J.D. Lung size mismatch and primary graft dysfunction after bilateral lung transplantation. *J. Heart Lung Transplant.* **2015**, *34*, 233–240. [CrossRef] [PubMed]
75. Neizer, H.; Singh, G.B.; Gupta, S.; Singh, S.K. Addressing donor-organ shortages using extended criteria in lung transplantation. *Ann. Cardiothorac. Surg.* **2019**, *9*, 49–50. [CrossRef] [PubMed]
76. D'Alessandro, D.; Schroder, J.; Meyer, D.M.; Vidic, A.; Shudo, Y.; Silvestry, S.; Leacche, M.; Sciortino, C.M.; Rodrigo, M.E.; Pham, S.M.; et al. Impact of controlled hypothermic preservation on outcomes following heart transplantation. *J. Heart Lung Transplant.* **2024**, *43*, 1153–1161. [CrossRef] [PubMed]
77. Hoetzenecker, K.; Ali, A.; Campo-Cañaveral de la Cruz, J.; Schwarz, S.; Crowley Carrasco, S.; Romero Roman, A.; Aladaileh, M.; Benazzo, A.; Jaksch, P.; Wakeam, E.; et al. Prolonged Preservation of up to 24 Hours at 10 °C Does Not Impact Outcomes after Lung Transplantation. *Ann. Surg.* **2025**, *281*, 664–670. [CrossRef]
78. Kukreja, J.; Campo-Canaveral de la Cruz, J.L.; Van Raemdonck, D.; Cantu, E.; Date, H.; D'Ovidio, F.; Hartwig, M.; Klapper, J.A.; Kelly, R.F.; Lindstedt, S.; et al. The 2024 American Association for Thoracic Surgery expert consensus document: Current standards in donor lung procurement and preservation. *J. Thorac. Cardiovasc. Surg.* **2025**, *169*, 484–504. [CrossRef]
79. Bobba, C.M.; Saha, B.; Stukov, Y.; Kugler, L.; Aladaileh, M.A.; Oduntan, O.; Weir, W.; Jacobs, J.P.; Gries, C.; Emtiazjoo, A.; et al. One-year clinical outcomes of an observational study of static lung preservation at 10° centigrade and semi-elective lung transplantation. *JHLT Open* **2025**, *9*, 100241. [CrossRef]
80. Abdelnour-Berchtold, E.; Ali, A.; Baciu, C.; Beroncal, E.L.; Wang, A.; Hough, O.; Kawashima, M.; Chen, M.; Zhang, Y.; Liu, M.; et al. Evaluation of 10 °C as the optimal storage temperature for aspiration-injured donor lungs in a large animal transplant model. *J. Heart Lung Transplant.* **2022**, *41*, 1679–1688. [CrossRef]
81. Ali, A.; Wang, A.; Ribeiro, R.V.P.; Beroncal, E.L.; Baciu, C.; Galasso, M.; Gomes, B.; Mariscal, A.; Hough, O.; Brambate, E.; et al. Static lung storage at 10 °C maintains mitochondrial health and preserves donor organ function. *Sci. Transl. Med.* **2021**, *13*, eabf7601. [CrossRef]
82. Wang, A.; Ali, A.; Baciu, C.; Bellissimo, C.; Siebiger, G.; Yamanashi, K.; Montagne, J.; Garza, G.; Goligher, E.; Keshavjee, S.; et al. Metabolomic studies reveal an organ-protective hibernation state in donor lungs preserved at 10 °C. *J. Thorac. Cardiovasc. Surg.* **2025**, *169*, 796–810.e791. [CrossRef]

83. Yamanashi, K.; Wang, A.; Bellissimo, C.A.; Siebiger, G.; Oliveira, P.; Zhang, Y.; Montagne, J.; Garza, G.; Furie, N.; Pal, P.; et al. Protective effects of 10 °C preservation on donor lungs with lipopolysaccharide-induced acute lung injury. *J. Thorac. Cardiovasc. Surg.* **2025**, *169*, e74–e87. [CrossRef]
84. Noda, K.; Philips, B.J.; Snyder, M.E.; Phillippi, J.A.; Sullivan, M.; Stolz, D.B.; Ren, X.; Luketich, J.D.; Sanchez, P.G. Heparanase inhibition preserves the endothelial glycocalyx in lung grafts and improves lung preservation and transplant outcomes. *Sci. Rep.* **2021**, *11*, 12265. [CrossRef]
85. Sladden, T.M.; Yerkovich, S.; Wall, D.; Tan, M.; Hunt, W.; Hill, J.; Smith, I.; Hopkins, P.; Chambers, D.C. Endothelial Glycocalyx Shedding Occurs during Ex Vivo Lung Perfusion: A Pilot Study. *J. Transplant.* **2019**, *2019*, 6748242. [CrossRef]
86. Ali, A.; Hoetzenecker, K.; Cruz, J.L.C.-C.d.l.; Schwarz, S.; Barturen, M.G., Tomlinson, G.; Yeung, J.; Donahoe, L.; Yasufuku, K.; Pierre, A.; et al. Extension of Cold Static Donor Lung Preservation at 10 °C. *NEJM Evid.* **2023**, *2*, EVIDoa2300008. [CrossRef] [PubMed]
87. Chouchani, E.T.; Pell, V.R.; Gaude, E.; Aksentijević, D.; Sundier, S.Y.; Robb, E.L.; Logan, A.; Nadtochiy, S.M.; Ord, E.N.J.; Smith, A.C.; et al. Ischaemic accumulation of succinate controls reperfusion injury through mitochondrial ROS. *Nature* **2014**, *515*, 431–435. [CrossRef] [PubMed]
88. Nguyen, D.C.; Loor, G.; Carrott, P.; Shafii, A. Review of donor and recipient surgical procedures in lung transplantation. *J. Thorac. Dis.* **2019**, *11*, S1810–S1816. [CrossRef]
89. Kuipers, M.T.; van der Poll, T.; Schultz, M.J.; Wieland, C.W. Bench-to-bedside review: Damage-associated molecular patterns in the onset of ventilator-induced lung injury. *Crit. Care* **2011**, *15*, 235. [CrossRef]
90. Mehew, J.D.; Hogg, R.; Clark, S.; Santhanakrishnan, K.; Catarino, P.; Mascaro, J.; Stock, U.; Dark, J. Risk of prolonged ischemic time linked to use of cardiopulmonary bypass during implantation for lung transplantation in the United Kingdom. *J. Heart Lung Transplant.* **2023**, *42*, 1378–1396. [CrossRef] [PubMed]
91. Iske, J.; Hinze, C.A.; Salman, J.; Haverich, A.; Tullius, S.G.; Ius, F. The potential of ex vivo lung perfusion on improving organ quality and ameliorating ischemia reperfusion injury. *Am. J. Transplant.* **2021**, *21*, 3831–3839. [CrossRef]
92. Casillan, A.J.; Zhou, A.L.; Ruck, J.M.; Larson, E.L.; Etchill, E.W.; Ha, J.S.; Shah, P.D.; Merlo, C.A.; Bush, E.L. The effect of allograft ischemic time on outcomes following bilateral, single, and reoperative lung transplantation. *J. Thorac. Cardiovasc. Surg.* **2024**, *167*, 556–565.e558. [CrossRef]
93. Ahmed, H.; Saez, D.G.; Zych, B.; Dunning, J.; Khoshbin, E. Moderately Prolonged Cold Ischemic Time. Does It Impact Outcome of Lung Transplantation. *J. Heart Lung Transplant.* **2023**, *42*, S527–S528. [CrossRef]
94. Elgharably, H.; Javorski, M.J.; McCurry, K.R. Bilateral sequential lung transplantation: Technical aspects. *J. Thorac. Dis.* **2021**, *13*, 6564–6575. [CrossRef] [PubMed]
95. Beller, J.P.; Byler, M.R.; Money, D.T.; Chancellor, W.Z.; Zhang, A.; Zhao, Y.; Stoler, M.H.; Narahari, A.K.; Shannon, A.; Mehaffey, J.H.; et al. Reduced-flow ex vivo lung perfusion to rehabilitate lungs donated after circulatory death. *J. Heart Lung. Transplant.* **2020**, *39*, 74–82. [CrossRef] [PubMed]
96. Barnes, L.; Reed, R.M.; Parekh, K.R.; Bhama, J.K.; Pena, T.; Rajagopal, S.; Schmidt, G.A.; Klesney-Tait, J.A.; Eberlein, M. Mechanical ventilation for the lung transplant recipient. *Curr. Pulmonol. Rep.* **2015**, *4*, 88–96. [CrossRef]
97. Rijn, R.v.; Schurink, I.J.; Vries, Y.d.; Berg, A.P.v.d.; Cerisuelo, M.C.; Murad, S.D.; Erdmann, J.I.; Gilbo, N.; Haas, R.J.d.; Heaton, N.; et al. Hypothermic Machine Perfusion in Liver Transplantation—A Randomized Trial. *N. Engl. J. Med.* **2021**, *384*, 1391–1401. [CrossRef]
98. Schlegel, A.; Porte, R.; Dutkowski, P. Protective mechanisms and current clinical evidence of hypothermic oxygenated machine perfusion (HOPE) in preventing post-transplant cholangiopathy. *J. Hepatol.* **2022**, *76*, 1330–1347. [CrossRef]
99. Minor, T.; von Horn, C.; Zlatev, H.; Saner, F.; Grawe, M.; Lüer, B.; Huessler, E.M.; Kuklik, N.; Paul, A. Controlled oxygenated rewarming as novel end-ischemic therapy for cold stored liver grafts. A randomized controlled trial. *Clin. Transl. Sci.* **2022**, *15*, 2918–2927. [CrossRef]
100. Hoyer, D.P.; Benkö, T.; Manka, P.; von Horn, C.; Treckmann, J.W.; Paul, A.; Minor, T. Long-term Outcomes After Controlled Oxygenated Rewarming of Human Livers Before Transplantation. *Transplant. Direct* **2020**, *6*, e542. [CrossRef]
101. Collins, M.G.; Chadban, S.J. Dealing With Delayed Graft Function. *Transplantation* **2024**, *108*, 1273–1274. [CrossRef]
102. Beyersdorf, F. The use of controlled reperfusion strategies in cardiac surgery to minimize ischaemia/reperfusion damage. *Cardiovasc. Res.* **2009**, *83*, 262–268. [CrossRef]
103. Schnickel, G.T.; Ross, D.J.; Beygui, R.; Shefizadeh, A.; Laks, H.; Saggar, R.; Lynch, J.P., 3rd; Ardehali, A. Modified reperfusion in clinical lung transplantation: The results of 100 consecutive cases. *J. Thorac. Cardiovasc. Surg.* **2006**, *131*, 218–223. [CrossRef]
104. Shaver, C.M.; Wickersham, N.; McNeil, J.B.; Nagata, H.; Miller, A.; Landstreet, S.R.; Kuck, J.L.; Diamond, J.M.; Lederer, D.J.; Kawut, S.M.; et al. Cell-free hemoglobin promotes primary graft dysfunction through oxidative lung endothelial injury. *JCI Insight* **2018**, *3*, e98546. [CrossRef] [PubMed]

105. Ellman, P.I.; Alvis, J.S.; Tache-Leon, C.; Singh, R.; Reece, T.B.; Kern, J.A.; Tribble, C.G.; Kron, I.L. Hyperoxic ventilation exacerbates lung reperfusion injury. *J. Thorac. Cardiovasc. Surg.* **2005**, *130*, 1440.e1–1440.e8. [CrossRef] [PubMed]
106. Beer, A.; Reed, R.M.; Bölükbas, S.; Budev, M.; Chaux, G.; Zamora, M.R.; Snell, G.; Orens, J.B.; Klesney-Tait, J.A.; Schmidt, G.A.; et al. Mechanical Ventilation after Lung Transplantation. An International Survey of Practices and Preferences. *Ann. Am. Thorac. Soc.* **2014**, *11*, 546–553. [CrossRef] [PubMed]
107. Dezube, R.; Arnaoutakis, G.J.; Reed, R.M.; Bolukbas, S.; Shah, A.S.; Orens, J.B.; Brower, R.G.; Eberlein, M. The effect of lung-size mismatch on mechanical ventilation tidal volumes after bilateral lung transplantation. *Interact. Cardiovasc. Thorac. Surg.* **2013**, *16*, 275–281. [CrossRef]
108. Chapin, K.C.; Dragnich, A.G.; Gannon, W.D.; Martel, A.K.; Bacchetta, M.; Erasmus, D.B.; Shaver, C.M.; Trindade, A.J. Risk factors and clinical consequences of early extubation failure in lung transplant recipients. *JHLT Open* **2024**, *4*, 100046. [CrossRef]
109. Habib, A.; Gouchoe, D.A.; Rosenheck, J.P.; Mokadam, N.A.; Henn, M.C.; Nunley, D.R.; Ramsammy, V.; Whitson, B.A.; Ganapathi, A.M. Early Extubation: Who Qualifies Postoperatively in Lung Transplantation? *J. Surg. Res.* **2024**, *299*, 303–312. [CrossRef]
110. Kao, C.C.; Parulekar, A.D. Postoperative management of lung transplant recipients. *J. Thorac. Dis.* **2019**, *11*, S1782–S1788. [CrossRef]
111. Duan, Q.; Zhang, Y.; Yang, D. Perioperative fluid management for lung transplantation is challenging. *Heliyon* **2023**, *9*, e14704. [CrossRef]
112. Currey, J.; Pilcher, D.V.; Davies, A.; Scheinkestel, C.; Botti, M.; Bailey, M.; Snell, G. Implementation of a management guideline aimed at minimizing the severity of primary graft dysfunction after lung transplant. *J. Thorac. Cardiovasc. Surg.* **2010**, *139*, 154–161. [CrossRef]
113. Laskey, D.; Housman, B.; Dawodu, G.; Scheinin, S. Intraoperative Extracorporeal Support during Lung Transplantation: Not Just for the High-Risk Patient. *J. Clin. Med.* **2024**, *13*, 192. [CrossRef]
114. Coster, J.N.; Loor, G. Extracorporeal life support during lung transplantation. *Indian J. Thorac. Cardiovasc. Surg.* **2021**, *37*, 476–483. [CrossRef]
115. Bermudez, C.A.; Shiose, A.; Esper, S.A.; Shigemura, N.; D'Cunha, J.; Bhama, J.K.; Richards, T.J.; Arlia, P.; Crespo, M.M.; Pilewski, J.M. Outcomes of Intraoperative Venoarterial Extracorporeal Membrane Oxygenation Versus Cardiopulmonary Bypass During Lung Transplantation. *Ann. Thorac. Surg.* **2014**, *98*, 1936–1943. [CrossRef]
116. Gray, A.L.; Mulvihill, M.S.; Hartwig, M.G. Lung transplantation at Duke. *J. Thorac. Dis.* **2016**, *8*, E185–E196. [CrossRef] [PubMed]
117. Luu, H.Y.; Santos, J.; Isaza, E.; Brzezinski, M.; Kukreja, J. Management of primary graft dysfunction after lung transplantation with extracorporeal life support: An evidence-based review. *J. Thorac. Dis.* **2023**, *15*, 4090–4100. [CrossRef] [PubMed]
118. Paulo, N.; Prunet, H.; Armoiry, X.; Hugon-Vallet, E.; Mocan, R.; Portran, P.; Sebbag, L.; Pozzi, M.; Baudry, G. Outcome of primary graft dysfunction rescued by venoarterial extracorporeal membrane oxygenation after heart transplantation. *Arch. Cardiovasc. Dis.* **2022**, *115*, 426–435. [CrossRef] [PubMed]
119. Boffini, M.; Simonato, E.; Ricci, D.; Scalini, F.; Marro, M.; Pidello, S.; Attisani, M.; Solidoro, P.; Lausi, P.O.; Fanelli, V.; et al. Extracorporeal membrane oxygenation after lung transplantation: Risk factors and outcomes analysis. *Ann. Cardiothorac. Surg.* **2019**, *8*, 54–61. [CrossRef]
120. Gulack, B.C.; Hirji, S.A.; Hartwig, M.G. Bridge to lung transplantation and rescue post-transplant: The expanding role of extracorporeal membrane oxygenation. *J. Thorac. Dis.* **2014**, *6*, 1070–1079.
121. Hatami, S.; Conway, J.; Freed, D.H.; Urschel, S. Thoracic organ donation after circulatory determination of death. *Transplant. Rep.* **2023**, *8*, 100125. [CrossRef]
122. Keshavamurthy, S.; Rodgers-Fischl, P. Donation after circulatory death (DCD)-lung procurement. *Indian J. Thorac. Cardiovasc. Surg.* **2021**, *37*, 425–432. [CrossRef]
123. Carteaux, G.; Parfait, M.; Combet, M.; Haudebourg, A.F.; Tuffet, S.; Mekontso Dessap, A. Patient-Self Inflicted Lung Injury: A Practical Review. *J. Clin. Med.* **2021**, *10*, 2738. [CrossRef] [PubMed]
124. Chi, Y.; Zhao, Z.; Frerichs, I.; Long, Y.; He, H. Prevalence and prognosis of respiratory pendelluft phenomenon in mechanically ventilated ICU patients with acute respiratory failure: A retrospective cohort study. *Ann. Intensive Care* **2022**, *12*, 22. [CrossRef] [PubMed]
125. Sklienka, P.; Frelich, M.; Burša, F. Patient Self-Inflicted Lung Injury-A Narrative Review of Pathophysiology, Early Recognition, and Management Options. *J. Pers. Med.* **2023**, *13*, 593. [CrossRef] [PubMed]
126. Stengl, M.; Ledvinova, L.; Chvojka, J.; Benes, J.; Jarkovska, D.; Holas, J.; Soukup, P.; Sviglerová, J.; Matejovic, M. Effects of clinically relevant acute hypercapnic and metabolic acidosis on the cardiovascular system: An experimental porcine study. *Crit. Care* **2013**, *17*, R303. [CrossRef]
127. Sylvester, J.T.; Shimoda, L.A.; Aaronson, P.I.; Ward, J.P. Hypoxic pulmonary vasoconstriction. *Physiol. Rev.* **2012**, *92*, 367–520. [CrossRef]

128. Prag, H.A.; Murphy, M.P.; Krieg, T. Preventing mitochondrial reverse electron transport as a strategy for cardioprotection. *Basic Res. Cardiol.* **2023**, *118*, 34. [CrossRef]
129. Gwoździńska, P.; Buchbinder, B.A.; Mayer, K.; Herold, S.; Morty, R.E.; Seeger, W.; Vadász, I. Hypercapnia Impairs ENaC Cell Surface Stability by Promoting Phosphorylation, Polyubiquitination and Endocytosis of β-ENaC in a Human Alveolar Epithelial Cell Line. *Front. Immunol.* **2017**, *8*, 591. [CrossRef]
130. Huppert, L.A.; Matthay, M.A. Alveolar Fluid Clearance in Pathologically Relevant Conditions: In Vitro and In Vivo Models of Acute Respiratory Distress Syndrome. *Front. Immunol.* **2017**, *8*, e00371. [CrossRef]
131. Vadász, I.; Sznajder, J.I. Gas Exchange Disturbances Regulate Alveolar Fluid Clearance during Acute Lung Injury. *Front. Immunol.* **2017**, *8*, 757. [CrossRef]
132. Alzahrani, A.; Noda, K.; Chan, E.G.; Ryan, J.P.; Furukawa, M.; Sanchez, P.G. The length of the warm ischemic interval in lung donation after circulatory death does not impact post-transplantation outcomes. *JHLT Open* **2025**, *8*, 100244. [CrossRef]
133. Berg, A.R.; Choi, A.Y.; Zhou, A.; MacArthur, J.W. From proxy to precision: The growing need to capture true warm ischemic time in donation-after-circulatory-death heart transplantation. *J. Heart Lung Transplant.* 2025, *in press*. [CrossRef] [PubMed]
134. Van Raemdonck, D.; Ceulemans, L.J.; Neyrinck, A.; Levvey, B.; Snell, G.I. Donation After Circulatory Death in lung transplantation. *Thorac. Surg. Clin.* **2022**, *32*, 153–165. [CrossRef] [PubMed]
135. Lazzeri, C.; Bonizzoli, M.; Di Valvasone, S.; Peris, A. Uncontrolled Donation after Circulatory Death Only Lung Program: An Urgent Opportunity. *J. Clin. Med.* **2023**, *12*, 6492. [CrossRef] [PubMed]
136. Bello, I.; Palleschi, A.; Cypel, M.; Argudo, E.; Sandiumenge, A. Unlocking the Potential of Uncontrolled DCD in Lung Transplantation: A Review of Two Decades of Experience. *JHLT Open* **2025**, *10*, 100374. [CrossRef]
137. Wong, A.; Liu, M. Inflammatory responses in lungs from donation after brain death: Mechanisms and potential therapeutic targets. *J. Heart Lung Transplant.* **2021**, *40*, 890–896. [CrossRef]
138. Baciu, C.; Sage, A.; Zamel, R.; Shin, J.; Bai, X.-H.; Hough, O.; Bhat, M.; Yeung, J.C.; Cypel, M.; Keshavjee, S.; et al. Transcriptomic investigation reveals donor-specific gene signatures in human lung transplants. *Eur. Respir. J.* **2021**, *57*, 2000327. [CrossRef]
139. Sommer, S.P.; Sommer, S.; Sinha, B.; Wiedemann, J.; Otto, C.; Aleksic, I.; Schimmer, C.; Leyh, R.G. Ischemia-reperfusion injury-induced pulmonary mitochondrial damage. *J. Heart Lung Transplant.* **2011**, *30*, 811–818. [CrossRef]
140. Baniene, R.; Trumbeckas, D.; Kincius, M.; Pauziene, N.; Raudone, L.; Jievaltas, M.; Trumbeckaite, S. Short ischemia induces rat kidney mitochondria dysfunction. *J. Bioenerg. Biomembr.* **2016**, *48*, 77–85. [CrossRef]
141. Zhang, L.; Zhang, S.N.; Li, L.; Zhang, X.B.; Wu, R.C.; Liu, J.H.; Huang, Z.Y.; Li, W.; Ran, J.H. Prolonged warm ischemia aggravates hepatic mitochondria damage and apoptosis in DCD liver by regulating Ca(2+)/CaM/CaMKII signaling pathway. *Int. J. Clin. Exp. Pathol.* **2019**, *12*, 217–228.
142. Parrilla, G.A.; Hunt, W.R.; Daneshmand, M.A. Lung transplantation following donation after circulatory death. *Transplant. Rep.* **2022**, *7*, 100110. [CrossRef]
143. Malas, J.; Chen, Q.; Thomas, J.; Emerson, D.; Megna, D.; Esmailian, F.; Bowdish, M.E.; Chikwe, J.; Catarino, P. The impact of thoracoabdominal normothermic regional perfusion on early outcomes in donation after circulatory death lung transplantation. *J. Heart Lung Transplant.* **2023**, *42*, 1040–1044. [CrossRef] [PubMed]
144. Chang, S.H.; Geraci, T.C.; Piper, G.L.; Chan, J.; James, L.; Paone, D.; Sommer, P.M.; Natalini, J.; Rudym, D.; Lesko, M.; et al. Outcomes of lung and heart-lung transplants utilizing donor after circulatory death with thoracoabdominal normothermic regional perfusion. *JHLT Open* **2024**, *4*, 100058. [CrossRef] [PubMed]
145. Alderete, I.S.; Pontula, A.; Halpern, S.E.; Patel, K.J.; Klapper, J.A.; Hartwig, M.G. Thoracoabdominal Normothermic Regional Perfusion and Donation After Circulatory Death Lung Use. *JAMA Netw. Open* **2025**, *8*, e2460033. [CrossRef]
146. Goff, R.R.; Daly, R.C.; Lease, E.D. Ex Vivo Lung Perfusion on Donor Lungs in the United States: National Trends and Post-Transplant Outcomes. *J. Heart Lung Transplant.* **2020**, *39*, S217. [CrossRef]
147. Divithotawela, C.; Cypel, M.; Martinu, T.; Singer, L.G.; Binnie, M.; Chow, C.-W.; Chaparro, C.; Waddell, T.K.; de Perrot, M.; Pierre, A.; et al. Long-term Outcomes of Lung Transplant With Ex Vivo Lung Perfusion. *JAMA Surg.* **2019**, *154*, 1143–1150. [CrossRef]
148. Abul Kashem, M.; Loor, G.; Hartwig, M.; Van Raemdonck, D.; Villavicencio, M.; Ius, F.; Ghadimi, K.; Salman, J.; Chandrashekaran, S.; Machuca, T.; et al. A multicenter analysis of lung transplantation outcomes comparing donation after circulatory death and donation after brain death. *JHLT Open* **2024**, *6*, 100132. [CrossRef]
149. Gandhi, N.N.; DeSantis, J.; Miskoff, J.A. Breathing New Life Into Donation After Circulatory Death (DCD) Lung Transplantation: The Role of Machine Perfusion. *Cureus* **2025**, *17*, e87196. [CrossRef]
150. Al Salihi, M.; Alsalihi, Y.; Cahill, J. Boosting lung transplantation, a narrative review of the impact of donor after cardiac death, organ care system and ex vivo lung perfusion in expanding donor pool. *Curr. Chall. Thorac. Surg.* **2022**, *5*, 19. [CrossRef]
151. Curley, G.F.; Laffey, J.G.; Zhang, H.; Slutsky, A.S. Biotrauma and Ventilator-Induced Lung Injury: Clinical Implications. *Chest* **2016**, *150*, 1109–1117. [CrossRef]

152. Lohser, J.; Slinger, P. Lung Injury After One-Lung Ventilation: A Review of the Pathophysiologic Mechanisms Affecting the Ventilated and the Collapsed Lung. *Anesth. Analg.* **2015**, *121*, 302–318. [CrossRef]
153. Sha, Y.; Xu, R.; Shao, S.; Yang, J.; Tang, B.; Liang, Q.; Wang, Z. Tailored single-lung ventilation approaches and postoperative pulmonary outcomes in thoracic surgery. *J. Thorac. Dis.* **2025**, *17*, 5371–5387. [CrossRef] [PubMed]
154. De Perrot, M.; McRae, K. Left ventricular lusitropy and primary graft dysfunction in lung transplantation. *J. Heart Lung Transplant.* **2019**, *38*, 719–720. [CrossRef] [PubMed]
155. Jin, Z.; Hana, Z.; Alam, A.; Rajalingam, S.; Abayalingam, M.; Wang, Z.; Ma, D. Review 1: Lung transplant-from donor selection to graft preparation. *J. Anesth.* **2020**, *34*, 561–574. [CrossRef] [PubMed]
156. Brower, R.G.; Matthay, M.A.; Morris, A.; Schoenfeld, D.; Thompson, B.T.; Wheeler, A. Ventilation with lower tidal volumes as compared with traditional tidal volumes for acute lung injury and the acute respiratory distress syndrome. *N. Engl. J. Med.* **2000**, *342*, 1301–1308. [CrossRef]
157. Briel, M.; Meade, M.; Mercat, A.; Brower, R.G.; Talmor, D.; Walter, S.D.; Slutsky, A.S.; Pullenayegum, E.; Zhou, Q.; Cook, D.; et al. Higher vs lower positive end-expiratory pressure in patients with acute lung injury and acute respiratory distress syndrome: Systematic review and meta-analysis. *JAMA* **2010**, *303*, 865–873. [CrossRef]
158. Ranieri, V.M.; Suter, P.M.; Tortorella, C.; De Tullio, R.; Dayer, J.M.; Brienza, A.; Bruno, F.; Slutsky, A.S. Effect of mechanical ventilation on inflammatory mediators in patients with acute respiratory distress syndrome: A randomized controlled trial. *JAMA* **1999**, *282*, 54–61. [CrossRef]
159. O'Croinin, D.; Ni Chonghaile, M.; Higgins, B.; Laffey, J.G. Bench-to-bedside review: Permissive hypercapnia. *Crit. Care* **2004**, *9*, 51. [CrossRef]
160. Peltekova, V.; Engelberts, D.; Otulakowski, G.; Uematsu, S.; Post, M.; Kavanagh, B.P. Hypercapnic acidosis in ventilator-induced lung injury. *Intensive Care Med.* **2010**, *36*, 869–878. [CrossRef]
161. Wu, S.Y.; Li, M.H.; Ko, F.C.; Wu, G.C.; Huang, K.L.; Chu, S.J. Protective effect of hypercapnic acidosis in ischemia-reperfusion lung injury is attributable to upregulation of heme oxygenase-1. *PLoS ONE* **2013**, *8*, e74742. [CrossRef]
162. Wu, S.Y.; Wu, C.P.; Kang, B.H.; Li, M.H.; Chu, S.J.; Huang, K.L. Hypercapnic acidosis attenuates reperfusion injury in isolated and perfused rat lungs. *Crit. Care Med* **2012**, *40*, 553–559. [CrossRef] [PubMed]
163. Steen, S.; Liao, Q.; Wierup, P.N.; Bolys, R.; Pierre, L.; Sjöberg, T. Transplantation of lungs from non-heart-beating donors after functional assessment ex vivo. *Ann. Thorac. Surg.* **2003**, *76*, 244–252; discussion 252. [CrossRef] [PubMed]
164. Steen, S.; Sjöberg, T.; Pierre, L.; Liao, Q.; Eriksson, L.; Algotsson, L. Transplantation of lungs from a non-heart-beating donor. *Lancet* **2001**, *357*, 825–829. [CrossRef] [PubMed]
165. Cypel, M.; Yeung, J.C.; Liu, M.; Anraku, M.; Chen, F.; Karolak, W.; Sato, M.; Laratta, J.; Azad, S.; Madonik, M.; et al. Normothermic Ex Vivo Lung Perfusion in Clinical Lung Transplantation. *N. Engl. J. Med.* **2011**, *364*, 1431–1440. [CrossRef]
166. Prasad, N.K.; Pasrija, C.; Talaie, T.; Krupnick, A.S.; Zhao, Y.; Lau, C.L. Ex Vivo Lung Perfusion: Current Achievements and Future Directions. *Transplantation* **2021**, *105*, 979–985. [CrossRef]
167. Kanou, T.; Nakahira, K.; Choi, A.M.; Yeung, J.C.; Cypel, M.; Liu, M.; Keshavjee, S. Cell-free DNA in human ex vivo lung perfusate as a potential biomarker to predict the risk of primary graft dysfunction in lung transplantation. *J. Thorac. Cardiovasc. Surg.* **2021**, *162*, 490–499.e492. [CrossRef]
168. Boffini, M.; Marro, M.; Simonato, E.; Scalini, F.; Costamagna, A.; Fanelli, V.; Barbero, C.; Solidoro, P.; Brazzi, L.; Rinaldi, M. Cytokines Removal During Ex-Vivo Lung Perfusion: Initial Clinical Experience. *Transpl. Int.* **2023**, *36*, 10777. [CrossRef]
169. Ponholzer, F.; Dumfarth, J.; Krapf, C.; Pircher, A.; Hautz, T.; Wolf, D.; Augustin, F.; Schneeberger, S. The impact and relevance of techniques and fluids on lung injury in machine perfusion of lungs. *Front. Immunol.* **2024**, *15*, e1358153. [CrossRef]
170. Hasenauer, A.; Bédat, B.; Parapanov, R.; Lugrin, J.; Debonneville, A.; Abdelnour-Berchtold, E.; Gonzalez, M.; Perentes, J.Y.; Piquilloud, L.; Szabo, C.; et al. Effects of cold or warm ischemia and ex-vivo lung perfusion on the release of damage associated molecular patterns and inflammatory cytokines in experimental lung transplantation. *J. Heart Lung Transplant.* **2021**, *40*, 905–916. [CrossRef]
171. Gouchoe, D.A.; Cui, E.Y.; Satija, D.; Henn, M.C.; Choi, K.; Rosenheck, J.P.; Nunley, D.R.; Mokadam, N.A.; Ganapathi, A.M.; Whitson, B.A. Ex Vivo Lung Perfusion and Primary Graft Dysfunction Following Lung Transplantation: A Contemporary United Network for Organ Sharing Database Analysis. *J. Clin. Med.* **2024**, *13*, 4440. [CrossRef]
172. Benazzo, A.; Peel, J.; Mariscal, A.; Yeung, J.; Aversa, M.; Keshavjee, S.; Cypel, M. Differential outcomes of ISHLT PGD 3 after ex-vivo lung perfusion compared to PGD 3 after direct transplantation. *J. Heart Lung Transplant.* 2025, *in press*. [CrossRef] [PubMed]
173. Lightle, W.; Daoud, D.; Loor, G. Breathing lung transplantation with the Organ Care System (OCS) Lung: Lessons learned and future implications. *J. Thorac. Dis.* **2019**, *11*, S1755–S1760. [CrossRef] [PubMed]

174. Warnecke, G.; Van Raemdonck, D.; Smith, M.A.; Massard, G.; Kukreja, J.; Rea, F.; Loor, G.; De Robertis, F.; Nagendran, J.; Dhital, K.K.; et al. Normothermic ex-vivo preservation with the portable Organ Care System Lung device for bilateral lung transplantation (INSPIRE): A randomised, open-label, non-inferiority, phase 3 study. *Lancet Respir. Med.* **2018**, *6*, 357–367. [CrossRef] [PubMed]
175. Gao, Q.; Kahan, R.; Gonzalez, T.J.; Zhang, M.; Alderete, I.S.; DeLaura, I.; Kesseli, S.J.; Song, M.; Asokan, A.; Barbas, A.S.; et al. Gene delivery followed by ex vivo lung perfusion using an adeno-associated viral vector in a rodent lung transplant model. *J. Thorac. Cardiovasc. Surg.* **2024**, *167*, e131–e139. [CrossRef]
176. Nykänen, A.I.; Mariscal, A.; Duong, A.; Estrada, C.; Ali, A.; Hough, O.; Sage, A.; Chao, B.T.; Chen, M.; Gokhale, H.; et al. Engineered mesenchymal stromal cell therapy during human lung ex vivo lung perfusion is compromised by acidic lung microenvironment. *Mol. Ther. Methods Clin. Dev.* **2021**, *23*, 184–197. [CrossRef]
177. Machuca, T.N.; Cypel, M.; Bonato, R.; Yeung, J.C.; Chun, Y.M.; Juvet, S.; Guan, Z.; Hwang, D.M.; Chen, M.; Saito, T.; et al. Safety and Efficacy of Ex Vivo Donor Lung Adenoviral IL-10 Gene Therapy in a Large Animal Lung Transplant Survival Model. *Hum. Gene Ther.* **2017**, *28*, 757–765. [CrossRef]
178. Oishi, H.; Juvet, S.C.; Martinu, T.; Sato, M.; Medin, J.A.; Liu, M.; Keshavjee, S. A novel combined ex vivo and in vivo lentiviral interleukin-10 gene delivery strategy at the time of transplantation decreases chronic lung allograft rejection in mice. *J. Thorac. Cardiovasc. Surg.* **2018**, *156*, 1305–1315. [CrossRef]
179. Nakata, K.; Alderete, I.S.; Hughes, B.A.; Hartwig, M.G. Ex vivo lung perfusion: Recent advancements and future directions. *Front. Immunol.* **2025**, *16*, e1513546. [CrossRef]
180. Coggins, M.P.; Bloch, K.D. Nitric Oxide in the Pulmonary Vasculature. *Arterioscler. Thromb. Vasc. Biol.* **2007**, *27*, 1877–1885. [CrossRef]
181. Klinger, J.R.; Kadowitz, P.J. The Nitric Oxide Pathway in Pulmonary Vascular Disease. *Am. J. Cardiol.* **2017**, *120*, S71–S79. [CrossRef]
182. Radi, R. Oxygen radicals, nitric oxide, and peroxynitrite: Redox pathways in molecular medicine. *Proc. Natl. Acad. Sci. USA* **2018**, *115*, 5839–5848. [CrossRef]
183. Kumar, A.; Noda, K.; Philips, B.; Velayutham, M.; Stolz, D.B.; Gladwin, M.T.; Shiva, S.; D'Cunha, J. Nitrite attenuates mitochondrial impairment and vascular permeability induced by ischemia-reperfusion injury in the lung. *Am. J. Physiol. Lung Cell. Mol. Physiol.* **2020**, *318*, L580–L591. [CrossRef]
184. Meade, M.O.; Granton, J.T.; Matte-Martyn, A.; McRae, K.; Weaver, B.; Cripps, P.; Keshavjee, S.H. A randomized trial of inhaled nitric oxide to prevent ischemia-reperfusion injury after lung transplantation. *Am. J. Respir. Crit. Care Med.* **2003**, *167*, 1483–1489. [CrossRef] [PubMed]
185. Cerier, E.; Lung, K.; Bharat, A. Role of Pulmonary Vasodilators in Ameliorating Primary Graft Dysfunction Following Lung Transplant. *JAMA Surg.* **2022**, *157*, e215857. [CrossRef] [PubMed]
186. Chin, B.Y.; Jiang, G.; Wegiel, B.; Wang, H.J.; Macdonald, T.; Zhang, X.C.; Gallo, D.; Cszimadia, E.; Bach, F.H.; Lee, P.J.; et al. Hypoxia-inducible factor 1alpha stabilization by carbon monoxide results in cytoprotective preconditioning. *Proc. Natl. Acad. Sci. USA* **2007**, *104*, 5109–5114. [CrossRef] [PubMed]
187. Kohmoto, J.; Nakao, A.; Kaizu, T.; Tsung, A.; Ikeda, A.; Tomiyama, K.; Billiar, T.R.; Choi, A.M.; Murase, N.; McCurry, K.R. Low-dose carbon monoxide inhalation prevents ischemia/reperfusion injury of transplanted rat lung grafts. *Surgery* **2006**, *140*, 179–185. [CrossRef]
188. Ryter, S.W.; Choi, A.M. Targeting heme oxygenase-1 and carbon monoxide for therapeutic modulation of inflammation. *Transl. Res.* **2016**, *167*, 7–34. [CrossRef]
189. Kang, I.S.; Kim, R.I.; Kim, C. Carbon Monoxide Regulates Macrophage Differentiation and Polarization toward the M2 Phenotype through Upregulation of Heme Oxygenase 1. *Cells* **2021**, *10*, 3444. [CrossRef]
190. Chhikara, M.; Wang, S.; Kern, S.J.; Ferreyra, G.A.; Barb, J.J.; Munson, P.J.; Danner, R.L. Carbon monoxide blocks lipopolysaccharide-induced gene expression by interfering with proximal TLR4 to NF-kappaB signal transduction in human monocytes. *PLoS ONE* **2009**, *4*, e8139. [CrossRef]
191. Rosas, I.O.; Goldberg, H.J.; Collard, H.R.; El-Chemaly, S.; Flaherty, K.; Hunninghake, G.M.; Lasky, J.A.; Lederer, D.J.; Machado, R.; Martinez, F.J.; et al. A Phase II Clinical Trial of Low-Dose Inhaled Carbon Monoxide in Idiopathic Pulmonary Fibrosis. *Chest* **2018**, *153*, 94–104. [CrossRef]
192. Goebel, U.; Wollborn, J. Carbon monoxide in intensive care medicine—time to start the therapeutic application?! *Intensive Care Med. Exp.* **2020**, *8*, 2. [CrossRef]
193. Li, H.; Zhou, R.; Liu, J.; Li, Q.; Zhang, J.; Mu, J.; Sun, X. Hydrogen-Rich Saline Attenuates Lung Ischemia-Reperfusion Injury in Rabbits. *J. Surg. Res.* **2012**, *174*, e11–e16. [CrossRef]

194. Kawamura, T.; Wakabayashi, N.; Shigemura, N.; Huang, C.S.; Masutani, K.; Tanaka, Y.; Noda, K.; Peng, X.; Takahashi, T.; Billiar, T.R.; et al. Hydrogen gas reduces hyperoxic lung injury via the Nrf2 pathway in vivo. *Am. J. Physiol. Lung Cell. Mol. Physiol.* **2013**, *304*, L646–L656. [CrossRef]
195. Yang, F.; Lei, Y.; Liu, R.; Luo, X.; Li, J.; Zeng, F.; Lu, S.; Huang, X.; Lan, Y. Hydrogen: Potential Applications in Solid Organ Transplantation. *Oxid. Med. Cell. Longev.* **2021**, *2021*, 6659310. [CrossRef]
196. Obara, T.; Naito, H.; Nojima, T.; Hirayama, T.; Hongo, T.; Ageta, K.; Aokage, T.; Hisamura, M.; Yumoto, T.; Nakao, A. Hydrogen in Transplantation: Potential Applications and Therapeutic Implications. *Biomedicines* **2024**, *12*, 118. [CrossRef] [PubMed]
197. Kayawake, H.; Chen-Yoshikawa, T.F.; Saito, M.; Yamagishi, H.; Yoshizawa, A.; Hirano, S.-i.; Kurokawa, R.; Date, H. Protective Effects of a Hydrogen-Rich Preservation Solution in a Canine Lung Transplantation Model. *Ann. Thorac. Surg.* **2021**, *111*, 246–252. [CrossRef] [PubMed]
198. Oesterle, A.; Laufs, U.; Liao, J.K. Pleiotropic Effects of Statins on the Cardiovascular System. *Circ. Res.* **2017**, *120*, 229–243. [CrossRef] [PubMed]
199. Raphael, J.; Collins, S.R.; Wang, X.-Q.; Scalzo, D.C.; Singla, P.; Lau, C.L.; Kozower, B.D.; Durieux, M.E.; Blank, R.S. Perioperative statin use is associated with decreased incidence of primary graft dysfunction after lung transplantation. *J. Heart Lung Transplant.* **2017**, *36*, 948–956. [CrossRef]
200. Bello, I.; Coll, E.; Sandiumenge, A.; Romero, L.; Jauregui, A.; Pérez, J.; Ochoa, J.; Peñafiel, S.; Sánchez, L.; Ascanio, F.; et al. Do the Pretransplant Use of Statins in a Recipient Reduce the Incidence of Primary Graft Dysfunction after Lung Transplant? *J. Heart Lung Transplant.* **2019**, *38*, S226. [CrossRef]
201. Dashti-Khavidaki, S.; Saidi, R.; Lu, H. Current status of glucocorticoid usage in solid organ transplantation. *World J. Transplant.* **2021**, *11*, 443–465. [CrossRef]
202. Araujo, L.F.; Holand, A.R.; Paludo Ade, O.; Silva É, F.; Forgiarini, L.A.; Forgiarini, L.F.; Barbachan, E.S.M.; Andrade, C.F. Effect of the systemic administration of methylprednisolone on the lungs of brain-dead donor rats undergoing pulmonary transplantation. *Clinics* **2014**, *69*, 128–133. [CrossRef] [PubMed]
203. Atkinson, B.J.; Sharma, N.S. Immunosuppression in lung transplantation: A narrative review. *Curr. Chall. Thorac. Surg.* **2023**, *5*, 21. [CrossRef]
204. Paulus, P.; Holfeld, J.; Urbschat, A.; Mutlak, H.; Ockelmann, P.A.; Tacke, S.; Zacharowski, K.; Reissig, C.; Stay, D.; Scheller, B. Prednisolone as Preservation Additive Prevents from Ischemia Reperfusion Injury in a Rat Model of Orthotopic Lung Transplantation. *PLoS ONE* **2013**, *8*, e73298. [CrossRef] [PubMed]
205. Van Zanden, J.E.; Leuvenink, H.G.D.; Verschuuren, E.A.M.; Veldhuis, Z.J.; Ottens, P.J.; Erasmus, M.E.; Hottenrott, M.C. Ex Vivo Perfusion With Methylprednisolone Attenuates Brain Death-induced Lung Injury in Rats. *Transplant. Direct* **2021**, *7*, e682. [CrossRef]
206. Birk, A.V.; Liu, S.; Soong, Y.; Mills, W.; Singh, P.; Warren, J.D.; Seshan, S.V.; Pardee, J.D.; Szeto, H.H. The mitochondrial-targeted compound SS-31 re-energizes ischemic mitochondria by interacting with cardiolipin. *J. Am. Soc. Nephrol.* **2013**, *24*, 1250–1261. [CrossRef]
207. Mitchell, W.; Pharaoh, G.; Tyshkovskiy, A.; Campbell, M.; Marcinek, D.J.; Gladyshev, V.N. The Mitochondria-Targeted Peptide Therapeutic Elamipretide Improves Cardiac and Skeletal Muscle Function During Aging Without Detectable Changes in Tissue Epigenetic or Transcriptomic Age. *Aging Cell* **2025**, *24*, e70026. [CrossRef]
208. Du, X.; Zeng, Q.; Luo, Y.; He, L.; Zhao, Y.; Li, N.; Han, C.; Zhang, G.; Liu, W. Application research of novel peptide mitochondrial-targeted antioxidant SS-31 in mitigating mitochondrial dysfunction. *Mitochondrion* **2024**, *75*, 101846. [CrossRef]
209. Prag, H.A.; Aksentijevic, D.; Dannhorn, A.; Giles, A.V.; Mulvey, J.F.; Sauchanka, O.; Du, L.; Bates, G.; Reinhold, J.; Kula-Alwar, D.; et al. Ischemia-Selective Cardioprotection by Malonate for Ischemia/Reperfusion Injury. *Circ. Res.* **2022**, *131*, 528–541. [CrossRef]
210. Jiang, T.; Liu, T.; Deng, X.; Ding, W.; Yue, Z.; Yang, W.; Lv, X.; Li, W. Adiponectin ameliorates lung ischemia-reperfusion injury through SIRT1-PINK1 signaling-mediated mitophagy in type 2 diabetic rats. *Respir. Res.* **2021**, *22*, 258. [CrossRef]
211. Lee, S.E.; Kim, I.H.; Kang, Y.C.; Kim, Y.; Yu, S.H.; Yeo, J.S.; Kwon, I.; Lim, J.H.; Kim, J.H.; Han, K.; et al. Mitochondrial transplantation attenuates lipopolysaccharide-induced acute respiratory distress syndrome. *BMC Pulm. Med.* **2024**, *24*, 477. [CrossRef]
212. Miao, X.; Jiang, P.; Wang, Z.; Kong, W.; Feng, L. Mitochondrial Transplantation: A Novel Therapeutic Approach for Treating Diseases. *MedComm (2020)* **2025**, *6*, e70253. [CrossRef] [PubMed]
213. Tian, D.; Zheng, X.; Tang, H.; Huang, H.; Wang, J.; Xu, L.; Li, C.; Yan, H.; Yu, R.; Nan, J.; et al. Metformin attenuates chronic lung allograft dysfunction: Evidence in rat models. *Respir. Res.* **2023**, *24*, 192. [CrossRef] [PubMed]
214. Liu, T.; Wei, H.; Zhang, L.; Ma, C.; Wei, Y.; Jiang, T.; Li, W. Metformin attenuates lung ischemia-reperfusion injury and necroptosis through AMPK pathway in type 2 diabetic recipient rats. *BMC Pulm. Med.* **2024**, *24*, 237. [CrossRef] [PubMed]

215. Nemeth, D.V.; Iannelli, L.; Gangitano, E.; D'Andrea, V.; Bellini, M.I. Energy Metabolism and Metformin: Effects on Ischemia-Reperfusion Injury in Kidney Transplantation. *Biomedicines* **2024**, *12*, 1534. [CrossRef]
216. Wei, H.; Liu, T.-H.; Zhang, L.-J.; Yan, W.; Ma, C.; Lv, S.-H.; Zeng, X.-Z.; Li, W.-Z. Metformin alleviates lung ischemia-reperfusion injury via the SIRT1 pathway following lung transplantation in diabetic rats. *Mol. Med. Rep.* **2025**, *32*, 287. [CrossRef]
217. Gazoni, L.M.; Walters, D.M.; Unger, E.B.; Linden, J.; Kron, I.L.; Laubach, V.E. Activation of A1, A2A, or A3 adenosine receptors attenuates lung ischemia-reperfusion injury. *J. Thorac. Cardiovasc. Surg.* **2010**, *140*, 440–446. [CrossRef]
218. Gazoni, L.M.; Laubach, V.E.; Mulloy, D.P.; Bellizzi, A.; Unger, E.B.; Linden, J.; Ellman, P.I.; Lisle, T.C.; Kron, I.L. Additive protection against lung ischemia-reperfusion injury by adenosine A2A receptor activation before procurement and during reperfusion. *J. Thorac. Cardiovasc. Surg.* **2008**, *135*, 156–165. [CrossRef]
219. Stone, M.L.; Sharma, A.K.; Mas, V.R.; Gehrau, R.C.; Mulloy, D.P.; Zhao, Y.; Lau, C.L.; Kron, I.L.; Huerter, M.E.; Laubach, V.E. Ex Vivo Perfusion With Adenosine A2A Receptor Agonist Enhances Rehabilitation of Murine Donor Lungs After Circulatory Death. *Transplantation* **2015**, *99*, 2494–2503. [CrossRef]
220. Mulloy, D.P.; Stone, M.L.; Crosby, I.K.; Lapar, D.J.; Sharma, A.K.; Webb, D.V.; Lau, C.L.; Laubach, V.E.; Kron, I.L. Ex vivo rehabilitation of non-heart-beating donor lungs in preclinical porcine model: Delayed perfusion results in superior lung function. *J. Thorac. Cardiovasc. Surg.* **2012**, *144*, 1208–1215. [CrossRef]
221. Wagner, C.E.; Pope, N.H.; Charles, E.J.; Huerter, M.E.; Sharma, A.K.; Salmon, M.D.; Carter, B.T.; Stoler, M.H.; Lau, C.L.; Laubach, V.E.; et al. Ex vivo lung perfusion with adenosine A2A receptor agonist allows prolonged cold preservation of lungs donated after cardiac death. *J. Thorac. Cardiovasc. Surg.* **2016**, *151*, 538–546. [CrossRef]
222. Fleischmann, E.; Conaway, M.; Rabin, J.; Vecere, K.; Masih, K.; Zhao, Y.; Zhang, A.; Khan, M.; Mas, V.; Krupnick, A.; et al. Regadenoson in the rehabilitation of marginal donor lungs on ex-vivo lung perfusion: A blinded multi-center randomized controlled clinical trial. *JTCVS Open* **2025**. [CrossRef]
223. Iyer, S.S.; Cheng, G. Role of interleukin 10 transcriptional regulation in inflammation and autoimmune disease. *Crit. Rev. Immunol.* **2012**, *32*, 23–63. [CrossRef] [PubMed]
224. Yeung, J.C.; Wagnetz, D.; Cypel, M.; Rubacha, M.; Koike, T.; Chun, Y.-M.; Hu, J.; Waddell, T.K.; Hwang, D.M.; Liu, M.; et al. Ex Vivo Adenoviral Vector Gene Delivery Results in Decreased Vector-associated Inflammation Pre- and Post–lung Transplantation in the Pig. *Mol. Ther.* **2012**, *20*, 1204–1211. [CrossRef] [PubMed]
225. Nykänen, A.I.; Keshavjee, S.; Liu, M. Creating superior lungs for transplantation with next-generation gene therapy during ex vivo lung perfusion. *J. Heart Lung Transplant.* **2024**, *43*, 838–848. [CrossRef]
226. Mulvihill, E.E.; Drucker, D.J. Pharmacology, physiology, and mechanisms of action of dipeptidyl peptidase-4 inhibitors. *Endocr. Rev.* **2014**, *35*, 992–1019. [CrossRef]
227. Zhang, T.; Tong, X.; Zhang, S.; Wang, D.; Wang, L.; Wang, Q.; Fan, H. The Roles of Dipeptidyl Peptidase 4 (DPP4) and DPP4 Inhibitors in Different Lung Diseases: New Evidence. *Front. Pharmacol.* **2021**, *12*, e731453. [CrossRef]
228. Zhai, W.; Cardell, M.; De Meester, I.; Augustyns, K.; Hillinger, S.; Inci, I.; Arni, S.; Jungraithmayr, W.; Scharpé, S.; Weder, W.; et al. Ischemia/reperfusion injury: The role of CD26/dipeptidyl-peptidase-IV-inhibition in lung transplantation. *Transplant. Proc.* **2006**, *38*, 3369–3371. [CrossRef]
229. Jungraithmayr, W.; De Meester, I.; Matheeussen, V.; Inci, I.; Augustyns, K.; Scharpé, S.; Weder, W.; Korom, S. Inhibition of CD26/DPP IV attenuates ischemia/reperfusion injury in orthotopic mouse lung transplants: The pivotal role of vasoactive intestinal peptide. *Peptides* **2010**, *31*, 585–591. [CrossRef]
230. Zhai, W.; Cardell, M.; De Meester, I.; Augustyns, K.; Hillinger, S.; Inci, I.; Arni, S.; Jungraithmayr, W.; Scharpé, S.; Weder, W.; et al. Intragraft DPP IV inhibition attenuates post-transplant pulmonary ischemia/reperfusion injury after extended ischemia. *J Heart Lung Transplant.* **2007**, *26*, 174–180. [CrossRef]
231. Delgado, M.; Ganea, D. Vasoactive intestinal peptide: A neuropeptide with pleiotropic immune functions. *Amino Acids* **2013**, *45*, 25–39. [CrossRef]
232. Zhou, Y.; Zhang, C.-Y.; Duan, J.-X.; Li, Q.; Yang, H.-H.; Sun, C.-C.; Zhang, J.; Luo, X.-Q.; Liu, S.-K. Vasoactive intestinal peptide suppresses the NLRP3 inflammasome activation in lipopolysaccharide-induced acute lung injury mice and macrophages. *Biomed. Pharmacother.* **2020**, *121*, 109596. [CrossRef]
233. Delgado, M.; Ganea, D. VIP and PACAP inhibit activation induced apoptosis in T lymphocytes. *Ann. N. Y. Acad. Sci.* **2000**, *921*, 55–67. [CrossRef] [PubMed]
234. Fadeel, B.; Åhlin, A.; Henter, J.-I.; Orrenius, S.; Hampton, M.B. Involvement of Caspases in Neutrophil Apoptosis: Regulation by Reactive Oxygen Species. *Blood* **1998**, *92*, 4808–4818. [CrossRef] [PubMed]
235. Lataillade, J.-J.; Clay, D.; Bourin, P.; Hérodin, F.i.; Dupuy, C.; Jasmin, C.; Le Bousse-Kerdilès, M.-C. Stromal cell–derived factor 1 regulates primitive hematopoiesis by suppressing apoptosis and by promoting G0/G1 transition in CD34+ cells: Evidence for an autocrine/paracrine mechanism. *Blood* **2002**, *99*, 1117–1129. [CrossRef] [PubMed]

236. Zhang, Y.; Liu, T.; Guo, H.; Shi, J.; Yang, J.; Fu, S.; Pan, X.; Li, F.; Zhang, H.; Zhang, D.; et al. Ex vivo lung perfusion with GLP-1R agonist mitigates ischemia/reperfusion injury through pyroptosis modulation in lung transplantation- an experimental study. *Int. J. Surg.* **2025**, *111*, 3781–3797. [CrossRef]
237. Mehdi, S.F.; Pusapati, S.; Anwar, M.S.; Lohana, D.; Kumar, P.; Nandula, S.A.; Nawaz, F.K.; Tracey, K.; Yang, H.; LeRoith, D.; et al. Glucagon-like peptide-1: A multi-faceted anti-inflammatory agent. *Front. Immunol.* **2023**, *14*, e1148209. [CrossRef]
238. Deacon, C.F. Physiology and Pharmacology of DPP-4 in Glucose Homeostasis and the Treatment of Type 2 Diabetes. *Front. Endocrinol.* **2019**, *10*, e00080. [CrossRef]
239. Fandiño, J.; Toba, L.; González-Matías, L.C.; Diz-Chaves, Y.; Mallo, F. GLP-1 receptor agonist ameliorates experimental lung fibrosis. *Sci. Rep.* **2020**, *10*, 18091. [CrossRef]
240. Shiraki, A.; Oyama, J.; Komoda, H.; Asaka, M.; Komatsu, A.; Sakuma, M.; Kodama, K.; Sakamoto, Y.; Kotooka, N.; Hirase, T.; et al. The glucagon-like peptide 1 analog liraglutide reduces TNF-α-induced oxidative stress and inflammation in endothelial cells. *Atherosclerosis* **2012**, *221*, 375–382. [CrossRef]
241. Steven, S.; Jurk, K.; Kopp, M.; Kröller-Schön, S.; Mikhed, Y.; Schwierczek, K.; Roohani, S.; Kashani, F.; Oelze, M.; Klein, T.; et al. Glucagon-like peptide-1 receptor signalling reduces microvascular thrombosis, nitro-oxidative stress and platelet activation in endotoxaemic mice. *Br. J. Pharmacol.* **2017**, *174*, 1620–1632. [CrossRef]
242. Steven, S.; Hausding, M.; Kröller-Schön, S.; Mader, M.; Mikhed, Y.; Stamm, P.; Zinßius, E.; Pfeffer, A.; Welschof, P.; Agdauletova, S.; et al. Gliptin and GLP-1 analog treatment improves survival and vascular inflammation/dysfunction in animals with lipopolysaccharide-induced endotoxemia. *Basic Res. Cardiol.* **2015**, *110*, 6. [CrossRef] [PubMed]
243. Sakanoue, I.; Nakajima, D. Mesenchymal stem cell therapy against ischemia-reperfusion injury in lung transplantation. *Curr. Opin. Organ. Transplant.* **2025**, *30*, 372–378. [CrossRef] [PubMed]
244. Park, K.-S.; Lässer, C.; Lötvall, J. Extracellular vesicles and the lung: From disease pathogenesis to biomarkers and treatments. *Physiol. Rev.* **2025**, *105*, 1733–1821. [CrossRef] [PubMed]
245. Wang, N.; Ma, F.; Song, H.; He, N.; Zhang, H.; Li, J.; Liu, Q.; Xu, C. Mesenchymal Stem Cell-Derived Extracellular Vesicles for Regenerative Applications and Radiotherapy. *Cell Transplant.* **2025**, *34*, 09636897241311019. [CrossRef]
246. Nykänen, A.I.; Liu, M.; Keshavjee, S. Mesenchymal Stromal Cell Therapy in Lung Transplantation. *Bioengineering* **2023**, *10*, 728. [CrossRef]
247. Matthay, M.A.; Calfee, C.S.; Zhuo, H.; Thompson, B.T.; Wilson, J.G.; Levitt, J.E.; Rogers, A.J.; Gotts, J.E.; Wiener-Kronish, J.P.; Bajwa, E.K.; et al. Treatment with allogeneic mesenchymal stromal cells for moderate to severe acute respiratory distress syndrome (START study): A randomised phase 2a safety trial. *Lancet Respir. Med.* **2019**, *7*, 154–162. [CrossRef]
248. Niroomand, A.; Hirdman, G.; Olm, F.; Lindstedt, S. Current Status and Future Perspectives on Machine Perfusion: A Treatment Platform to Restore and Regenerate Injured Lungs Using Cell and Cytokine Adsorption Therapy. *Cells* **2022**, *11*, 91. [CrossRef]
249. Yang, X.; Hong, S.; Yan, T.; Liu, M.; Liu, M.; Zhao, J.; Yue, B.; Wu, D.; Shao, J.; Huang, M.; et al. MiR-146a engineered extracellular vesicles derived from mesenchymal stromal cells more potently attenuate ischaemia–reperfusion injury in lung transplantation. *Clin. Transl. Med.* **2025**, *15*, e70298. [CrossRef]
250. Egan, T.M.; Haithcock, B.E.; Lobo, J.; Mody, G.; Love, R.B.; Requard III, J.J.; Espey, J.; Ali, M.H. Donation after circulatory death donors in lung transplantation. *J. Thorac. Dis.* **2021**, *13*, 6536–6549. [CrossRef]
251. Motoyama, H.; Chen, F.; Ohsumi, A.; Hijiya, K.; Okita, K.; Nakajima, D.; Sakamoto, J.; Yamada, T.; Sato, M.; Aoyama, A.; et al. Protective effect of plasmin in marginal donor lungs in an ex vivo lung perfusion model. *J. Heart Lung Transplant.* **2013**, *32*, 505–510. [CrossRef]
252. Liersch-Nordqvist, A.; Fakhro, M.; Pierre, L.; Hlebowicz, J.; Malmsjo, M.; Ingemansson, R.; Lindstedt, S. The impact of alteplase on pulmonary graft function in donation after circulatory death—An experimental study. *Ann. Med. Surg.* **2017**, *22*, 1–6. [CrossRef]
253. Van Raemdonck, D.; Neyrinck, A.; Cypel, M.; Keshavjee, S. Ex-vivo lung perfusion. *Transpl. Int.* **2015**, *28*, 643–656. [CrossRef]
254. Morgan, M.J.; Kim, Y.-S. Roles of RIPK3 in necroptosis, cell signaling, and disease. *Exp. Mol. Med.* **2022**, *54*, 1695–1704. [CrossRef] [PubMed]
255. Dong, L.; Liang, F.; Lou, Z.; Li, Y.; Li, J.; Chen, Y.; Ding, J.; Jiang, B.; Wu, C.; Yu, H.; et al. Necrostatin-1 Alleviates Lung Ischemia-Reperfusion Injury via Inhibiting Necroptosis and Apoptosis of Lung Epithelial Cells. *Cells* **2022**, *11*, 3139. [CrossRef] [PubMed]
256. Ueda, S.; Chen-Yoshikawa, T.F.; Tanaka, S.; Yamada, Y.; Nakajima, D.; Ohsumi, A.; Date, H. Protective effect of necrosulfonamide on rat pulmonary ischemia-reperfusion injury via inhibition of necroptosis. *J. Thorac. Cardiovasc. Surg.* **2022**, *163*, e113–e122. [CrossRef] [PubMed]
257. Teke, Z.; Kabay, B.; Ozden, A.; Yenisey, C.; Bir, F.; Demirkan, N.C.; Bicakci, T.; Erdem, E. Effects of tempol, a membrane-permeable radical scavenger, on local and remote organ injuries caused by intestinal ischemia/reperfusion in rats. *J. Surg. Res.* **2008**, *149*, 259–271. [CrossRef]

258. Baltalarli, A.; Ozcan, V.; Bir, F.; Aybek, H.; Sacar, M.; Onem, G.; Goksin, I.; Demir, S.; Teke, Z. Ascorbic acid (vitamin C) and iloprost attenuate the lung injury caused by ischemia/reperfusion of the lower extremities of rats. *Ann. Vasc. Surg.* **2006**, *20*, 49–55. [CrossRef]
259. Inci, I.; Zhai, W.; Arni, S.; Hillinger, S.; Vogt, P.; Weder, W. N-acetylcysteine attenuates lung ischemia-reperfusion injury after lung transplantation. *Ann. Thorac. Surg.* **2007**, *84*, 240–246; discussion 246. [CrossRef]
260. Rega, F.R.; Wuyts, W.A.; Vanaudenaerde, B.M.; Jannis, N.C.; Neyrinck, A.P.; Verleden, G.M.; Lerut, T.E.; Van Raemdonck, D.E. Nebulized N-acetyl cysteine protects the pulmonary graft inside the non-heart-beating donor. *J. Heart Lung Transplant.* **2005**, *24*, 1369–1377. [CrossRef]
261. Okamoto, T.; Tang, X.; Janocha, A.; Farver, C.F.; Gladwin, M.T.; McCurry, K.R. Nebulized nitrite protects rat lung grafts from ischemia reperfusion injury. *J. Thorac. Cardiovasc. Surg.* **2013**, *145*, 1108–1116.e1101. [CrossRef]
262. Sugimoto, R.; Okamoto, T.; Nakao, A.; Zhan, J.; Wang, Y.; Kohmoto, J.; Tokita, D.; Farver, C.F.; Tarpey, M.M.; Billiar, T.R.; et al. Nitrite reduces acute lung injury and improves survival in a rat lung transplantation model. *Am. J. Transplant.* **2012**, *12*, 2938–2948. [CrossRef]
263. Egemnazarov, B.; Sydykov, A.; Schermuly, R.T.; Weissmann, N.; Stasch, J.-P.; Sarybaev, A.S.; Seeger, W.; Grimminger, F.; Ghofrani, H.A. Novel soluble guanylyl cyclase stimulator BAY 41-2272 attenuates ischemia-reperfusion-induced lung injury. *Am. J. Physiol.-Lung Cell. Mol. Physiol.* **2009**, *296*, L462–L469. [CrossRef]
264. Zhang, Y.; Ding, S.; Li, C.; Wang, Y.; Chen, Z.; Wang, Z. Effects of N-acetylcysteine treatment in acute respiratory distress syndrome: A meta-analysis. *Exp. Ther. Med.* **2017**, *14*, 2863–2868. [CrossRef]
265. Liu, X.; Pan, B.; Wang, X.; Xu, J.; Wang, X.; Song, Z.; Zhang, E.; Wang, F.; Wang, W. Ischemia/reperfusion-activated ferroptosis in the early stage triggers excessive inflammation to aggregate lung injury in rats. *Front. Med.* **2023**, *10*, 1181286. [CrossRef]
266. Deng, P.; Wu, Y.; Wan, L.; Sun, X.; Sun, Q. Maresin1 Alleviates Ischemia Reperfusion Injury After Lung Transplantation by Inhibiting Ferroptosis via the PKA-Hippo-YAP Signaling Pathway. *Biomedicines* **2025**, *13*, 1594. [CrossRef]
267. Zhao, J.; Li, J.; Wei, D.; Gao, F.; Yang, X.; Yue, B.; Xiong, D.; Liu, M.; Xu, H.; Hu, C.; et al. Liproxstatin-1 Alleviates Lung Transplantation-induced Cold Ischemia-Reperfusion Injury by Inhibiting Ferroptosis. *Transplantation* **2023**, *107*, 2190–2202. [CrossRef]

antioxidants

MDPI

Review

Feedback Loops Shape Oxidative and Immune Interactions in Hepatic Ischemia–Reperfusion Injury

Kenneth J. Dery *, Richard Chiu, Aanchal Kasargod and Jerzy W. Kupiec-Weglinski

Division of Liver and Pancreas Transplantation, Department of Surgery, The Dumont-UCLA Transplantation Center, David Geffen School of Medicine at UCLA, Los Angeles, CA 90095, USA; rchiu2003@g.ucla.edu (R.C.); akasargod@g.ucla.edu (A.K.); jkupiec@mednet.ucla.edu (J.W.K.-W.)

* Correspondence: kdery@mednet.ucla.edu

Abstract

Reactive oxygen species (ROS) play a dual role as both essential signaling molecules and harmful mediators of damage. Imbalances in the redox state of the liver can overwhelm antioxidant defenses and promote mitochondrial dysfunction, oxidative damage, and inflammation. Complex feedback loops between ROS and immune signaling pathways are a hallmark of pathological liver conditions, such as hepatic ischemia–reperfusion injury (IRI). This is a major cause of liver transplant failure and is of increasing significance due to the increased use of marginally discarded livers for transplantation. This review outlines the major enzymatic and metabolic sources of ROS in hepatic IRI, including mitochondrial reverse electron transport, NADPH oxidases, cytochrome P450 enzymes, and endoplasmic reticulum stress. Hepatocyte injury activates redox feedback loops that initiate immune cascades through DAMP release, toll-like receptor signaling, and cytokine production. Emerging regulatory mechanisms, such as succinate accumulation and cytosolic calcium–CAMKII signaling, further shape oxidative dynamics. Pharmacological therapies and the use of antioxidant and immunomodulatory approaches, including nanoparticles and redox-sensitive therapeutics, are discussed as protective strategies. A deeper understanding of how redox and immune feedback loops interact is an exciting and active area of research that warrants further clinical investigation.

Keywords: hepatocytes; cross-talk; inflammation; ischemia–reperfusion injury; Kupffer cells; organ transplantation; oxidative stress; ROS

1. Introduction

In the past, liver research focused mainly on elucidating how the dysregulation of the metabolic and detoxifying functions of hepatocytes contributes to systemic disease [1]. Some well-researched liver pathologies include ischemia–reperfusion injury (IRI), metabolic syndrome, nonalcoholic fatty liver disease (NAFLD), viral hepatitis, and hepatocellular carcinoma [2]. Hepatic IRI occurs during organ transplantation when donor tissues are exposed to a period of ischemia or lack of oxygen, initiating a cascade of events upon reperfusion that includes the release of pro-inflammatory cytokines [3] (Figure 1). Initially, mitochondrial dysfunction leads to the rapid generation of reactive oxygen species (ROS), which leads to oxidative stress, tissue inflammation, and cell death, contributing significantly to graft dysfunction and poor transplant outcomes [4,5]. Despite diverse etiologies, these liver conditions are unified by a common pathogenic feature: the overproduction of ROS, which drives oxidative stress and cellular dysfunction [2].

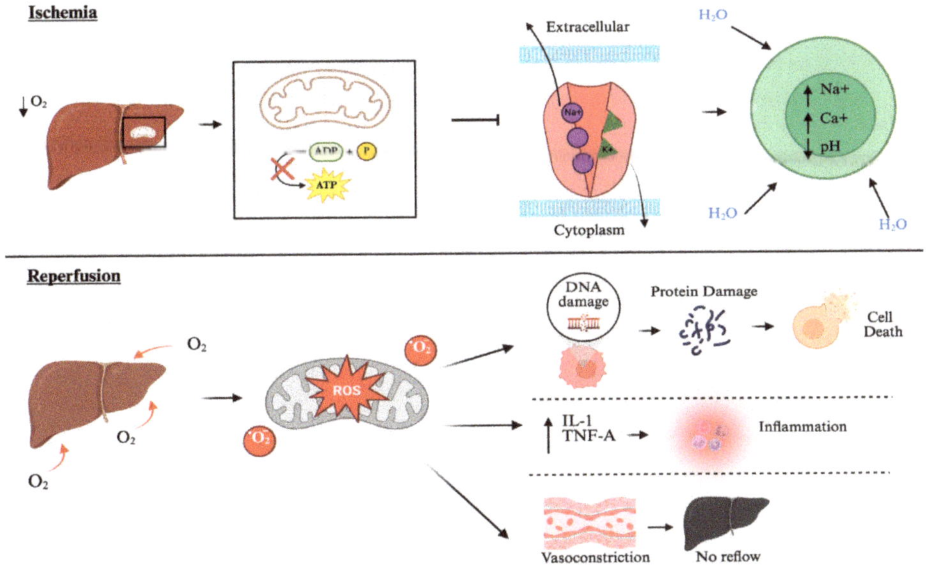

Figure 1. Mechanism of hepatic IRI. Liver injury begins with the oxygen-depleted ischemic phase, where a lack of blood flow to the liver creates an oxygen-poor environment. This environment then inhibits mitochondrial production of ATP, which in turn inhibits the Na^+/K^+ ATPase pump, leading to an increased ion concentration in the cells and swelling. This sets the stage for the reperfusion phase, where oxygen is reintroduced to the liver, but is turned into oxygen free radicals. ROS have multiple damaging effects, including DNA and protein degradation, leading to cell death, increased inflammation, and vasoconstriction, preventing the reflow of blood back into the liver. Created by Biorender.com.

ROS are highly reactive molecules generated as the byproducts of normal metabolism or induced by inflammatory stimuli [6]. They are generated through multiple cellular pathways, and their detrimental effects have been extensively documented [7]. During oxidative stress, especially under conditions such as IRI, enzymatic pathways, including xanthine oxidase and NADPH oxidase, generate excessive levels of ROS, which exacerbate cellular damage and contribute to mitochondrial dysfunction [8].

Under physiological conditions, low to moderate ROS levels serve as signaling molecules that modulate hepatocyte function, immune cell activation, and tissue remodeling [9]. However, excessive ROS overwhelms antioxidant defenses, leading to oxidative damage, mitochondrial dysfunction, and the activation of inflammatory cascades [10]. For example, ROS production leads to the recruitment of neutrophils to the cellular environment, furthering the damage to hepatocytes [11]. In response to stress, the damaged liver cells release damage-associated molecular patterns (DAMPs), which then activate toll-like receptor (TLR) pathways, expressing myeloid differentiation genes such as MyD88, and eventually neutrophil extracellular traps (NETs) [12]. This signaling cascade exacerbates liver IRI by activating cytokine-releasing Kupffer cells, initiating the release of interleukins, tumor necrosis factor-alpha (TNFA), increasing the sequestration of CD4+ T cells, and promoting apoptosis [13]. Figure 2 details how Kupffer cells undergo phenotypic changes during oxidative stress.

As a leading cause of organ dysfunction and failure, IRI warrants continued investigation into its oxidant mechanisms [14,15]. Despite decades of intense research, the therapeutic options for many of these liver pathologies remain limited to supportive or symptom-based approaches. Although the importance of oxidative stress in liver disease is well recognized, the complexity of redox-regulated hepatocyte–immune interactions remains incompletely understood. Emerging evidence suggests that intrinsic and therapeutically modulated antioxidant mechanisms can disrupt this damaging feedback loop and restore immunological hemostasis and metabolic balance. This review explores the mechanistic foundations of ROS generation and antioxidant defenses in the liver, specifically focusing on efforts to mitigate IRI but also on understanding how redox dynamics govern hepatocyte–immune cell crosstalk in health and disease.

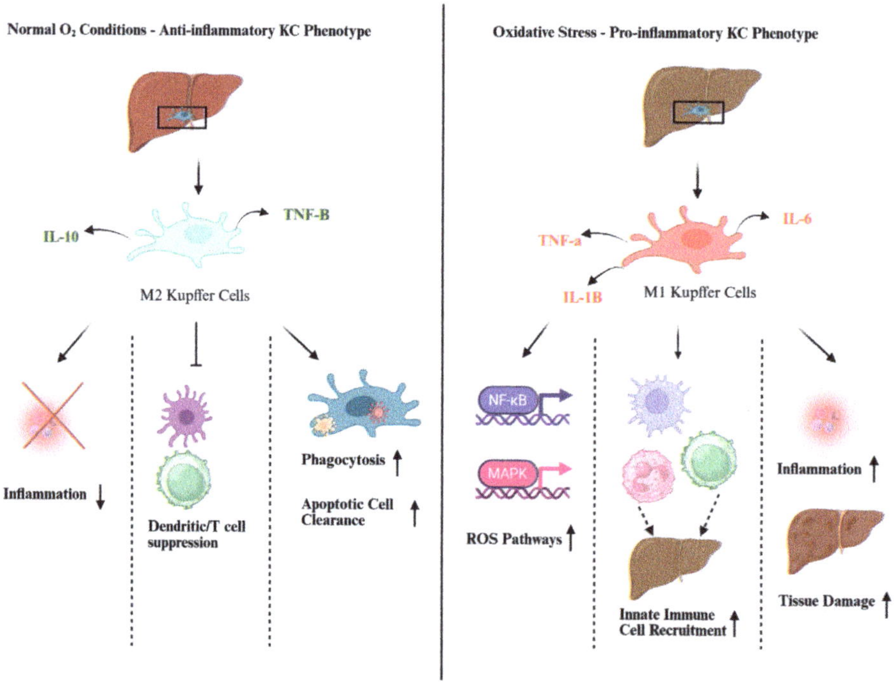

Figure 2. Kupffer cell phenotype changes during oxidative stress. Under normoxic conditions, Kupffer cells exhibit M2 macrophage qualities, performing typical functions such as releasing anti-inflammatory cytokines like IL-10 and TNF-β, suppressing dendritic cell and T cell activation, and clearing immune debris and pathogens. However, under oxidative stress, Kupffer cells display M1 macrophage qualities, releasing pro-inflammatory cytokines like TNF-α, IL-1β, and IL-6, recruiting innate immune cells to the liver, and causing tissue damage. Arrows indicate possible Kupffer cell differentiation fates and downstream effects under normal oxygen (anti-inflammatory M2 phenotype) and oxidative stress (pro-inflammatory M1 phenotype) conditions. Created by Biorender.com.

2. Oxidant Mechanisms That Contribute to ROS in Hepatic IRI

2.1. Major Sources of ROS

ROS produced by mitochondria can benefit the cellular environment by activating therapeutic antioxidant processes in the event of cellular stress. ROS regulate cell proliferation and differentiation at controlled levels, modulate immune responses, influence autophagy and apoptosis, and act as secondary messengers in signal transduction pathways [16]. Hydrogen peroxide (H_2O_2) and superoxide ($O_2^{-}\cdot$) are specific oxidants that function as redox signaling agents. They occur in normally metabolizing cells at a steady-state level and are formed continuously. However, its excess accumulation within hepatocytes can often lead to liver damage [17]. Maintaining cellular homeostasis and overall liver health critically depends on a balanced interplay between oxidative stress mechanisms and antioxidant defense systems [18]. Table 1 highlights some representative studies that focus on oxidative stress-related pathways and their key findings from 2024 to 2025.

Table 1. Representative oxidative stress-related pathways and key findings from the period of 2024–2025.

Liver Disease	Gene/Pathway	Key Findings	Ref.
Iron Overload-Induced Liver Damage	TGF-β/Smad	Ellagic acid mitigates ferroptosis, alleviating liver damage.	[19]
Alcohol-Related Liver Disease (ALD)	TLR4/NF-κB/NLRP3	*H. pylori* FMT exacerbates ALD via LPS-induced pathway activation.	[20]
Liver Transplant-Related Biliary Injury	Nrf-2/HO-1, JNK	Nanomedicine inhibits ROS and modulates macrophages via Nrf-2/HO-1.	[21]
Hepatic Ischemia–Reperfusion Injury	ROS scavenging enzymes	Copper-based nanozymes scavenge ROS and protect liver.	[22]
Hepatic Ischemia–Reperfusion Injury	Keap1/Nrf2/HO-1	Crocetin preconditioning activates Nrf2/HO-1 by disrupting Keap1.	[23]
Fatty Liver and Ischemia–Reperfusion Injury	PI3K/AKT	Puerarin regulates PI3K/AKT to reduce liver IR injury.	[24]
Diabetic Liver Disease	RAGE, TGF-β, TNF-α	Crocin and losartan reduce fibrosis-related gene expression.	[25]
NASH	FXR	ROS-scavenging nanobubbles treat NASH via FXR activation.	[26]
NALFD	AMPK/ACC/SREBP1	Codonopsis polysaccharides reduce lipid accumulation and inflammation.	[27]
Alcoholic Liver Injury	NRF1-TFAM	Nobiletin preserves mitochondria via NRF1-TFAM signaling.	[28]
Alcoholic Steatosis	PCSK9	FAF2 silencing modulates PCSK9 to reduce steatosis.	[29]
Liver Fibrosis	miR-3667-3P/ACSL4	circ_0074763 regulates ACSL4 via miRNA axis in fibrosis.	[30]
CCl_4-Induced Fibrosis	TGF-β1-Smad	Umbelliferone inhibits fibrosis through TGF-β1-Smad.	[31]
Chronic Liver Injury	Nrf2	COX-2 inhibition upregulates Nrf2 to reduce ferroptosis.	[32]
Hepatocarcinoma	PI3K/AKT, ROS	FDX1 downregulation activates mitophagy, promotes HCC.	[33]
Hepatocarcinoma	TRIM7/Nrf2	Fangchinoline inhibits HCC by regulating ROS via TRIM7/Nrf2.	[34]
Hepatocarcinoma	SHP2/PI3K	Hypoxia-induced ROS promotes HCC growth via SHP2/PI3K.	[35]
Hepatocarcinoma	HEXB	ROS induces EV release by up-regulating HEXB to promote HCC.	[36]

Recent evidence has underscored the importance of temporal and spatial ROS dynamics as a critical driver of downstream inflammatory and cell death pathways [37]. During ischemic stress, following orthotopic liver transplantation (OLT), mitochondrial metabolism becomes impaired, leading to the accumulation of succinate because of stalled tricarboxylic acid (TCA) cycle activity (Figure 3). The key event occurs during reperfusion; the sudden reintroduction of oxygen enables the rapid oxidation of the accumulated succinate by mitochondrial complex II (succinate dehydrogenase). This process drives electrons into the electron transport chain, creating a highly reduced ubiquinone pool that facilitates reverse electron transport (RET) at complex I [38]. RET is a major source of mitochondrial ROS generation, contributing to oxidative stress, mitochondrial dysfunction, and tissue injury associated with ischemia–reperfusion injury [39].

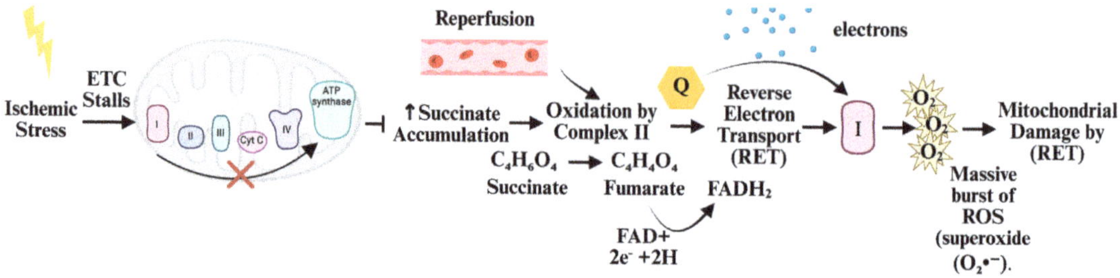

Figure 3. Generation of ROS in the mitochondria from Reverse Electron Transport (RET). Ischemic stress causes stalling in the electron transport chain. Upon reperfusion in the recipient during liver transplantation, mitochondrial succinate levels increase. This causes rapid oxidation to fumarate by succinate dehydrogenase (complex II), driving a surge of electrons into the electron transport chain (ETC). This process, known as reverse electron transport (RET), leads to excessive superoxide ($O_2\cdot^-$) production at complex I. RET is triggered by metabolic stress, such as ischemia–reperfusion, and contributes to oxidative damage and redox signaling. Created by Biorender.com.

Studies on succinate show that it is not associated with metabolic syndrome and liver dysfunction, however [40]. One recent study used mice with muscle-specific ablation of succinate dehydrogenase to show that knockout mice demonstrate normal liver histology and oxidative capacity, suggesting that additional regulatory mechanisms beyond succinate accumulation may govern mitochondrial ROS production and tissue damage during IRI. For example, a recent study showed that hepatic mitochondrial fat oxidation, lipolysis, and TCA cycle activity are enhanced independent of mitochondrial calcium levels through cytosolic calcium–CAMKII signaling [41]. The authors used a liver-specific mitochondrial calcium uniporter knockout mouse model (MCU KO) to reduce mitochondrial calcium ($[Ca^{2+}]$mt) while elevating cytosolic calcium ($[Ca^{2+}]$cyt). Using in vivo metabolic flux analysis, radiolabeled $[^{14}C_{16}]$ palmitate oxidation assays, liver slice studies, and CAMKII modulation (activation and knockdown) showed that increased $[Ca^{2+}]$cyt activates CAMKII, driving enhanced hepatic fat oxidation and reduced triacylglycerol accumulation. Whether elevated $[Ca^{2+}]$cyt-CAMKII activity may promote substrate flux through the TCA cycle to reduce succinate accumulation during ischemia, thereby limiting RET-driven ROS upon reperfusion, remains to be determined.

Another major source of ROS in hepatic IRI comes from the NADPH oxidase family of NOX enzymes, particularly during reperfusion [42]. NOX enzymes transfer electrons from NADPH inside the cell to oxygen-rich membranes, generating H_2O_2 and superoxide O_2^- species. During reperfusion, the sudden influx of oxygen supply on toll-like receptors (TLRs) on Kupffer cells, endothelial cells, and hepatocytes upregulate NOX expression and activity. Subsequent ROS production can influence lipid peroxidation, protein oxidation, and DNA damage and act as pro-inflammatory signaling molecules that amplify cytokine production and immune cell recruitment [43]. A recent study strengthened our understanding of how NOX enzymes amplify oxidative stress and inflammation [44]. The authors showed that rapamycin reduction in NOX enzymes depressed pro-inflammatory cytokine levels and apoptotic markers in a murine fibrotic liver IRI model. Cytochrome P450 is another source of ROS, particularly in monooxygenases that catalyze the oxidation of various substrates (drugs, toxins, fatty acids) using molecular oxygen (O_2) and NADPH [45]. In a recent study, the authors showed that iridoid glycoside aucubin, a natural plant-derived compound from *Plantago asiatica*, reduces the ROS in liver IRI by suppressing key inflammatory and oxidative stress pathways. Their key data showed that aucubin inhibited the signaling pathways that involved High Mobility Group Box 1 (HMGB1), TLR-4, and

Nuclear Factor kappa-light-chain-enhancer of activated B cells (NF-κB) [46]. Moreover, aucubin reduced mitochondrial dysfunction, apoptosis, and Cytochrome P450 expression, which are all directly associated with lowering ROS levels and protecting hepatic tissue.

Finally, recent studies have focused on the unfolded protein response as a mechanism of generating ROS [47]. During cellular stress, such as oxygen deprivation during the ischemic IRI phase, ATP levels drop, and protein folding halts. This causes unfolded protein accumulation in the endoplasmic reticulum (ER) and hyperactivates enzymes such as Ero1 and protein disulfide isomerase, leading to excess H_2O_2 formation. Indeed, a recent study showed that hypothermic oxygenated perfusion (HOPE) effectively mitigated ER stress by modulating unfolded protein response (UPR) signaling [47]. The authors showed that HOPE activated the Janus kinase 2 (JAK2)/ Signal Transducer and Activator of Transcription 3 (STAT3) pathway, leading to the upregulation of the Hematopoietic Cell-Specific Lyn Substrate 1-Associated Protein X-1 (HAX1). This multifunctional protein has been shown to be involved in regulating apoptosis, calcium homeostasis, and cell survival, particularly under stress conditions. These studies show that hepatic ROS arises from metabolic, enzymatic, and signaling disruptions during I/R stress. A thorough understanding of ROS production's temporal and spatial mechanisms may provide the foundation for identifying strategies to mitigate hepatic injury and improve clinical outcomes.

2.2. *Key Hepatic and Immune Cell Players*

As the principal parenchymal cells of the liver, hepatocytes act as the central regulators of IR-triggered oxidative stress [48]. Not only are they responsible for metabolic homeostasis, detoxification, and protein synthesis, but they also interact with other liver cells, like Kupffer cells and stellate cells, to maintain local homeostasis and responses to injury [49]. Hepatocytes are equipped with endogenous antioxidant systems such as glutathione, superoxide dismutase, and catalase to play a dual role as both sources and targets of ROS [50]. Hepatocytes adapt to rising ROS levels by activating redox-sensitive transcription factors such as nuclear factor erythroid 2–2-related factor 2 (NRF2) [51]. A high oxygen tension initiates a mechanism in hepatocytes that causes NRF2 dissociation from its cytoplasmic inhibitor KEAP1 [52]. This causes its translocation to the nucleus, where it promotes the expression of over 200 genes involved in antioxidant defense, detoxification, and metabolic regulation, including heme oxygenase-1 (HO-1), NAD(P)H quinone dehydrogenase 1 (NQO1), and GSH synthesis enzymes [53,54].

The relationship between mitochondrial ROS-driven inflammation and lipid accumulation in hepatocytes was recently interrogated using primary cultured hepatocytes in a model of NAFLD [55]. Zaluzanin C, a sesquiterpene lactone [56], protected hepatocytes from mitochondrial ROS by preventing Tumor Necrosis Factor Receptor 1 (TNFR1) induction. This study also showed that mitophagy, a specialized type of autophagy that targets the mitochondria [57], induces and upregulates Peroxisome proliferator-activated receptor gamma coactivator 1-alpha (PGC1α), Mitochondrial Transcription Factor A (TFAM), Nrf1, and β-oxidation gene expression, indicating its dual antioxidant and metabolic benefit. In a related investigation, it was demonstrated that hepatocytes respond to LPS-induced oxidative stress by increasing ROS production and cytokine expression, contributing to hepatic inflammation [58]. Rocaglamide-A, a natural bioactive compound extracted from plants of the genus *Aglaia* with known potent pharmacological properties, was shown to be able to reduce ROS levels in hepatocytes by upregulating antioxidant genes and inhibiting the phosphorylation of c-Jun N-terminal kinase (JNK) and Activator Protein-1 (AP-1), key signaling molecules activated by LPS. Rocaglamide-A was able to mitigate nitrosative (e.g., reactive nitrogen species (RNS), such as nitric oxide (NO)) and oxidative stress, highlighting hepatocytes as both sources and targets of ROS-mediated inflammatory signaling in liver injury.

Liver sinusoidal endothelial cells (LSECs) and hepatic stellate cells also play important roles in modulating redox balance and mediating the progression of hepatic IRI [59]. LSECs line the walls of the hepatic sinusoids, which are the specialized capillary-like blood vessels in the liver [60]. During IRI, LSECs experience oxidative stress marked by mitochondrial dysfunction and NADPH oxidase activation, leading to excessive ROS generation [61]. This disrupts the fenestrated architecture of the sinusoids, impairs barrier integrity, and facilitates leukocyte adhesion and transmigration. By comparison, hepatic stellate cells are located in the narrow Disse space between hepatocytes and LSECs [62]. These cells store vitamin A as part of their quiescent (non-activated) state and become activated upon liver injury or I/R stress [63]. Notably, hepatic stellate cells transform upon activation into myofibroblast-like cells that secrete ECM components such as collagen, contributing to fibrosis [64].

Both LSECs and hepatic stellate cells were recently interrogated using single-cell RNA sequencing and transcriptome RNA sequencing in a hepatic model of IRI following transplantation [65]. The clustering analyses revealed 11 distinct cell types across 25 clusters, including 5 non-immune and 6 immune populations. Non-immune cells included hepatocytes, endothelial cells, stellate cells, cholangiocytes [66], and erythroid cells, while immune cells consisted of macrophages, monocytes, NK/T cells [67], B cells [68], and plasma cells [69]. Differential gene expression analysis between pre-perfusion (PP) and post-reperfusion (PR) tissues identified key dysregulated genes in both immune and non-immune liver cell populations. Among the immune-modulating non-parenchymal cells, LSECs showed 14 upregulated and 3 downregulated genes in PR tissue. Several upregulated genes, such as the Heat Shock Protein Family E Member 1 (HSPE1), were associated with the heat shock protein (HSP) signaling pathway. Additional genes, such as BCL2-associated athanogene 3 (BAG3), are implicated in cell cycle control and LSEC homeostasis disruptions. Inflammatory mediators like Annexin A1 (ANXA1) were suggestive of endothelial dysfunction and liver transplant-associated injury. Notably, this study demonstrated a novel function of LSECs in the bidirectional crosstalk between cells of the liver and monocytes. Intercellular communication analysis using CellPhoneDB (Wellcome Sanger Institute, Hinxton, United Kingdom) [70], a database designed to analyze cell–cell communication using single-cell transcriptomic data, revealed the upregulation of the ANXA1-Formyl Peptide Receptor 2 (FPR2) signaling axis. This study used immunofluorescence, flow cytometry, and Western blot analyses to validate their transcriptomic data in a murine IRI model and strengthen their bioinformatics data. These findings point to a mechanism where the LSEC–monocyte ANXA1–FPR2 axis may suggest a feed-forward loop in which LSEC activation enhances monocyte recruitment and inflammatory activity, potentially amplifying liver injury during reperfusion. This study also places this interaction within broader immune regulatory networks, including TLR signaling, NET formation, and Notch1-mediated pathways, which may amplify oxidative stress and immunopathology during IRI.

Besides hepatocytes, LSECs, and hepatic stellate cells, other liver cells, like the Kupffer cells and infiltrating neutrophils, greatly influence hepatocyte metabolism during I/R oxidative stress [71]. Located in the liver sinusoids, Kupffer cells clear cellular debris and harmful substances and detect and remove pathogens. These resident macrophages serve as the first responders to inflammation and injury following activation by DAMPs. Kupffer cells become active during I/R stress, when endogenous molecules like mitochondrial DNA, HMGB1, or ATP, serving as DAMPs, signal tissue damage [72]. Following this,

Kupffer cells produce ROS as part of the inflammatory response, leading to sustained liver injury, due to its role as signaling molecules to amplify inflammation by activating transcription factors like NF-κB, promoting the production of pro-inflammatory cytokines (e.g., TNF-α, IL-1β).

Their role in shaping the redox landscape of the hepatic microenvironment is an area of active research [73,74]. For example, a recent study explored how Kupffer cells use Peroxisome Proliferator-Activated Receptor Gamma (PPARγ)-mediated metabolic reprogramming to regulate oxidative stress and inflammation in NAFLD. PPARγ is a nuclear receptor and transcription factor that regulates lipid metabolism, glucose homeostasis, and anti-inflammatory responses [75]. The authors found that PPARγ activation enhanced fatty acid oxidation, reduced ROS production, and suppressed pro-inflammatory cytokine secretion. By linking the antioxidant effect to activation of the Keap1-Nrf2 pathway, the study showed a link between Kupffer cell ROS regulation and hepatocyte inflammatory response [76].

As the most abundant white blood cell type in the bloodstream, neutrophils form an integral line of innate defense following I/R stress. These granulocytic leukocytes rapidly respond to infection or tissue injury by migrating to affected sites. Neutrophils engulf pathogens and debris by phagocytosis, release ROS to kill microbes, and form neutrophil extracellular traps (NETs), web-like structures of DNA and proteins, to trap and neutralize pathogens. Notably, the characterization of NETs in the context of hepatic I/R oxidative stress has recently been an area of active investigation. For example, our group recently showed that neutrophils regulate bioactive lipid sphingosine-1-phosphate (S1P) and its receptors S1PR2 and S1PR3 following hepatic IRI caused by OLT [77]. The S1P–S1PR2/3 signaling axis act in concert as part of a group of G-protein-coupled receptors (GPCRs). Notably, the study identified the long isoform of Carcinoembryonic Antigen–Related Cell Adhesion Molecule 1 (CEACAM1), a transmembrane glycoprotein with extracellular Ig-like domains and variable cytoplasmic tails generated by alternative splicing [78–80], as the regulator of S1P–S1PR2/3-dependent NETosis [77]. In another recent study, the authors used microarray, bulk RNA-seq, and single-cell RNA-seq datasets from the Gene Expression Omnibus database [81]. The study's novelty was that patients stratified by expression levels of NET-related genes exhibited distinct clinical profiles, with high or low expressers correlating with different post-transplant outcomes. Moreover, specific NET-associated gene signatures were predictive biomarkers for early allograft dysfunction following liver transplantation. A recent separate investigation also showed that during hepatic IRI, crosstalk between neutrophils and macrophage-derived Spleen tyrosine kinase (SYK) drives poor postoperative outcomes and tumor recurrence. The administration of pharmacologic SYK inhibitors significantly attenuated tissue damage by reducing neutrophil recruitment, NETs formation, NLRP3 inflammasome assembly, and liver inflammation [82]. These collective studies reveal a dynamic interplay among the native and non-parenchymal cells of the liver in terms of orchestrating the redox balance and immune response during hepatic IRI. Working towards understanding how their intercommunication drives liver injury may provide multiple potential targets for antioxidants and immunomodulatory intervention.

3. Immune–Hepatic Crosstalk in Response to Oxidative Stress

3.1. Innate Immune Responses

The bidirectional communication between parenchymal and immune cells and how it interacts through the duality of amplifying oxidative injury yet initiates repair mechanisms is not well defined [83,84]. Some historical studies have shown that Kupffer cells sense DAMPs during I/R oxidative stress and respond by producing ROS, TNF-α, IL-1β, and chemokines (e.g., CCL2) [85]. These mediators comprise hepatocyte mitochondrial function in a feed-forward loop that polarizes Kupffer cells away from pro-inflammatory (M1-like) and towards reparative (M2-like) phenotypes depending on the state of the redox balance [86] (Figure 4). We recently uncovered divergent functions for T cell immunoglobulin and mucin domain containing 4 (Tim4 signaling) depending on whether its source derives from donor liver or recipient-derived tissue [87]. More specifically, we showed that the disruption of donor Tim4 markedly attenuated IRI, whereas the loss of recipient Tim4 unexpectedly increased the hepatocellular damage, ER stress, disturbed lipid metabolism, and increased pro-inflammatory gene program (e.g., CD36, C/EBP Homologous Protein (CHOP), and IL-10). In thc clinical cohort, we reported that high hepatic TIM4 levels in transplant patients correlated with a higher BMI, increased ER stress and apoptotic markers, innate/adaptive immune activation, and higher early allograft dysfunction, suggesting worse graft survival. These findings suggest that targeting donor-derived TIM4 signaling, while preserving recipient TIM4 function, may be a viable strategy to preserve postoperative outcomes in liver transplantation.

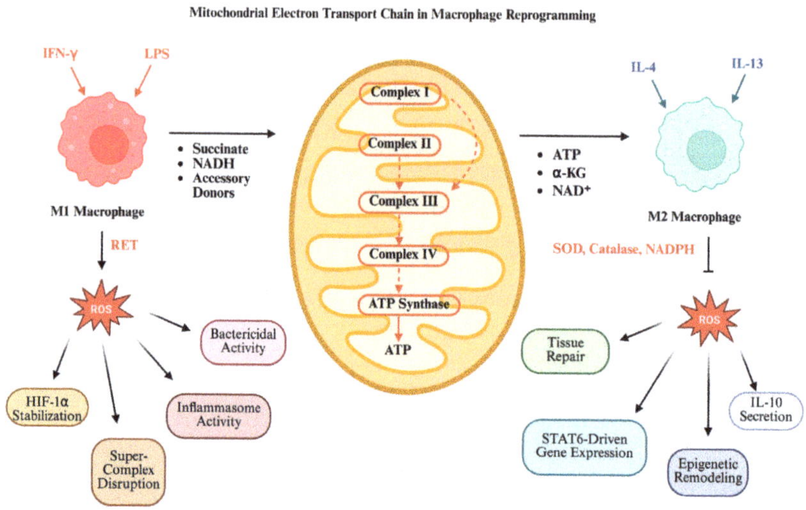

Figure 4. The mitochondrial ETC guides macrophage polarization into pro-inflammatory (M1) and anti-inflammatory (M2) states. In M1 macrophages, stimuli such as LPS and IFN-γ drive glycolysis and succinate accumulation, fueling reverse electron transport (RET) and mitochondrial ROS (mtROS) production. This promotes HIF-1α stabilization, inflammasome activation, and bactericidal activity. M2 macrophages, activated by IL-4/IL-13, rely on oxidative phosphorylation, fatty acid oxidation, and efficient ETC function with minimal ROS. The ETC supplies ATP, α-ketoglutarate, and NAD^+, supporting IL-10 secretion, tissue repair, and epigenetic remodeling. M2-derived antioxidants such as SOD, catalase, and NADPH further inhibit ROS, reinforcing an anti-inflammatory phenotype. Created in Biorender.com.

3.2. *Adaptive Immune Involvement*

Beyond the innate immune system, the liver regulates adaptive immune responses to hepatic I/R oxidative stress through T cell modulation [87]. In chronic inflammatory conditions such as Hepatitis B virus (HBV) infection, the liver functions as a rheostat, dampening $CD8^+$ T cell effector activity to prevent excessive immune-mediated tissue damage [88]. In this study, the authors demonstrated that liver-specific T cells, particularly CXCR6+ CD8 T cells, exhibit signs of exhaustion due to increased cyclic adenosine monophosphate (cAMP)-Protein Kinase A (PKA)-cAMP Response Element Modulator (CREM) signaling, which suppresses T cell activation (Figure 5). While protective in chronic infections, this mechanism may hinder effective immune responses under oxidative stress conditions, impairing the liver's ability to clear damaged cells and resolve inflammation. In a related recent report, it was demonstrated that hypothermic oxygenated machine perfusion (HOPE) impacts both the oxidative stress response and adaptive alloimmunity, leading to a shift toward immunoregulation [89]. Specifically, HOPE-treated liver grafts showed reduced intrahepatic immune cells and lower activation of ROS pathways compared with static cold storage in 27 patients evaluated in two randomized controlled trials. Mechanistically, perfused livers showed increased circulating and donor-specific regulatory $CD4^{+}FOXP3^{+}CD127^{lo}$ T cells two weeks post transplant, and decreased $CD8^{+}$ T cell alloreactivity at 3 months. The novelty of this study may implicate pre-transplant conditioning as an active way to modulate the host immune response, offering a new immunological rationale for the clinical benefits of machine perfusion strategies [1].

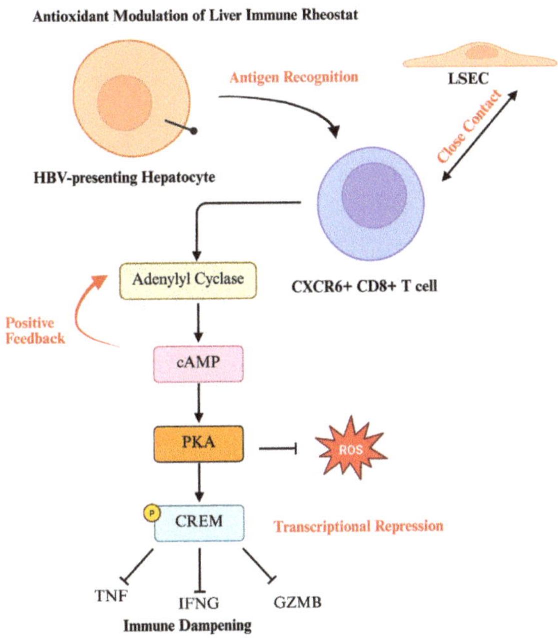

Figure 5. LSEC mediates cAMP Signaling of T cell activity in the liver. The liver maintains immune quiescence through a local rheostat mechanism involving HBV-presenting hepatocytes, liver sinusoidal endothelial cells (LSECs), and $CXCR6^{+}$ $CD8^{+}$ T cells. Antigen recognition leads to LSEC-mediated activation of adenylyl cyclase in T cells, triggering the cAMP–PKA–CREM pathway. This signaling cascade represses effector gene expression (IFNG, GZMB, TNF) and reduces mitochondrial ROS production, collectively dampening T cell activity. This results in a tunable immunosuppressive environment that prevents excessive inflammation and preserves tissue integrity. Created in Biorender.com.

Building on these observations of the adaptive immune response in hepatic IRI, a recent study showed that monoclonal therapy using anti-TIM1 monoclonal antibodies offered substantial protection against inflammation and apoptosis following administration [68]. The authors attribute the mechanism to the expansion of $TIM1^{+}$ regulatory B cells (Bregs) that increased the secretion of the anti-inflammatory cytokine IL-10. Notably, the protective effects of anti-TIM1 were lost upon B cell depletion with anti-CD20, underscoring the central role of Bregs as a critical immune population in regulating liver inflammation during transplant-related injury.

3.3. Feedback Loops Between ROS and Immune Activation

The dysregulation of feedback loops between oxidative stress and immune signaling intensifies the inflammatory cascade during hepatic IRI. Their coordination of complex physiological responses due to ROS build-up is partly responsible for ensuing hepatocyte apoptosis, endothelial dysfunction, and, in severe cases, graft failure following liver transplantation. In the past few years, several representative research studies have addressed the transcriptional regulation, immune signaling, and metabolic stress involved in feedback loops resulting from hepatic IRI. Sun et al. investigated a transcriptional regulatory feedback loop involving Small Nucleolar RNA Host Gene 1 (SNHG1), miR-186-5p, and the transcription factor YY1, which together promoted the survival and proliferation of murine hepatocytes. Notably, the ability of SNHG1 to titrate away the inhibitory regulation of miR-186-5p contributed to a positive feedback loop that ultimately reduced hepatocyte apoptosis [90].

Building on this, a recent study investigated pathological feedback loops where ischemia causes primary cilia shortening in biliary epithelial cells, triggering transcriptional regulation and cellular senescence following liver transplantation [91]. In a related recent report, the authors investigated the positive feedback loop involving murine HMGB1 release, which activates TLR4, leading to NF-κB-driven neutrophil recruitment and further ROS generation, perpetuating liver injury [92]. Mechanistically, the authors show that the active peptide (Ac2-26) of Annexin A1 can be used therapeutically to target feedback loops that lead to neutrophil immune activation, inflammatory cytokine cascades (like TNF-α, IL-1β, IL-6), and ROS amplification. These limited studies highlight how feedback loops confer stability, precision, and adaptability to biological systems. In the future, we will need to understand how multiple feedback loops (hepatocytes -> Kupffer cells, neutrophils -> hepatocytes, T cells -> macrophages) all interact together to mitigate liver damage by modulating both oxidative stress while integrating immune feedback mechanisms.

4. Recent Antioxidant Efforts to Mitigate ROS in Hepatic IRI

4.1. Targeted Delivery Systems

Nanomedicine has benefited dramatically from the interdisciplinary collaboration of biomedical sciences, physics, and engineering that has led to the design of nanoscale materials that can deliver therapeutic agents with high precision to the liver. New studies using targeted nanoparticles continue to expand our appreciation of how antioxidant strategies can be modulated and tested in preclinical models. Nanoparticles are being designed to target damaged hepatic tissue during IRI, where they can scavenge ROS, modulate immune responses, and release anti-inflammatory drugs [93]. Surface modifications, like Polyethylene glycol (PEG)ylation and ligand targeting, continue to be optimized to enhance controlled-release mechanisms that alter bioavailability while minimizing systemic toxicity [94,95]. PEGylation provides a hydrophilic layer that prevents rapid clearance by the reticuloendothelial system [96], allowing for a longer time in circulation and more particles to accumulate in ischemic liver tissue. This was demonstrated in a recent study by Gao et al. (2025), which used PEGylated catalase (CAT-PEG) to mitigate oxidative stress and inflammation following hepatic IRI [97]. Similarly, a recent study showed how surface modifications using 1,2-distearoyl-sn-glycero-3-phosphoethanolamine (DSPE)-PEG2000-Galactose significantly alleviated a mouse model of hepatic IRI [98].

Specifically, the authors engineered DSPE-PEG2000-Galactose to target mesenchymal stem cell-derived exosomes to the liver. Antioxidant nanoparticles are often modified with targeting ligands such as N-acetylgalactosamine (GalNAc), mannose, and aptamers to improve specificity further. A separate recent investigation found that strategic surface engineering techniques to exploit natural ligand receptor interactions in a model of partial liver warm ischemia [99]. More specifically, mannose receptors (CD206) were coupled to Receptor-Interacting Protein Kinase 3 (RIPK3) siRNA as a part of the delivery system. RIPK3 is a serine/threonine protein kinase critical in regulating necroptosis, whereas mannose receptors are highly expressed on Kupffer cells. In this way, macrophages preferentially took up mannose-decorated nanoparticles via receptor-mediated endocytosis, leading to the knockdown of ROS production in Kupffer cells. Another study demonstrating how surface modifications reduce ROS production in IRI is based on delivering Ceria@Apt, a cerium oxide type of nanoparticles, to the liver [100]. The authors showed that by conjugating cerium oxide to anti-C5a, a natural neutrophil/macrophage chemoattractant that is part of the complement system, nanoparticles could simultaneously scavenge ROS and block C5a-mediated inflammation. While offering a hint to their therapeutic potential, future studies may benefit from determining whether anti-inflammatory nanoparticles used in hepatic IRI would be as versatile for other systemic ischemic disorders.

4.2. *Enzyme-Based Nano-Therapies*

Some recent examples of studies that exploit nanomedicine in hepatic IRI models include one report on the synthesis of ultrasmall cerium (CE)–manganese nanoclusters that exhibit superoxide dismutase (SOD)- and catalase (CAT)-mimetic activity, enabling the efficient scavenging of key ROS including $OH^{\cdot}$, $O_2^{-\cdot}$, and H_2O_2 [101]. The authors showed that cerium–manganese nanoclusters demonstrate strong biocompatibility, preferential liver accumulation, and significant therapeutic efficacy in reducing oxidative stress, hepatocellular injury, and inflammation in a murine model of hepatic IRI. Mechanistically, the dual-valent Ce^{3+}/Ce^{4+}-dependent redox activity coupled with MnO_2-mediated catalysis enabled ROS reduction and inflammatory responses by suppressing Kupffer cell and neutrophil activation. The following year, a study showed that cerium oxide (Co) acts as a potent ROS scavenger when administered via laparotomy to rats prior to ischemic/reperfusion stress (I/R) injury [102]. The authors showed that Co therapy leads to lower levels of lipid peroxidation, higher levels of antioxidant enzyme catalase, and detoxification enzyme glutathione S-transferase.

4.3. *Redox Signaling Modulators Targeting Hepatic IRI Using Nanomedicine*

Recent advancements in nanomedicine highlight how redox-sensitive delivery platforms are used to engage metabolic and immune pathways implicated in liver injury. For example, a multifunctional nanodrug, A-MPDA@Fe_3O_4@PVP, was recently developed to scavenge ROS to alleviate hepatic ischemia–reperfusion injury [103]. Notably, this nanoplatform combines L-arginine-doped mesoporous polydopamine with ferric oxide and a PVP coating, enabling enzymatic ROS scavenging and immunomodulation. In their preclinical models, A-MPDA@Fe_3O_4@PVP lowered oxidative damage and preserved liver function through a mechanism that involved the activation of the PPARγ/NF-κB pathway [103]. Another group developed a ROS-responsive liposomal nanocarrier (RLLs) co-loaded with LY294002 and oridonin to target key signaling pathways in NAFLD. LY294002 is a broad-spectrum inhibitor of phosphoinositide 3-kinases (PI3Ks), while oridonin is a natural Chinese medicinal herb known to have anti-inflammatory, anti-tumor, antioxidant, and anti-fibrotic properties [104,105]. The RLLs were shown to be effective ROS scavengers, could enhance hepatic delivery via Cluster of Differentiation 44 (CD44)-mediated targeting, and stabilize CYP450 activity, leading to improved insulin sensitivity and reduced inflammation and fibrosis in a CCl_4-induced NAFLD mouse model [95]. CD44 is a transmembrane glycoprotein that functions as a receptor for various ligands, most notably hyaluronic acid, an extracellular matrix component [106]. Cytochrome P450 belongs to the superfamily of heme-containing liver enzymes essential for metabolizing drugs, toxins, and endogenous compounds like hormones and fatty acids [107]. By integrating ROS-responsive materials, immunomodulatory capabilities, and surface modifications like CD44-mediated targeting, nanoparticles may soon offer clinicians the opportunity to deliver drugs actively participating in redox regulation and tissue repair.

Many recent studies have built on the therapeutic potential of flavonoid compounds to mitigate hepatic IRI. For example, hydroxysafflor yellow A (HSYA), a water-soluble flavonoid derived from safflower, was shown to reduce and suppress intracellular ROS and apoptosis. It could also lead to decreased markers of DNA damage and lipid peroxidation, indicating potent antioxidant and cytoprotective effects [108]. Reducing oxidative stress was attributed to lower key inflammatory cytokines such as TNF-α, IL-1β, and IL-6, suggesting that its hepatoprotective function involves direct redox regulation and the modulation of inflammatory signaling pathways. Table 2 shows synthetic antioxidant enhancements to mitigate hepatic IRI.

Table 2. Synthetic antioxidant enhancements to mitigate hepatic IRI.

Antioxidant	Structure/Category	Mechanism	Clinical Applications	Ref.
Targeted Delivery				
(PEG)ylation	Hydrophilic Polymer	Promotes particle circulation and therapeutic effects.	Use of PEGylated catalase (CAT-PEG) reduced hepatic IRI.	[97,98]
GalNAc	Amino Disaccharide	Binding with hepatocyte ASGPR enables nanoparticle targeting to liver cells.	Enhanced CRISPR gene editing therapy with specificity to the liver.	[109]
Mannose	Monosaccharide	Modifications taken up by Kupffer cells to reduce ROS.	Mannose-conjugated RIPK3 siRNA delivery improves treatment of atherosclerosis.	[99,110]
Aptamers	Single-stranded nucleic acid sequences	High-affinity aptamer sequences guide nanoparticles to desired location.	Aptamer conjugation to gold nanoparticles (AuNPs) as a targeted treatment for cancer.	[111–113]
Enzyme-Based				
Ultrasmall Cerium (CE)–Manganese Nanoclusters	Nanozyme	Displayed (SOD)- and (CAT)-mimetic activity promoted ROS scavenging activity.	Use of CE–Manganese nanoclusters reduced oxidative stress in a murine hepatic injury model.	[101]
Cerium Oxide	Metal Oxide	Reduces lipid peroxidation; increases catalase and GST activity; acts as a potent ROS scavenger.	Administration of cerium oxide via laparotomy prior to IRI improved outcomes in rat model.	[102]
Redox Signaling Modulators				
A-MPDA@Fe_3O_4@PVP	Polydopamine Nanodrug	Prevents Fe_3O_4 accumulation; mimics CAT and SOD activity; activates PPARγ/NF-κB pathway to reduce oxidative stress.	When administered under hepatic IRI conditions, promoted ROS scavenging, immunomodulation, and liver function.	[103]

Table 2. *Cont.*

Antioxidant	Structure/Category	Mechanism	Clinical Applications	Ref.
RLLs + LY294002 and Oridonin	Liposomal Nanocarrier	LY294002 inhibits PI3Ks; Oridonin provides antioxidant and anti-inflammatory effects; RLLs enhance liver delivery via CD44 targeting and stabilize CYP450, reducing inflammation and injury.	The use of this combination treatment improved insulin sensitivity and lowered inflammation and fibrosis in NAFLD mouse.	[95]
Flavonoid Compounds	Polyphenol	Reduces hepatic IRI and OxS through nanoparticle scavenging and suppression of pro-inflammatory cytokines TNF-α, IL-1β, and IL-6.	Hydroxysafflor yellow A (HSYA) was shown to reduce intracellular ROS, apoptosis, DNA damage, and lipid peroxidation.	[108]

Abbreviations: Asialoglycoprotein Receptor (ASGPR), Catalase (CAT), Cluster of Differentiation 44 (CD44), 1,2-distearoyl-sn-glycero-3-phosphoethanolamine (DSPE), Ischemia–Reperfusion Injury (IRI), N-acetylgalactosamine (GalNAc), Nonalcoholic Fatty Liver Disease (NAFLD), Nuclear Factor Kappa B (NF- κB), Oxidative Stress (OxS), Peroxisome Proliferator-Activated Receptor Gamma (PPARγ), Phosphoinositide 3-Kinases (P13Ks), Polyethylene Glycol (PEG), Reactive Oxygen Species (ROS), Receptor-Interacting Protein Kinase 3 (RIPK3), ROS-responsive Liposomal Nanocarriers (RLLs), Small Interfering RNA (SiRNA), Superoxide Dismutase (SOD).

5. Challenges and Future Directions

The grand challenge for the future of liver transplantation translational research lies in bridging the complexity of immune cascades with intricate molecular cross-regulation among diverse hepatic cell populations [114]. Our inability to integrate all the molecular pathways involved in hepatic IRI cascade into a unified framework remains a significant block to therapeutic progress. While these may present limitations for clinical organ transplantation, ample opportunities for insightful and ground-breaking basic research remain. The drive towards improving the donor organ supply represents the most challenging global problem, with the number of patients awaiting life-saving transplant increasing six-fold [114]. Impaired donor tissue quality remains the major contributing factor to the organ shortage. Our aging population, with its pre-existing diseases (e.g., nonalcoholic steatohepatitis, NASH), is particularly susceptible to innate immune-driven tissue damage during cadaver organ harvesting. A stepwise bench-to-bedside translational approach is warranted to promote inflammation-resolving defenses by targeting excessive ROS generation. This will require renewed focus on "rejuvenating" donor organs in the peri-transplant period so as to improve their tissue quality and promote tissue regeneration via specific antioxidant molecular signaling pathways [114].

Antioxidant molecular tools, like nanoparticles, must overcome inherent challenges before translational success is achieved. For example, biological barriers that prevent the intracellular delivery of antioxidants/anti-inflammatory therapeutics by inefficient endosomal escape will need to be overcome to enhance bioactivity at target sites. Reproducibility and scale-up synthesis remain formidable hurdles. Translating antioxidants or anti-inflammatory therapeutics into clinically viable products will require robust manufacturing pipelines, the standardization of surface modifications, and regulatory-compliant quality control. Another concern that must be considered is whether future antioxidants/anti-inflammatory therapeutics trigger immunogenicity or provoke unintended immune responses. The risk is heightened in hepatic IRI, where immune sensitivity is elevated. Moreover, the growing appreciation for differences in redox and immune states among patients needing liver transplantation will require personalized approaches that tailor treatments to individual oxidative stress profiles, immune status, or genetic predispositions. Finally, more studies need to focus on developing reliable biomarkers to measure the status of ROS, cytokines, or danger signals in real time. In this way, clinicians may use the dynamic modulation of feedback loops and better control immune–redox balance to manage hepatic IRI. Table 3 shows several representative clinical studies focused on therapeutic targets for ROS, collected from the years 2022–2025.

Table 3. Representative clinical studies focused on therapeutic targets for ROS, collected from years 2022–2025.

Study Focus	Therapy	Study Design Phase, N, Year	Novelty	Outcome	Ref.
Oxidative Stress					
ALD	CYP2EI inhibitor CMZ	RCT, P2, 60, 2023	Inhibition of ethanol metabolism pathway in decreasing liver toxicity and damage	CMZ treatment significantly decreased hepatic steatosis more effectively than no treatment or CZP treatment only.	[115]
Skin Damage	GSH synthesis booster GAP	RCT, 21, 2024	Increased stability of topical GSH protection through GAP formulation	Topical GAP application induced higher GSH expression in human keratinocytes and mitigated damaged-induced oxidative stress and ROS production.	[116]
Chronic Pain	Phytocannabinoid, omega-3 fatty acids, glucosinolates	RCT, 25, 2023	Decrease in ROS through dietary changes involving nutrients in hemp oil, calamari oil, and broccoli	Participants who received the multi-ingredient therapeutic supplement experienced significantly reduced ROS production and pain levels due to OxS.	[117]
Immune Cells					
Fanconi Anemia	Quercetin	CT, P1, 30, 2025	Treatment of immune-deficiency disorder through oral quercetin interventions	Some patients showed less ROS in blood and bone marrow stem cell regions, increase in platelet count, decrease in neutrophil and hemoglobin levels.	[118]
Myocardial Infarction	CoQ10	RCT, 131, 2024	CoQ10 as a therapeutic recovery agent post MI	MI patients who received CoQ10 experienced improved cardiac function recovery, and animal studies indicated decreased pro-inflammatory immune cell recruitment as the cause.	[119]
Cancer Immunotherapy	OX40 agonist GSK3174998	CT, P1, 138, 2023	Use of antibody GSK3174998 alone or in combination regimen with PD-1 blocker to inhibit cancer growth	While treatment was tolerated by patients, there was little success in inducing immune cell activation in controlling disease progression using either regimen.	[120]
IRI					
Aneurysm Repair	Sevoflurane and Desflurane	RCT, 80, 2024	Use of volatile anesthetics in avoiding OxS/IRI and ROS production during surgery	While individual biomarkers for OxS/antioxidant effect were not significantly different in treatment groups, there was an improved OXY-SCORE in patients who received Desflurane post aneurysm repair.	[121]
Myocardial Infarction	Pentoxifylline	RCT, P2, 161, 2023	Pentoxifylline intravenous pre-treatment ahead of PCI to avoid IRI	While treatment was tolerated by patients, there was no significant difference between treatment group and control.	[122]
Nerve cell recovery	miR-106a Nanoparticles carrying DEX	RCT, 2022	Use of combination treatment in nanoparticles to attenuate IRI in hippocampal neurons	Pro-inflammatory and apoptotic activity, as well as IRI reduced through treatment with miR-106a nanoparticles and DEX.	[123]

Abbreviations: Alcohol-associated Liver Disease (ALD), Clinical Trial (CT), Clomethiazole (CMZ), Clorazepate (CZP), Coenzyme Q10 (CoQ10), Cytochrome P450 2E1 (CYP2E1), Dexmedetomidine (DEX),Glutathione (GSH), Glutathione Amino Acid Precursor (GAP), Ischemia–Reperfusion Injury (IRI), MicroRNA-106a (miR-106a), Myocardial Infarction (MI), Oxidative Stress (OxS), Percutaneous Coronary Intervention (PCI), Phase (P), Programmed Cell-Death Protein 1 (PD-1), Randomized Controlled Trial (RCT), Reactive Oxygen Species (ROS).

6. Conclusions

The interplay between oxidative stress, immune crosstalk, and feedback loops in hepatic IRI remains poorly understood. Understanding how these multiple feedback loops converge and influence each other may be key to identifying precise intervention points and improving outcomes in liver transplantation. Accumulating evidence suggests that managing ROS in the stressed liver may protect hepatocytes from damage and suppress immune activation through DAMP release and inflammatory signaling cascades. Integrating a systems biology approach that includes emerging antioxidants and immunomodulatory therapies could provide new avenues for personalized and more effective treatments.

Author Contributions: Conceptualization—K.J.D.; Writing—original draft—K.J.D.; Figures and Tables—R.C. and A.K.; Writing—review and editing—J.W.K.-W. and K.J.D.; Project Administration—J.W.K.-W. All authors have read and agreed to the published version of the manuscript.

Funding: This work was supported by NIH Grants P01 AI120944, R01 DK062357, and R01 AI155856-01.

Acknowledgments: All authors have seen the manuscript and consented to be included here. Figures 1–5 were created with Biorender.com. There was no assistance in the preparation of the manuscript.

Conflicts of Interest: The authors declare no conflicts of interest.

References

1. Dery, K.J.; Kaldas, F.; Kupiec-Weglinski, J.W. Targeting Ischemia-reperfusion injury in liver transplant rejuvenation. *Transplant. Rep.* **2025**, *10*, 100176. [CrossRef]
2. Mansouri, A.; Gattolliat, C.H.; Asselah, T. Mitochondrial Dysfunction and Signaling in Chronic Liver Diseases. *Gastroenterology* **2018**, *155*, 629–647. [CrossRef] [PubMed]
3. Dery, K.J.; Yao, S.; Cheng, B.; Kupiec-Weglinski, J.W. New therapeutic concepts against ischemia-reperfusion injury in organ transplantation. *Expert Rev. Clin. Immunol.* **2023**, *19*, 1205–1224. [CrossRef]
4. Dery, K.J.; Kupiec-Weglinski, J.W. New insights into ischemia-reperfusion injury signaling pathways in organ transplantation. *Curr. Opin. Organ Transpl.* **2022**, *27*, 424–433. [CrossRef]
5. Dery, K.J.; Kojima, H.; Kageyama, S.; Kadono, K.; Hirao, H.; Cheng, B.; Zhai, Y.; Farmer, D.G.; Kaldas, F.M.; Yuan, X.; et al. Alternative splicing of CEACAM1 by hypoxia-inducible factor-1α enhances tolerance to hepatic ischemia in mice and humans. *Sci. Transl. Med.* **2023**, *15*, eadf2059. [CrossRef] [PubMed]
6. Che, Z.; Zhou, Z.; Li, S.Q.; Gao, L.; Xiao, J.; Wong, N.K. ROS/RNS as molecular signatures of chronic liver diseases. *Trends Mol. Med.* **2023**, *29*, 951–967. [CrossRef] [PubMed]
7. Shields, H.J.; Traa, A.; Van Raamsdonk, J.M. Beneficial and Detrimental Effects of Reactive Oxygen Species on Lifespan: A Comprehensive Review of Comparative and Experimental Studies. *Front. Cell Dev. Biol.* **2021**, *9*, 628157. [CrossRef]
8. Ben-Mahdi, M.H.; Dang, P.M.; Gougerot-Pocidalo, M.A.; O'Dowd, Y.; El-Benna, J.; Pasquier, C. Xanthine Oxidase-Derived ROS Display a Biphasic Effect on Endothelial Cells Adhesion and FAK Phosphorylation. *Oxid. Med. Cell Longev.* **2016**, *2016*, 9346242. [CrossRef]
9. Wei, Y.; Jia, S.; Ding, Y.; Xia, S.; Giunta, S. Balanced basal-levels of ROS (redox-biology), and very-low-levels of pro-inflammatory cytokines (cold-inflammaging), as signaling molecules can prevent or slow-down overt-inflammaging, and the aging-associated decline of adaptive-homeostasis. *Exp. Gerontol.* **2023**, *172*, 112067. [CrossRef]
10. Palma, F.R.; Gantner, B.N.; Sakiyama, M.J.; Kayzuka, C.; Shukla, S.; Lacchini, R.; Cunniff, B.; Bonini, M.G. ROS production by mitochondria: Function or dysfunction? *Oncogene* **2024**, *43*, 295–303. [CrossRef]
11. Lu, J.; Liu, J.; Li, A. Roles of neutrophil reactive oxygen species (ROS) generation in organ function impairment in sepsis. *J. Zhejiang Univ. Sci. B* **2022**, *23*, 437–450. [CrossRef]
12. Yang, L.; Shi, F.; Cao, F.; Wang, L.; She, J.; He, B.; Xu, X.; Kong, L.; Cai, B. Neutrophils in Tissue Injury and Repair: Molecular Mechanisms and Therapeutic Targets. *MedComm* **2025**, *6*, e70184. [CrossRef]
13. Fang, S.; Jiang, M.; Jiao, J.; Zhao, H.; Liu, D.; Gao, D.; Wang, T.; Yang, Z.; Yuan, H. Unraveling the ROS-Inflammation-Immune Balance: A New Perspective on Aging and Disease. *Aging Dis.* **2025**, *17*, 1–21. [CrossRef]
14. Kupiec-Weglinski, J.W. Grand Challenges in Organ Transplantation. *Front. Transpl.* **2022**, *1*, 897679. [CrossRef]

15. Dery, K.J.; Najjar, S.M.; Beauchemin, N.; Shively, J.E.; Kupiec-Weglinski, J.W. Mechanism and function of CEACAM1 splice isoforms. *Eur. J. Clin. Investig.* **2024**, *54* (Suppl. S2), e14350. [CrossRef]
16. Sies, H.; Belousov, V.V.; Chandel, N.S.; Davies, M.J.; Jones, D.P.; Mann, G.E.; Murphy, M.P.; Yamamoto, M.; Winterbourn, C. Defining roles of specific reactive oxygen species (ROS) in cell biology and physiology. *Nat. Rev. Mol. Cell Biol.* **2022**, *23*, 499–515. [CrossRef]
17. Li, S.; Tan, H.Y.; Wang, N.; Zhang, Z.J.; Lao, L.; Wong, C.W.; Feng, Y. The Role of Oxidative Stress and Antioxidants in Liver Diseases. *Int. J. Mol. Sci.* **2015**, *16*, 26087–26124. [CrossRef]
18. Allameh, A.; Niayesh-Mehr, R.; Aliarab, A.; Sebastiani, G.; Pantopoulos, K. Oxidative Stress in Liver Pathophysiology and Disease. *Antioxidants* **2023**, *12*, 1653. [CrossRef] [PubMed]
19. Fu, H.; Li, W.; Cheng, Q.; Weng, Z.; Huang, Z.; Zhu, L.; Ding, T.; Ding, B. Ellagic acid alleviates iron overload-induced liver damage by mitigating ferroptosis through modulation of the TGFβ/Smad signaling pathway. *Food Res. Int.* **2025**, *214*, 116590. [CrossRef] [PubMed]
20. Gao, H.; Bai, H.; Su, Y.; Gao, Y.; Fang, H.; Li, D.; Yu, Y.; Lu, X.; Xia, D.; Mao, D.; et al. Fecal microbiota transplantation from Helicobacter pylori carriers following bismuth quadruple therapy exacerbates alcohol-related liver disease in mice via LPS-induced activation of hepatic TLR4/NF-κB/NLRP3 signaling. *J. Transl. Med.* **2025**, *23*, 627. [CrossRef]
21. Dong, T.; Zhang, C.; Wu, Z.; Shuai, L.; Fu, N.; Zhang, Y.; Zhang, L.; Xiong, X. A biomimetic nanomedicine alleviates liver transplant-related biliary injury by sequentially inhibiting oxidative stress and regulating macrophage polarization via Nrf-2/HO-1 and JNK pathways. *Mater. Today Bio* **2025**, *32*, 101797. [CrossRef] [PubMed]
22. Lin, C.S.; He, M.Q.; An, M.Y.; Zhao, Q.H.; Zhang, Z.H.; Deng, K.Y.; Ai, Y.; Xin, H.B. Ultra-Small Copper-Based Multienzyme-Like Nanoparticles Protect Against Hepatic Ischemia-Reperfusion Injury Through Scavenging Reactive Oxygen Species in Mice. *Small* **2024**, *20*, e2403313. [CrossRef] [PubMed]
23. Hui, B.; Zhang, X.; Wang, S.; Shu, Y.; Li, R.; Yang, Z. Crocetin preconditioning attenuates ischemia reperfusion-induced hepatic injury by disrupting Keap1/Nrf2 interaction and activating Nrf2/HO-1 pathway. *Tissue Cell* **2024**, *88*, 102411. [CrossRef]
24. Yang, F.; Gao, H.; Niu, Z.; Ni, Q.; Zhu, H.; Wang, J.; Lu, J. Puerarin protects the fatty liver from ischemia-reperfusion injury by regulating the PI3K/AKT signaling pathway. *Braz. J. Med. Biol. Res.* **2024**, *57*, e13229. [CrossRef] [PubMed]
25. Rajabi, S.; Mohammadi, Y.; Kabiri-Rad, H.; Rajabi-Moghaddam, M.; Farimani, A.R. Comparative Effects of Crocin and Losartan on RAGE, TGF-β, TNF-α Gene Expression and Histopathological Changes of the Liver Tissue in Rats With Diabetes. *Endocrinol. Diabetes Metab.* **2025**, *8*, e70016. [CrossRef] [PubMed]
26. Lin, J.; Chen, J.; Wang, M.; He, K.; Lin, C.; Cao, X.; Lai, J.; Zeng, B.; Guo, X. Ultrasound-driven ROS-scavenging nanobubbles for synergistic NASH treatment via FXR activation. *Ultrason. Sonochem.* **2025**, *118*, 107352. [CrossRef]
27. Chen, Q.; Lin, H.; Huang, X.; Yu, W. Codonopsis pilosula polysaccharides attenuate lipid accumulation and inflammatory response in the NAFLD mouse by regulating AMPK/ACC/SREBP1 signaling pathway. *Tissue Cell* **2025**, *96*, 102984. [CrossRef]
28. Lu, D.; Huang, A.; Tong, X.; Zhang, X.; Li, S.; Yu, X. Nobiletin protects against alcohol-induced mitochondrial dysfunction and liver injury by regulating the hepatic NRF1-TFAM signaling pathway. *Redox Rep.* **2024**, *29*, 2395779. [CrossRef]
29. Huda, N.; Kusumanchi, P.; Jiang, Y.; Gao, H.; Thoudam, T.; Zeng, G.; Skill, N.J.; Sun, Z.; Liangpunsakul, S.; Ma, J.; et al. Silencing FAF2 mitigates alcohol-induced hepatic steatosis by modulating lipolysis and PCSK9 pathway. *Hepatol. Commun.* **2025**, *9*, e0641. [CrossRef]
30. Cheng, Y.; Song, T.; Yao, J.; Wang, Q.; Meng, C.; Feng, F. Study on the mechanism of hsa_circ_0074763 regulating the miR-3667-3P/ACSL4 axis in liver fibrosis. *Sci. Rep.* **2025**, *15*, 10548. [CrossRef]
31. Liang, L.; Dong, Z.; Shen, Z.; Zang, Y.; Yang, W.; Wu, L.; Bao, L. Inhibitory effects of umbelliferone on carbon tetrachloride-induced hepatic fibrosis in rats through the TGF-β1-Smad signaling pathway. *Mol. Med. Rep.* **2025**, *32*, 171. [CrossRef] [PubMed]
32. Yang, Z.; Tai, Y.; Lan, T.; Zhao, C.; Gao, J.H.; Tang, C.W.; Tong, H. Inhibition of Cyclooxygenase-2 Upregulates the Nuclear Factor Erythroid 2-related Factor 2 Signaling Pathway to Mitigate Hepatocyte Ferroptosis in Chronic Liver Injury. *J. Clin. Transl. Hepatol.* **2025**, *13*, 409–417. [CrossRef] [PubMed]
33. Sun, B.; Ding, P.; Song, Y.; Zhou, J.; Chen, X.; Peng, C.; Liu, S. FDX1 downregulation activates mitophagy and the PI3K/AKT signaling pathway to promote hepatocellular carcinoma progression by inducing ROS production. *Redox Biol.* **2024**, *75*, 103302. [CrossRef]
34. Liu, Y.; Wang, Y.; Wang, J.; Wang, X.; Chen, L.; Han, T.; Lian, H.; Gan, M.; Wang, J. Fangchinoline suppresses hepatocellular carcinoma by regulating ROS accumulation via the TRIM7/Nrf2 signaling pathway. *Phytomedicine* **2024**, *135*, 156143. [CrossRef]
35. Niu, Z.; Zhao, Q.; Cao, H.; Yang, B.; Wang, S. Hypoxia-activated oxidative stress mediates SHP2/PI3K signaling pathway to promote hepatocellular carcinoma growth and metastasis. *Sci. Rep.* **2025**, *15*, 4847. [CrossRef]

36. Duan, J.; Huang, Z.; Qin, S.; Li, B.; Zhang, Z.; Liu, R.; Wang, K.; Nice, E.C.; Jiang, J.; Huang, C. Oxidative stress induces extracellular vesicle release by upregulation of HEXB to facilitate tumour growth in experimental hepatocellular carcinoma. *J. Extracell. Vesicles* **2024**, *13*, e12468. [CrossRef]
37. Chouchani, E.T.; Kazak, L.; Jedrychowski, M.P.; Lu, G.Z.; Erickson, B.K.; Szpyt, J.; Pierce, K.A.; Laznik-Bogoslavski, D.; Vetrivelan, R.; Clish, C.B.; et al. Mitochondrial ROS regulate thermogenic energy expenditure and sulfenylation of UCP1. *Nature* **2016**, *532*, 112–116. [CrossRef]
38. Zhao, R.Z.; Jiang, S.; Zhang, L.; Yu, Z.B. Mitochondrial electron transport chain, ROS generation and uncoupling (Review). *Int. J. Mol. Med.* **2019**, *44*, 3–15. [CrossRef]
39. Liao, F.H.; Chen, S.P.; Yao, C.N.; Wu, T.H.; Liu, M.T.; Hsu, C.S.; Chen, H.M.; Lin, S.Y. Oxygen-Binding Sites of Enriched Gold Nanoclusters for Capturing Mitochondrial Reverse Electrons. *Nano Lett.* **2024**, *24*, 11202–11209. [CrossRef]
40. Balnis, J.; Jackson, E.L.; Drake, L.A.; Vincent, C.E.; Hwajeong, L.; Singer, H.A.; Jaitovich, A. Chronic succinate exposure does not cause liver injury. *Am. J. Physiol. Endocrinol. Metab.* **2025**, *329*, E39–E45. [CrossRef] [PubMed]
41. LaMoia, T.E.; Hubbard, B.T.; Guerra, M.T.; Nasiri, A.; Sakuma, I.; Kahn, M.; Zhang, D.; Goodman, R.P.; Nathanson, M.H.; Sancak, Y.; et al. Cytosolic calcium regulates hepatic mitochondrial oxidation, intrahepatic lipolysis, and gluconeogenesis via CAMKII activation. *Cell Metab.* **2024**, *36*, 2329–2340.e4. [CrossRef]
42. Tang, S.P.; Mao, X.L.; Chen, Y.H.; Yan, L.L.; Ye, L.P.; Li, S.W. Reactive Oxygen Species Induce Fatty Liver and Ischemia-Reperfusion Injury by Promoting Inflammation and Cell Death. *Front. Immunol.* **2022**, *13*, 870239. [CrossRef]
43. Matuz-Mares, D.; Vázquez-Meza, H.; Vilchis-Landeros, M.M. NOX as a Therapeutic Target in Liver Disease. *Antioxidants* **2022**, *11*, 2038. [CrossRef]
44. Kang, S.W.; Ban, J.Y.; Park, M.S. Protective Role of Rapamycin in Fibrotic Liver Ischemia/Reperfusion Injury (C57bl/6 Mouse). *Transpl. Proc.* **2024**, *56*, 672–677. [CrossRef]
45. An, X.; Yu, W.; Liu, J.; Tang, D.; Yang, L.; Chen, X. Oxidative cell death in cancer: Mechanisms and therapeutic opportunities. *Cell Death Dis.* **2024**, *15*, 556. [CrossRef]
46. Zhang, S.; Feng, Z.; Gao, W.; Duan, Y.; Fan, G.; Geng, X.; Wu, B.; Li, K.; Liu, K.; Peng, C. Aucubin Attenuates Liver Ischemia-Reperfusion Injury by Inhibiting the HMGB1/TLR-4/NF-κB Signaling Pathway, Oxidative Stress, and Apoptosis. *Front. Pharmacol.* **2020**, *11*, 544124. [CrossRef] [PubMed]
47. Yue, P.; Lv, X.; You, J.; Zou, Y.; Luo, J.; Lu, Z.; Cao, H.; Liu, Z.; Fan, X.; Ye, Q. Hypothermic oxygenated perfusion attenuates DCD liver ischemia-reperfusion injury by activating the JAK2/STAT3/HAX1 pathway to regulate endoplasmic reticulum stress. *Cell Mol. Biol. Lett.* **2023**, *28*, 55. [CrossRef] [PubMed]
48. Liu, J.; Luo, R.; Zhang, Y.; Li, X. Current status and perspective on molecular targets and therapeutic intervention strategy in hepatic ischemia-reperfusion injury. *Clin. Mol. Hepatol.* **2024**, *30*, 585–619. [CrossRef]
49. Zhou, Z.; Xu, M.-J.; Gao, B. Hepatocytes: A key cell type for innate immunity. *Cell. Mol. Immunol.* **2016**, *13*, 301–315. [CrossRef]
50. Yabe, Y.; Koyama, Y.; Nishikawa, M.; Takakura, Y.; Hashida, M. Hepatocyte-specific distribution of catalase and its inhibitory effect on hepatic ischemia/reperfusion injury in mice. *Free Radic. Res.* **1999**, *30*, 265–274. [CrossRef]
51. Gan, L.; Wang, W.; Jiang, J.; Tian, K.; Liu, W.; Cao, Z. Dual role of Nrf2 signaling in hepatocellular carcinoma: Promoting development, immune evasion, and therapeutic challenges. *Front. Immunol.* **2024**, *15*, 1429836. [CrossRef] [PubMed]
52. Ong, A.J.S.; Bladen, C.E.; Tigani, T.A.; Karamalakis, A.P.; Evason, K.J.; Brown, K.K.; Cox, A.G. The KEAP1-NRF2 pathway regulates TFEB/TFE3-dependent lysosomal biogenesis. *Proc. Natl. Acad. Sci. USA* **2023**, *120*, e2217425120. [CrossRef] [PubMed]
53. Hirao, H.; Dery, K.J.; Kageyama, S.; Nakamura, K.; Kupiec-Weglinski, J.W. Heme Oxygenase-1 in liver transplant ischemia-reperfusion injury: From bench-to-bedside. *Free Radic. Biol. Med.* **2020**, *157*, 75–82. [CrossRef] [PubMed]
54. Fuertes-Agudo, M.; Luque-Tévar, M.; Cucarella, C.; Martín-Sanz, P.; Casado, M. Advances in Understanding the Role of NRF2 in Liver Pathophysiology and Its Relationship with Hepatic-Specific Cyclooxygenase-2 Expression. *Antioxidants* **2023**, *12*, 1491. [CrossRef] [PubMed]
55. Jung, J.W.; Wang, F.; Turk, A.; Park, J.S.; Ma, H.; Ma, Y.; Noh, H.R.; Sui, G.; Shin, D.S.; Lee, M.K.; et al. Zaluzanin C Alleviates Inflammation and Lipid Accumulation in Kupffer Cells and Hepatocytes by Regulating Mitochondrial ROS. *Molecules* **2023**, *28*, 7484. [CrossRef]
56. Michalska, K.; Szneler, E.; Kisiel, W. Sesquiterpene lactones from Lactuca canadensis and their chemotaxonomic significance. *Phytochemistry* **2013**, *90*, 90–94. [CrossRef]
57. Yang, M.; Wei, X.; Yi, X.; Jiang, D.-S. Mitophagy-related regulated cell death: Molecular mechanisms and disease implications. *Cell Death Dis.* **2024**, *15*, 505. [CrossRef]
58. Ha, Y.S.; Kim, T.K.; Heo, J.; Oh, J.; Kim, S.K.; Kim, J.; Lee, J.; Yang, S.R.; Hwang, S.; Kim, S.J. Rocaglamide-A mitigates LPS-induced hepatic inflammation by modulating JNK/AP-1 signaling cascade and ROS production in hepatocytes. *Toxicol. Res.* **2025**, *41*, 47–59. [CrossRef] [PubMed]

59. Dai, Q.; Ain, Q.; Seth, N.; Rooney, M.; Zipprich, A. Liver sinusoidal endothelial cells: Friend or foe in metabolic dysfunction-associated steatotic liver disease/metabolic dysfunction-associated steatohepatitis. *Dig. Liver Dis.* **2025**, *57*, 943–953. [CrossRef]
60. He, Q.; He, W.; Dong, H.; Guo, Y.; Yuan, G.; Shi, X.; Wang, D.; Lu, F. Role of liver sinusoidal endothelial cell in metabolic dysfunction-associated fatty liver disease. *Cell Commun. Signal.* **2024**, *22*, 346. [CrossRef]
61. Yinzhi, D.; Jianhua, H.; Hesheng, L. The roles of liver sinusoidal endothelial cells in liver ischemia/reperfusion injury. *J. Gastroenterol. Hepatol.* **2024**, *39*, 224–230. [CrossRef] [PubMed]
62. Ma, X.; Huang, T.; Chen, X.; Li, Q.; Liao, M.; Fu, L.; Huang, J.; Yuan, K.; Wang, Z.; Zeng, Y. Molecular mechanisms in liver repair and regeneration: From physiology to therapeutics. *Signal Transduct. Target. Ther.* **2025**, *10*, 63. [CrossRef]
63. Czuba, L.C.; Wu, X.; Huang, W.; Hollingshead, N.; Roberto, J.B.; Kenerson, H.L.; Yeung, R.S.; Crispe, I.N.; Isoherranen, N. Altered vitamin A metabolism in human liver slices corresponds to fibrogenesis. *Clin. Transl. Sci.* **2021**, *14*, 976–989. [CrossRef]
64. Kisseleva, T.; Ganguly, S.; Murad, R.; Wang, A.; Brenner, D.A. Regulation of Hepatic Stellate Cell Phenotypes in Metabolic Dysfunction–Associated Steatohepatitis. *Gastroenterology* **2025**, *20*, S0016-5085(25)00528-1. [CrossRef]
65. Sun, C.; Li, L.; Li, D.; Wang, Z. Discovery of Endothelial-Monocyte Crosstalk in Ischemic-Reperfusion Injury Following Liver Transplantation Based on Integration of Single-Cell RNA and Transcriptome RNA Sequencing. *J. Cell Mol. Med.* **2025**, *29*, e70336. [CrossRef]
66. Rejas, C.; Junger, H. Cholangiocyte Organoids in Liver Transplantation; a Comprehensive Review. *Transpl. Int.* **2024**, *37*, 12708. [CrossRef] [PubMed]
67. Richards, J.A.; Wigmore, S.J.; Anderton, S.M.; Howie, S.E.M. NKT cells are important mediators of hepatic ischemia-reperfusion injury. *Transpl. Immunol.* **2017**, *45*, 15–21. [CrossRef]
68. Zhang, Y.; Zhang, C.; Yang, B.; Peng, C.; Zhou, J.; Ren, S.; Hu, Z. The effect of TIM1(+) Breg cells in liver ischemia-reperfusion injury. *Cell Death Dis.* **2025**, *16*, 171. [CrossRef]
69. Wang, L.; Li, J.; He, S.; Liu, Y.; Chen, H.; He, S.; Yin, M.; Zou, D.; Chen, S.; Luo, T.; et al. Resolving the graft ischemia-reperfusion injury during liver transplantation at the single cell resolution. *Cell Death Dis.* **2021**, *12*, 589. [CrossRef] [PubMed]
70. Efremova, M.; Vento-Tormo, M.; Teichmann, S.A.; Vento-Tormo, R. CellPhoneDB: Inferring cell–cell communication from combined expression of multi-subunit ligand–receptor complexes. *Nat. Protoc.* **2020**, *15*, 1484–1506. [CrossRef]
71. Dixon, L.J.; Barnes, M.; Tang, H.; Pritchard, M.T.; Nagy, L.E. Kupffer cells in the liver. *Compr. Physiol.* **2013**, *3*, 785–797. [CrossRef]
72. Kaltenmeier, C.; Wang, R.; Popp, B.; Geller, D.; Tohme, S.; Yazdani, H.O. Role of Immuno-Inflammatory Signals in Liver Ischemia-Reperfusion Injury. *Cells* **2022**, *11*, 2222. [CrossRef]
73. Zhao, M.; Huang, H.; He, F.; Fu, X. Current insights into the hepatic microenvironment and advances in immunotherapy for hepatocellular carcinoma. *Front. Immunol.* **2023**, *14*, 1188277. [CrossRef]
74. Zhou, M.; Lv, J.; Chen, X.; Shi, Y.; Chao, G.; Zhang, S. From gut to liver: Exploring the crosstalk between gut-liver axis and oxidative stress in metabolic dysfunction-associated steatotic liver disease. *Ann. Hepatol.* **2025**, *30*, 101777. [CrossRef] [PubMed]
75. Asgharzadeh, F.; Memarzia, A.; Alikhani, V.; Beigoli, S.; Boskabady, M.H. Peroxisome proliferator-activated receptors: Key regulators of tumor progression and growth. *Transl. Oncol.* **2024**, *47*, 102039. [CrossRef] [PubMed]
76. Chen, Y.X.; Wu, Y.P.; Zhang, Y.; Ji, P.X.; Hua, J. Modulation of Lipid Metabolism and Keap1-Nrf2 Pathway Activation in Macrophages by Targeting PPARγ Affects NAFLD Progression. *J. Gastroenterol. Hepatol.* **2025**. [CrossRef] [PubMed]
77. Hirao, H.; Kojima, H.; Dery, K.J.; Nakamura, K.; Kadono, K.; Zhai, Y.; Farmer, D.G.; Kaldas, F.M.; Kupiec-Weglinski, J.W. Neutrophil CEACAM1 determines susceptibility to NETosis by regulating the S1PR2/S1PR3 axis in liver transplantation. *J. Clin. Investig.* **2023**, *133*, e162940. [CrossRef]
78. Dery, K.J.; Wong, Z.; Wei, M.; Kupiec-Weglinski, J.W. Mechanistic Insights into Alternative Gene Splicing in Oxidative Stress and Tissue Injury. *Antioxid. Redox Signal.* **2023**, *41*, 890–909. [CrossRef]
79. Dery, K.J.; Silver, C.; Yang, L.; Shively, J.E. Interferon regulatory factor 1 and a variant of heterogeneous nuclear ribonucleoprotein L coordinately silence the gene for adhesion protein CEACAM1. *J. Biol. Chem.* **2018**, *293*, 9277–9291. [CrossRef]
80. Dery, K.J.; Gaur, S.; Gencheva, M.; Yen, Y.; Shively, J.E.; Gaur, R.K. Mechanistic control of carcinoembryonic antigen-related cell adhesion molecule-1 (CEACAM1) splice isoforms by the heterogeneous nuclear ribonuclear proteins hnRNP L, hnRNP A1, and hnRNP M. *J. Biol. Chem.* **2011**, *286*, 16039–16051. [CrossRef]
81. Xie, M.; He, Z.; Bin, B.; Wen, N.; Wu, J.; Cai, X.; Sun, X. Bulk and single-cell RNA sequencing analysis with 101 machine learning combinations reveal neutrophil extracellular trap involvement in hepatic ischemia-reperfusion injury and early allograft dysfunction. *Int. Immunopharmacol.* **2024**, *131*, 111874. [CrossRef]
82. Chen, X.; Jiang, C.; Chen, M.; Li, X.; Yu, W.; Qiu, A.; Sun, L.; Pu, L.; Shi, Y. SYK promotes the formation of neutrophil extracellular traps by inducing PKM2 nuclear translocation and promoting STAT3 phosphorylation to exacerbate hepatic ischemia-reperfusion injury and tumor recurrence. *Mol. Med.* **2024**, *30*, 146. [CrossRef]

83. Zhao, Y.; Zhao, S.; Liu, S.; Ye, W.; Chen, W.-d. Kupffer cells, the limelight in the liver regeneration. *Int. Immunopharmacol.* **2025**, *146*, 113808. [CrossRef]
84. Duan, Y.; Yang, Y.; Zhao, S.; Bai, Y.; Yao, W.; Gao, X.; Yin, J. Crosstalk in extrahepatic and hepatic system in NAFLD/NASH. *Liver Int.* **2024**, *44*, 1856–1871. [CrossRef]
85. Tsung, A.; Klune, J.R.; Zhang, X.; Jeyabalan, G.; Cao, Z.; Peng, X.; Stolz, D.B.; Geller, D.A.; Rosengart, M.R.; Billiar, T.R. HMGB1 release induced by liver ischemia involves Toll-like receptor 4 dependent reactive oxygen species production and calcium-mediated signaling. *J. Exp. Med.* **2007**, *204*, 2913–2923. [CrossRef] [PubMed]
86. Wynn, T.A.; Vannella, K.M. Macrophages in Tissue Repair, Regeneration, and Fibrosis. *Immunity* **2016**, *44*, 450–462. [CrossRef] [PubMed]
87. Hirao, H.; Kageyama, S.; Nakamura, K.; Kadono, K.; Kojima, H.; Siyuan, Y.; Farmer, D.G.; Kaldas, F.M.; Dery, K.J.; Kupiec-Weglinski, J.W. Recipient TIM4 signaling regulates ischemia reperfusion-induced ER stress and metabolic responses in liver transplantation: From mouse-to-human. *Front. Transpl.* **2023**, *2*, 1176384. [CrossRef]
88. Bosch, M.; Kallin, N.; Donakonda, S.; Zhang, J.D.; Wintersteller, H.; Hegenbarth, S.; Heim, K.; Ramirez, C.; Fürst, A.; Lattouf, E.I.; et al. A liver immune rheostat regulates CD8 T cell immunity in chronic HBV infection. *Nature* **2024**, *631*, 867–875. [CrossRef] [PubMed]
89. Elgosbi, M.; Kurt, A.S.; Londoño, M.C.; Caballero-Marcos, A.; Lim, T.Y.; Lozano, J.J.; Dave, M.; Heaton, N.; Sánchez-Fueyo, A.; Cortes-Cerisuelo, M. Hypothermic oxygenated machine perfusion influences the immunogenicity of donor livers in humans. *Liver Transpl.* **2025**, *31*, 311–322. [CrossRef]
90. Sun, Q.; Gong, J.; Wu, J.; Hu, Z.; Zhang, Q.; Zhu, X. SNHG1-miR-186-5p-YY1 feedback loop alleviates hepatic ischemia/reperfusion injury. *Cell Cycle* **2022**, *21*, 1267–1279. [CrossRef]
91. Esser, H.; Kilpatrick, A.M.; Man, T.Y.; Aird, R.; Rodrigo-Torres, D.; Buch, M.L.; Boulter, L.; Walmsley, S.; Oniscu, G.C.; Schneeberger, S.; et al. Primary cilia as a targetable node between biliary injury, senescence and regeneration in liver transplantation. *J. Hepatol.* **2024**, *81*, 1005–1022. [CrossRef] [PubMed]
92. Bai, C.; Jiang, Z.; Jiang, H.; Yu, S.; Li, M.; Chu, F.; Sheng, Y.; Li, J.; Jiang, J.; Li, W. Ac2-26 alleviates hepatic ischemia-reperfusion injury based on inhibiting the positive feedback loop of HMGB1/TLR4/NF-κB/neutrophils. *Exp. Ther. Med.* **2022**, *24*, 673. [CrossRef]
93. Padmanaban, S.; Pully, D.; Samrot, A.V.; Gosu, V.; Sadasivam, N.; Park, I.K.; Radhakrishnan, K.; Kim, D.K. Rising Influence of Nanotechnology in Addressing Oxidative Stress-Related Liver Disorders. *Antioxidants* **2023**, *12*, 1405. [CrossRef]
94. Pasut, G.; Panisello, A.; Folch-Puy, E.; Lopez, A.; Castro-Benítez, C.; Calvo, M.; Carbonell, T.; García-Gil, A.; Adam, R.; Roselló-Catafau, J. Polyethylene glycols: An effective strategy for limiting liver ischemia reperfusion injury. *World, J. Gastroenterol.* **2016**, *22*, 6501–6508. [CrossRef]
95. Xin, X.; Li, J.; Wu, W.; Zhao, P.; Yang, Y.; Zhu, Y.; Ren, L.; Qin, C.; Yin, L. ROS-scavenging nanomedicine for "multiple crosstalk" modulation in non-alcoholic fatty liver disease. *Biomater. Sci.* **2023**, *11*, 3709–3725. [CrossRef]
96. Li, S.D.; Huang, L. Nanoparticles evading the reticuloendothelial system: Role of the supported bilayer. *Biochim. Biophys. Acta* **2009**, *1788*, 2259–2266. [CrossRef]
97. Gao, S.; Li, F.; Wu, D.; Ma, R.; Li, Y.; Zhang, Y.; Han, Z.; He, Q.; Li, J.; Liu, C.; et al. Poly(Ethylene Glycol)-Modified Catalase Blocking Reactive Oxygen Species for the Treatment of Hepatic Ischemia. *Macromol. Rapid Commun.* **2025**, e2500367. [CrossRef]
98. Lu, X.; Hu, H.; Zhou, Y.; Zhang, H.; Xie, C.; Sun, Y.; Shao, Z.; Tang, L.; Ren, Y.; Chen, J.; et al. One-step engineered mesenchymal stem cell-derived exosomes against hepatic ischemia-reperfusion injury. *Int. J. Pharm.* **2025**, *672*, 125292. [CrossRef]
99. Xu, D.; Qu, X.; Tian, Y.; Jie, Z.; Xi, Z.; Xue, F.; Ma, X.; Zhu, J.; Xia, Q. Macrophage Notch1 inhibits TAK1 function and RIPK3-mediated hepatocyte necroptosis through activation of β-catenin signaling in liver ischemia and reperfusion injury. *Cell Commun. Signal.* **2022**, *20*, 144. [CrossRef] [PubMed]
100. Zhang, X.; Hu, J.; Becker, K.V.; Engle, J.W.; Ni, D.; Cai, W.; Wu, D.; Qu, S. Antioxidant and C5a-blocking strategy for hepatic ischemia-reperfusion injury repair. *J. Nanobiotechnol.* **2021**, *19*, 107. [CrossRef] [PubMed]
101. Zhang, S.; Cao, Y.; Xu, B.; Zhang, H.; Zhang, S.; Sun, J.; Tang, Y.; Wang, Y. An antioxidant nanodrug protects against hepatic ischemia-reperfusion injury by attenuating oxidative stress and inflammation. *J. Mater. Chem. B* **2022**, *10*, 7563–7569. [CrossRef] [PubMed]
102. Gobut, H.; Erel, S.; Ozdemir, C.; Mortas, T.; Arslan, M.; Kucuk, A.; Kasapbasi, E.; Kavutcu, M. Effects of cerium oxide on liver tissue in liver ischemia-reperfusion injury in rats undergoing sevoflurane anesthesia. *Exp. Ther. Med.* **2023**, *25*, 164. [CrossRef] [PubMed]
103. Mo, D.; Cui, W.; Chen, L.; Meng, J.; Sun, Y.; Cai, K.; Zhang, J.; Zhang, J.; Wang, K.; Luo, X. Activation of the PPARγ/NF-κB pathway by A-MPDA@Fe(3)O(4)@PVP via scavenging reactive oxygen species to alleviate hepatic ischemia-reperfusion injury. *J. Mater. Chem. B* **2024**, *12*, 5722–5733. [CrossRef] [PubMed]
104. Duarte, A.; Silveira, G.G.; Soave, D.F.; Costa, J.P.O.; Silva, A.R. The Role of the LY294002—A Non-Selective Inhibitor of Phosphatidylinositol 3-Kinase (PI3K) Pathway- in Cell Survival and Proliferation in Cell Line SCC-25. *Asian Pac. J. Cancer Prev.* **2019**, *20*, 3377–3383. [CrossRef]

105. Li, X.; Zhang, C.T.; Ma, W.; Xie, X.; Huang, Q. Oridonin: A Review of Its Pharmacology, Pharmacokinetics and Toxicity. *Front. Pharmacol.* **2021**, *12*, 645824. [CrossRef]
106. Pashkina, E.; Bykova, M.; Berishvili, M.; Lazarev, Y.; Kozlov, V. Hyaluronic Acid-Based Drug Delivery Systems for Cancer Therapy. *Cells* **2025**, *14*, 61. [CrossRef]
107. Zhang, Y.; Zhang, G.; Wang, T.; Chen, Y.; Wang, J.; Li, P.; Wang, R.; Su, J. Understanding Cytochrome P450 Enzyme Substrate Inhibition and Prospects for Elimination Strategies. *Chembiochem* **2024**, *25*, e202400297. [CrossRef]
108. Liao, J.; Meng, C.; Cheng, J.; Liu, B.; Shao, Y. HSYA from safflower mitigates oxidative stress, inflammation, and apoptosis in liver ischemia-reperfusion injury. *Xenobiotica* **2025**, *55*, 239–245. [CrossRef]
109. Kasiewicz, L.N.; Biswas, S.; Beach, A.; Ren, H.; Dutta, C.; Mazzola, A.M.; Rohde, E.; Chadwick, A.; Cheng, C.; Garcia, S.P.; et al. GalNAc-Lipid nanoparticles enable non-LDLR dependent hepatic delivery of a CRISPR base editing therapy. *Nat. Commun.* **2023**, *14*, 2776. [CrossRef]
110. He, H.; Yuan, Q.; Bie, J.; Wallace, R.L.; Yannie, P.J.; Wang, J.; Lancina, M.G., 3rd; Zolotarskaya, O.Y.; Korzun, W.; Yang, H.; et al. Development of mannose functionalized dendrimeric nanoparticles for targeted delivery to macrophages: Use of this platform to modulate atherosclerosis. *Transl. Res.* **2018**, *193*, 13–30. [CrossRef]
111. Nimjee, S.M.; White, R.R.; Becker, R.C.; Sullenger, B.A. Aptamers as Therapeutics. *Annu. Rev. Pharmacol. Toxicol.* **2017**, *57*, 61–79. [CrossRef]
112. Rabiee, N.; Chen, S.; Ahmadi, S.; Veedu, R.N. Aptamer-engineered (nano)materials for theranostic applications. *Theranostics* **2023**, *13*, 5183–5206. [CrossRef]
113. Deng, G.; Zha, H.; Luo, H.; Zhou, Y. Aptamer-conjugated gold nanoparticles and their diagnostic and therapeutic roles in cancer. *Front. Bioeng. Biotechnol.* **2023**, *11*, 1–15. [CrossRef] [PubMed]
114. Kojima, H.; Nakamura, K.; Kupiec-Weglinski, J.W. Therapeutic targets for liver regeneration after acute severe injury: A preclinical overview. *Expert Opin. Ther. Targets* **2020**, *24*, 13–24. [CrossRef]
115. Hohmann, N.; Schröder, F.; Moreira, B.; Teng, H.; Burhenne, J.; Bruckner, T.; Mueller, S.; Haefeli, W.E.; Seitz, H.K. Effect of Clomethiazole Vs. Clorazepate on Hepatic Fat and Serum Transaminase Activities in Alcohol-Associated Liver Disease: Results from a Randomized, Controlled Phase II Clinical Trial. *Alcohol. Alcohol.* **2023**, *58*, 134–141. [CrossRef]
116. Cui, X.; Mi, T.; Xiao, X.; Zhang, H.; Dong, Y.; Huang, N.; Gao, P.; Lee, J.; Guelakis, M.; Gu, X. Topical glutathione amino acid precursors protect skin against environmental and oxidative stress. *J. Eur. Acad. Dermatol. Venereol.* **2024**, *38* (Suppl. S3), 3–11. [CrossRef] [PubMed]
117. Carlisle, C.; Polley, K.; Panda, C.; Barron, K.; Hamrock, M.; Dominique, A.; Metzger, B.; Le Brun-Blashka, S.; Komarnytsky, S. Alleviation of Pain, PAIN Interference, and Oxidative Stress by a Novel Combination of Hemp Oil, Calamari Oil, and Broccoli: A Randomized, Double-Blind, Placebo-Controlled Trial. *Nutrients* **2023**, *15*, 2654. [CrossRef]
118. Mehta, P.A.; Nelson, A.; Loveless, S.; Lane, A.; Fukuda, T.; Teusink-Cross, A.; Elder, D.; Lagory, D.; Miller, E.; Cancelas, J.A.; et al. Phase 1 study of quercetin, a natural antioxidant for children and young adults with Fanconi anemia. *Blood Adv.* **2025**, *9*, 1927–1939. [CrossRef]
119. Pan, W.; Zhou, G.; Hu, M.; Li, G.; Zhang, M.; Yang, H.; Li, K.; Li, J.; Liu, T.; Wang, Y.; et al. Coenzyme Q10 mitigates macrophage mediated inflammation in heart following myocardial infarction via the NLRP3/IL1β pathway. *BMC Cardiovasc. Disord.* **2024**, *24*, 76.
120. Postel-Vinay, S.; Lam, V.K.; Ros, W.; Bauer, T.M.; Hansen, A.R.; Cho, D.C.; Stephen Hodi, F.; Schellens, J.H.M.; Litton, J.K.; Aspeslagh, S.; et al. First-in-human phase I study of the OX40 agonist GSK3174998 with or without pembrolizumab in patients with selected advanced solid tumors (ENGAGE-1). *J. Immunother. Cancer* **2023**, *11*, e005301. [CrossRef]
121. Burgos-Santamaría, A.; Rodríguez-Rodríguez, P.; Arnalich-Montiel, A.; Arribas, S.M.; Fernández-Riveira, C.; Barrio-Pérez, I.M.; Río, J.; Ligero, J.M.; Quintana-Villamandos, B. OXY-SCORE and Volatile Anesthetics: A New Perspective of Oxidative Stress in EndoVascular Aneurysm Repair-A Randomized Clinical Trial. *Int. J. Mol. Sci.* **2024**, *25*, 10770. [CrossRef] [PubMed]
122. Kakavand, H.; Saadatagah, S.; Naderian, M.; Aghakouchakzadeh, M.; Jalali, A.; Sadri, F.; Amoli, A.I.; Hosseini, S.H.; Jenab, Y.; Pourhosseini, H.; et al. Evaluating the role of intravenous pentoxifylline administration on primary percutaneous coronary intervention success rate in patients with ST-elevation myocardial infarction (PENTOS-PCI). *Naunyn Schmiedebergs Arch. Pharmacol.* **2023**, *396*, 557–565. [CrossRef] [PubMed]
123. Yang, S.; Guo, L.; Wang, D.; Yang, Y.; Wang, J. Research on Mechanism of *miR*-106a Nanoparticles Carrying Dexmedetomidine in Regulating Recovery and Metabolism of Nerve Cells in Hypoxia-Reoxygenation Injury. *J. Biomed. Nanotechnol.* **2022**, *18*, 343–351. [CrossRef] [PubMed]

antioxidants

MDPI

Review

Involvement of Oxidative Stress and Antioxidants in Modification of Cardiac Dysfunction Due to Ischemia–Reperfusion Injury

Naranjan S. Dhalla [1,*], Petr Ostadal [2] and Paramjit S. Tappia [3]

[1] St. Boniface Hospital Albrechtsen Research Centre, Institute of Cardiovascular Sciences, Department of Physiology & Pathophysiology, Max Rady College of Medicine, University of Manitoba, Winnipeg, MB R2H 2A6, Canada
[2] Department of Cardiology, 2nd Faculty of Medicine, Charles University, Motol University Hospital, V Uvalu 84, 15000 Prague, Czech Republic; ostadal.petr@gmail.com
[3] Asper Clinical Research Institute, St. Boniface Hospital, Winnipeg, MB R2H 2A6, Canada; ptappia@sbrc.ca
* Correspondence: nsdhalla@sbrc.ca

Abstract: Delayed reperfusion of the ischemic heart (I/R) is known to impair the recovery of cardiac function and produce a wide variety of myocardial defects, including ultrastructural damage, metabolic alterations, subcellular Ca^{2+}-handling abnormalities, activation of proteases, and changes in cardiac gene expression. Although I/R injury has been reported to induce the formation of reactive oxygen species (ROS), inflammation, and intracellular Ca^{2+} overload, the generation of oxidative stress is considered to play a critical role in the development of cardiac dysfunction. Increases in the production of superoxide, hydroxyl radicals, and oxidants, such as hydrogen peroxide and hypochlorous acid, occur in hearts subjected to I/R injury. In fact, mitochondria are a major source of the excessive production of ROS in I/R hearts due to impairment in the electron transport system as well as activation of xanthine oxidase and NADPH oxidase. Nitric oxide synthase, mainly present in the endothelium, is also activated due to I/R injury, leading to the production of nitric oxide, which, upon combination with superoxide radicals, generates nitrosative stress. Alterations in cardiac function, sarcolemma, sarcoplasmic reticulum Ca^{2+}-handling activities, mitochondrial oxidative phosphorylation, and protease activation due to I/R injury are simulated upon exposing the heart to the oxyradical-generating system (xanthine plus xanthine oxidase) or H_2O_2. On the other hand, the activation of endogenous antioxidants such as superoxide dismutase, catalase, glutathione peroxidase, and the concentration of a transcription factor (Nrf2), which modulates the expression of various endogenous antioxidants, is depressed due to I/R injury in hearts. Furthermore, pretreatment of hearts with antioxidants such as catalase plus superoxide dismutase, N-acetylcysteine, and mercaptopropionylglycerine has been observed to attenuate I/R-induced subcellular Ca^{2+} handling and changes in Ca^{2+}-regulatory activities; additionally, it has been found to depress protease activation and improve the recovery of cardiac function. These observations indicate that oxidative stress is intimately involved in the pathological effects of I/R injury and different antioxidants attenuate I/R-induced subcellular alterations and improve the recovery of cardiac function. Thus, we are faced with the task of developing safe and effective antioxidants as well as agents for upregulating the expression of endogenous antioxidants for the therapy of I/R injury.

Keywords: ischemia–reperfusion injury; cardiac dysfunction; oxidative stress; antioxidants; subcellular defects; Ca^{2+}-handling abnormalities

 https://doi.org/10.3390/antiox14030340

1. Introduction

It is now well known that myocardial ischemia induces marked alterations in contractile function, cellular metabolism, and cardiac ultrastructure due to the lack of both oxygen and substrates. Although the reperfusion of the ischemic myocardium is beneficial in improving cardiac function and myocardial changes, delayed reperfusion, after a certain critical time of ischemic insult, has been shown to impair the recovery of cardiac function and exacerbate metabolic alterations, induce Ca^{2+}-handling abnormalities, and promote damage to the myocardial structure [1–15]. The effects of delayed reperfusion are superimposed upon those for myocardial ischemia and are termed as ischemia–reperfusion (I/R) injury. Although the nature of defects due to I/R injury is not fully understood, this condition is generally associated with several adverse events such as arrhythmias, diverse signal transduction defects, mitochondrial dysfunction, microvascular damage, and cellular death. Furthermore, I/R injury is invariably seen in clinical conditions including acute coronary syndrome, angioplasty, thrombolysis, coronary-bypass surgery, cardiac transplantation, and stroke [16–35]. It should be mentioned that I/R injury is a complex health hazard, and the mechanisms of I/R-induced cardiac dysfunction are similar to those for hypoxia reoxygenation.

Cardiac dysfunction in hearts subjected to I/R injury has also been shown to involve oxidative stress, inflammation, endoplasmic reticulum stress, intracellular Ca^{2+}-overload, and defects in subcellular organelles such as sarcolemma (SL), sarcoplasmic reticulum (SR), mitochondria (MT), and myofibrils (MF) [36–51]. However, oxidative stress is considered to play a critical role in the development of impaired cardiac performance due to I/R injury, because several defects associated with this pathological condition are elicited as its consequence. Furthermore, different antioxidants have been reported to attenuate the I/R-induced alterations in the heart [7,11,15,36,41,44,48,50–52]. It is therefore the objective of this article to provide an updated comprehensive review of various sources for the generation of oxidative stress as well as the role of endogenous antioxidants during the development of I/R injury. It is also planned to discuss the implications of oxidative stress in inducing cardiac dysfunction due to I/R injury. Furthermore, this study was undertaken with the intention of including evidence for the involvement of oxidative stress in I/R-induced subcellular alterations, particularly with respect to Ca^{2+}-handling defects and the subsequent impairment of cardiac performance. In addition, the pharmacotherapy of I/R injury with both endogenous and exogenous antioxidant systems will be described for improving cardiac function in pathological conditions. Accordingly, an appropriate literature search was conducted on MEDLINE via PubMed using the following search terms: cardiac ischemia–reperfusion injury, reactive oxygen species, oxidative stress, antioxidants, Ca^{2+} handling, intracellular Ca^{2+} overload, and combination thereof was undertaken and the articles quoted in this review were selected to provide support of our hypothesis.

2. Generation of Oxidative Stress and Status of Antioxidant Systems in I/R Hearts

Oxidative stress is associated with an increase in the production of reactive oxygen species (ROS) and/or a decrease in the activities of antioxidant defense systems due to I/R injury in the heart [8,9,14,15,43,44,51]. There are five major types of ROS (superoxide radicals, hydroxyl radicals, hydrogen peroxide (H_2O_2), hypochlorous acid, and peroxynitrite) which are increased in the heart upon the induction of I/R injury. ROS are mainly generated by the impairment of electron transport in mitochondria, xanthine (X) + xanthine oxidase (XO) reaction, and arachidonic acid metabolism, as well as by the activation of monoamine oxidase, NADPH oxidase, the endothelium, and neutrophils. It should be mentioned that superoxide radicals are rapidly converted into H_2O_2, which is a precursor of hydroxyl ions in the presence of iron and copper, as well as hypochlorous acid (HOCl) in the presence of myeloperoxidases and chloride ions. Superoxide radicals also react with nitric oxide (produced upon the activation of endothelium) to form peroxynitrite. Although all members of the ROS family are inter-related, hydroxyl radicals are considered to be the most reactive, with a very short half-life. It should also be pointed out that low concentrations of ROS produce beneficial effects on the heart by activating different redox-sensitive signal transduction pathways, whereas high concentrations of ROS (oxidative stress) produce harmful effects by reacting with cellular proteins, lipids, carbohydrates, and DNA. Thus, I/R injury is known to produce changes in membrane permeability, protein thiol group oxidation, and lipid peroxidation, which are considered to be mediated through the generation of oxidative stress.

Excessive generation of ROS by mitochondrial defects and other sources have been demonstrated to be associated with the activation of transient receptor potential melastatin 2 (TRPM2), the production of endoplasmic reticulum stress (ER stress), DNA damage, and the upregulation of NADPH oxidase, heme oxygenases, and cyclooxygenases [53–66]. ROS have also been shown to produce ventricular arrhythmias, alter the apelinergic system and ubiquitin–proteosome axis, and induce different types of cell death, such as necrosis, apoptosis, necroptosis, pyroptosis, and ferroptosis [67–78]. Different endogenous proteins such as perilipin, SESTRIN2, heat shock protein 22, and humanin, as well as exosomes and microRNAs with antioxidant properties, have been reported to protect against the harmful effects of ROS in the heart [79–85]. Various enzymes, including superoxide dismutase (SOD), catalase, and glutathione peroxidases, as well as vitamins such as vitamin E, vitamin A, and vitamin C, are known to serve as endogenous antioxidants [8,44,49–51]. These antioxidants are considered to act through mechanisms involved in either scavenging ROS or inhibiting the generation of ROS in the myocardium. The levels of these antioxidants are not only decreased upon the reperfusion of an ischemic heart; these interventions are also effective in attenuating I/R injury to the heart upon pretreatment. These observations support the view that the generation of ROS and the development of oxidative stress are intimately involved in the pathogenesis of I/R injury to the heart [8,49–51,86,87].

3. Mechanisms of I/R-Injury-Induced Subcellular Defects and Cardiac Dysfunction

The status of cardiac function is determined by the coordinated Ca^{2+}-handling activities of different subcellular organelles, including SL, SR, and MT, as well as the Ca^{2+}-regulated activity of MF [11,88–90]; thus, it has been suggested that abnormalities in subcellular function due to oxidative stress play an important role in the development of cardiac dysfunction as a consequence of I/R injury [8,41,51]. It should be pointed out that myocardial ischemia upon occluding the coronary arteries is associated with a lack of oxygen, the inability of MT to oxidize substrates, and the accumulation of hydrogen in cardiomyocytes; these alterations result in an increase in the intracellular concentration of Ca^{2+} upon the stimulation of SL Na^+-H^+ exchange and SL Na^+-Ca^{2+} exchange systems. The increased levels of Ca^{2+} in the ischemic myocardium activate XO and produce ROS through a reaction with X. Furthermore, the inability of MT to oxidize substrate in the ischemic heart is known to depress oxidative phosphorylation, impair the MT electron transport system, generate ROS, and produce the cessation of contractile activity. All these changes that are attributable to myocardial ischemia are reversible upon reperfusion; however, delayed reperfusion results in marked defects in cardiomyocytes, myocardial interstitium, endothelium, and coronary vasculature for the induction of ultrastructural abnormalities, as well as the impairment of contractile function recovery as a consequence of ROS production [1–11,41,43,51]. Such alterations in cardiomyocytes due to reperfusion of the ischemic heart are associated with a further increase in the entry of Ca^{2+} due to an increase in membrane permeability as well as depressions in SL Na^{+}-K^{+} ATPase and SL Na^{+}- Ca^{2+} exchange activities. In addition, there occurs a depression in the SR Ca^{2+} pump activity and leakage of Ca^{2+} from the SR tubular system due to ROS-induced alterations in the SR membrane. These Ca^{2+}-handling abnormalities in SL and SR lead to the development of intracellular Ca^{2+} overload and subsequent MT Ca^{2+} overload, which is known to induce further defects in the MT electron transport system, oxidative phosphorylation activity, and energy production; in addition, it leads to the generation of oxidative stress, the opening of MT pores, and the release of cytotoxic substances for the induction of programmed cell death.

Although oxidative stress is considered to be mainly generated by MT upon inducing I/R injury, the involvement of other systems cannot be overlooked. Examples of these include the following: Ca^{2+}-handling abnormalities in SL and SR for the occurrence of MT Ca^{2+} overload; endothelium nitric oxide synthase for the production of nitric oxide; peroxynitrite, macrophages, and leukocytes for the release of proinflammatory cytokines such as tumor necrosis factor-α (TNF-α) and interleukins (IL-1β and IL-6); long noncoding RNA–RNA axis and thioredoxin-interacting protein for the generation of oxidative stress during the development of I/R injury [91–99]. Furthermore, the activation of both SL- and MT-associated NADPH oxidases and glucose homeostasis, as well as the oxidation of free fatty acids and arachidonic acid metabolic pathways, have been demonstrated to play a critical role in the development of oxidative stress during the initiation and progression of I/R injury to the heart [20,21,51,100]. It is also noteworthy that the concentrations of different ROS and oxidants are increased in the heart upon inducing I/R injury, whereas those for endogenous antioxidant enzymes are decreased [49–51,101–103]; these observations provide strong evidence for the occurrence of oxidative stress during the development of oxidative stress. Several in vivo studies have also shown that the activities of different transcription factors such as nuclear factor erythroid 2-related factor 2 (Nrf2) and Kelch-like ECH-associated protein 1 (Keap 1), which modulate the levels of various antioxidants, are depressed due to I/R injury [104–112]. Accordingly, the upregulation of both transcription factors (Nrf2 and Keap1) is considered to be an excellent strategy for reducing oxidative stress responses, subcellular Ca^{2+}-handling defects, and the development of intracellular Ca^{2+} overload due to I/R injury.

4. Pharmacotherapy and Cardioprotection of I/R-Induced Injury

Extensive experimental work in the area of pharmacotherapy and cardioprotection has been carried out to investigate the beneficial effects of several interventions in preventing I/R injury to the heart [8,44,51,113]. Different pharmacologic agents such as hypoglycemic drugs [114,115], aldosterone inhibitors [116], regulatory interventions (including SIRT1 (regulator of autophagy), STING (stimulator of interferon genes), and AMP-activated protein kinase [117–119]), and nanomedicines [120] have been found to attenuate I/R injury. Likewise, some interventions, such as nitric oxide, heme oxygenase 1, propofal, and adiponectin (which affects diverse molecular targets), were observed to partially prevent I/R injury in the heart [121–124]. Furthermore, different types of RNAs (circular RNA, noncoding RNA, and microRNA) have also been reported to exert beneficial effects in attenuating I/R injury through some complex mechanisms [125–127]. Some phytochemicals, natural products, and micronutrients have been claimed to protect against I/R injury by improving antioxidant status [128–130]. It may well be the case that all the interventions indicated in this section partially depress I/R injury by reducing the formation of ROS or increasing the concentrations of different antioxidants; however, the involvement of other mechanisms, such as alterations in inflammation, reduction in intracellular Ca^{2+} overload, or the inhibition of protease activation, cannot be ruled out with any certainty.

In view of the depressed endogenous antioxidant levels in the I/R hearts, several investigators have used redox sensitive therapy for preventing I/R injury. In this regard, supplementation with exogenous antioxidant preparations [51,52,126,131,132] and the administration of interventions which upregulate the transcription factor Nrf2 [107,110,111], through increasing antioxidant status, have been shown to exert beneficial effects against I/R injury. Various proteins, such as humanin, berberine, sestrin, taurine, fisetin, quercetin, and polydatin, all with antioxidant properties, have also been observed to attenuate I/R injury in the heart [81,122,133–137]. Different vitamins, such as vitamins A, C, and E, with antioxidant activities, have also been shown to exert beneficial effects against I/R injury [138,139]. Some gases, such as molecular hydrogen and hydrogen sulfide [109,131,140–143], as well as ischemic preconditioning [90,144], have also been reported to exert beneficial actions. All these observations, showing cardioprotective effects of various interventions in I/R hearts due to their antioxidant activities, support the view that oxidative stress plays a pivotal role in the development of I/R injury.

5. Evidence for the Involvement of Oxidative Stress in I/R-Induced Cardiac Dysfunction

The intention here is to provide further evidence for the occurrence of oxidative stress in the impairment of cardiac function recovery upon the reperfusion of the ischemic heart. Accordingly, we have analyzed some information from some experiments which were carried out by inducing I/R injury in isolated perfused rat hearts that were pretreated in the absence and presence of some antioxidants. It should be mentioned that isolated heats were subjected to 30 min of global ischemia before inducing reperfusion for 30 to 60 min. Furthermore, the effects of I/R-induced injury were compared with those obtained from rat hearts perfused with or without oxyradical-generating system (X plus XO) as well as H_2O_2, a well-known oxidant, for 30 min. We have shown that the reperfusion of the ischemic heart results in a depression of the left ventricular developed pressure, while the left ventricular end diastolic pressure is markedly increased, demonstrating that reperfusion of the ischemic heart impairs the recovery of cardiac function [87]. We have further reported an increase in the biomarkers of oxidative stress (H_2O_2 content and malondialdehyde) in hearts subjected to I/R [87]. Treatment of hearts with an antioxidant mixture (SOD–catalase) was observed to attenuate the I/R-induced changes in cardiac function and biomarkers of oxidative stress [87]. In addition, the myocardial Ca^{2+} contents in control, I/R, and SOD–catalase-treated I/R hearts were reported to be 8.4 ± 1.2, 22.6 ± 2.9, and 9.8 ± 1.6 µmol/g dry wt., respectively [87]. These data revealed the impact of oxidative stress and intracellular Ca^{2+} overload and the beneficial actions of antioxidants on cardiac function.

The I/R-induced myocardial functional changes were demonstrated to be associated with a marked reduction in SL Na^+-K^+ ATPase activity as well as an increase in matrix metalloproteinase (MMP) and calpain activities upon the reperfusion of ischemic hearts [145]. The protective role of antioxidants was further demonstrated by the attenuation of these I/R-induced effects when the reperfusion of ischemic hearts was carried out in the presence of well-known antioxidants, namely N-acetylcysteine (NAC) or mercaptopropionyl glycine (MPG) [145]. On the other hand, the perfusion of hearts with X plus XO was also shown to be associated with reduced Na^+-K^+ ATPase activities as well as increased activities of both MMP and calpain. Other subcellular activities, including SL Na^+-Ca^{2+} exchange, ATP-dependent Ca^{2+} uptake, and Ca^{2+}-stimulated ATP activities were depressed upon reperfusing ischemic hearts or when hearts are perfused with a medium containing X plus

XO. These changes in the SL enzyme or Ca^{2+}-handling activities in I/R hearts or in hearts exposed to an oxyradical-generating system were shown to be partially normalized in the presence of SOD–catalase [146–148].

It was also shown that, while SR Ca^{2+} uptake, Ca^{2+}-stimulated ATPase, Ca^{2+} release, and ryanodine-binding activities were depressed in I/R hearts, the reperfusion of ischemic hearts in the presence of SOD–catalase attenuate these alterations (except that for Ca^{2+}-stimulated ATPase) [149]. Furthermore, the perfusion of hearts with X plus XO or H_2O_2 [149] followed by reperfusion also depressed SR Ca^{2+} uptake, Ca^{2+}-stimulated ATPase, Ca^{2+} release, and ryanodine binding activities [149]. Taken together, these observations indicated that defects in both SL and SR organelles due to I/R injury can not only be prevented by antioxidant mixtures, but are simulated when hearts are exposed to ROS-generating systems.

The effects of I/R injury and ROS-generating systems on other subcellular organelles, such as mitochondria (MT) and myofibrils (MF), have also been examined. In this regard, depressions in MT state 3 respiration and ADP/O ratio index were reported upon subjection of the heart to I/R injury; these were attenuated by SOD–catalase [150]. Similarly, perfusion of the rat heart with X+XO or H_2O_2 [150] also reduces MT state 3 respiration and the ADP/O ratio index. In addition, the I/R-induced depression observed for MF Ca^{2+}-stimulated ATPase activity was prevented in the presence of SOD–catalase or N-acetylcysteine [151,152]. It was also noted that MF Mg^{2+}-ATPase activity was increased when perfusing the isolated rat hearts with X+XO or H_2O_2, whereas MF Ca^{2+}-stimulated ATPase activity was depressed. Although the exact reason for the difference in the responses of MF Mg^{2+}-ATPase to I/R injury and oxidative stress is not clear, MF Ca^{2+}-stimulated ATPase activity was depressed under both experimental conditions. These observations suggest that both I/R injury and the ROS-generating system produce similar changes in the MT and MF and the effects of I/R injury were attenuated by antioxidants.

In view of the critical role of SR Ca^{2+} handling as well as the involvement of oxidative stress in the development of intracellular Ca^{2+} overload upon the induction of I/I injury, the effects of NAC and MPG on I/R-induced and X–XO-induced changes in SR Ca^{2+} uptake and SR Ca^{2+} release activities were examined in isolated rat heart [48]. In this regard, I/R-induced depressions in Ca^{2+} uptake and SR Ca^{2+} release activities were attenuated by both NAC and MPG treatments. Likewise, treatments of hearts with NAC or MPG mitigated the X–XO-induced alterations in cardiac Ca^{2+} uptake and SR Ca^{2+} release activities [48]. These data, with exogenous antioxidants (NAC and MPG), support observations regarding the beneficial effects of endogenous antioxidant mixtures (SOD plus CAT) on I/R-induced decreases in SR Ca^{2+} transport activities.

Although the role of oxidative stress and intracellular Ca^{2+} overload in I/R injury has been demonstrated in experimental studies by employing different animal models, the beneficial effects of various antioxidants in the clinical setting remain to be conclusively established [48,51,87,153]. Nonetheless, the lower sensitivity of female hearts to I/R injury in comparison to male hearts has been attributed to the reduction in Ca^{2+} handling as well as oxidative stress [154–160]. A schematic representation of the complex relationship involved in the development of oxidative stress and intracellular Ca^{2+} overload, as well as the occurrence of subcellular Ca^{2+}-handling abnormalities, is depicted in Figure 1. It should be mentioned that the mechanisms for the reduction of antioxidant levels in I/R injury are not understood, whereas the depression in transcription factors such as Nrf2 under in vivo conditions may be involved in reducing endogenous antioxidant levels and activities.

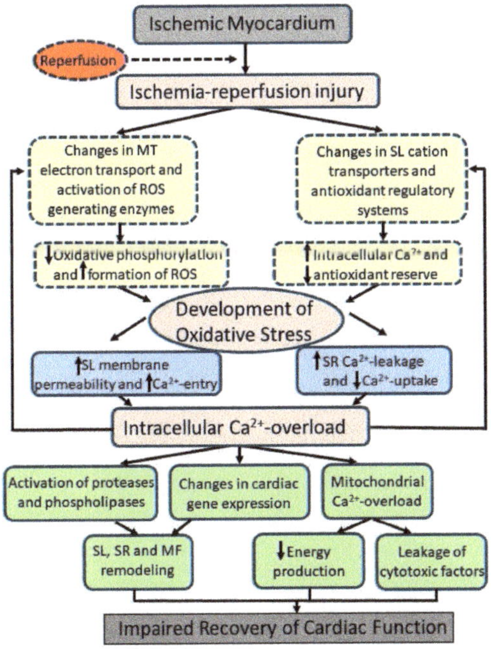

Figure 1. Schematic representation of reperfusion-induced events in ischemic myocardium (ischemia–reperfusion injury) involving subcellular alterations for the generation of oxidative stress, development of intracellular Ca^{2+} overload, and impaired recovery of cardiac function. MT = mitochondria, SL = sarcolemma; ROS = reactive oxygen species; SR = sarcoplasmic reticulum; Ca^{2+} = calcium; MF = myofibrils.

It can be argued that we have provided the above evidence in support of the involvement of oxidative stress and the beneficial effects of antioxidants on I/R injury from the data obtained in our laboratory. However, it is pointed out that there is a real lack of information from other laboratories on I/R-induced alterations in subcellular organelles and Ca^{2+}-handling activities that can be attributed to oxidative stress; thus, it is essential to emphasize the involvement of the interaction of oxidative stress, antioxidants, and subcellular Ca^{2+}-handling activities. Nonetheless, there is a wealth of information regarding the role of oxidative stress in I/R-induced changes in cardiac function [161–167] as well as structural factors [168–174], metabolic factors [175–177], apoptosis [178–180], signal transduction [32,181–185], and arrhythmias [186–189]. These observations support our viewpoint indirectly.

6. Perspectives and Conclusions

From the foregoing discussion, it is evident that both oxidative stress and intracellular Ca^{2+} overload induce I/R injury to the heart. Since both these pathogenic factors are inter-related, it is difficult to determine the sequence of their development as well as their cause–effect relationship for inducing I/R injury. In this regard, it should be mentioned that changes occur in the MT electron transport system and in energy production due to myocardial ischemia; moreover, a large amount of H_2 is accumulated in the ischemic myocardium. Reperfusion of the ischemic heart removes H_2 from cardiomyocytes upon stimulating the SL Na^+-H^+ and SL Na^+-Ca^{2+} exchange systems, which increases the intracellular concentration of Ca^{2+} and subsequently activates different proteases and phospholipases. These changes will depress SR Ca^{2+} pump activity to further promote the elevation of intracellular Ca^{2+}. In addition, the increased protease and phospholipase activities will increase the permeability of both SL and SR mechanisms for increasing the entry of extracellular Ca^{2+} and leakage of Ca^{2+} from SR stores, respectively. Such defects in Ca^{2+} handling by SL and SR will result in the occurrence of intracellular Ca^{2+} overload and marked accumulation of Ca^{2+} in MT. Thus, MT Ca^{2+} overload will be associated with the generation of ROS due to further derangement of the electron transport system as well as activation of different enzymes, including XO and NADPH oxidase, leading to the generation of ROS. This excessive production of ROS will result in the occurrence of oxidative stress, the intensity of which will be further promoted by a depression in the level of endogenous antioxidants.

It is now well known that the delayed reperfusion of the ischemic heart produces marked alterations in myocardial metabolism and cardiac ultrastructure in addition to impairing the recovery of cardiac function. Such changes in I/R hearts are associated with the increased formation of ROS. It is noteworthy that MT are the major source of ROS production due to defects in the electron transport system; another major source is the activation of XO and NADPH oxidase, as a consequence of reperfusion of ischemic hearts. The activation of endothelium nitric oxide synthase and the formation of nitric oxide also occur; these combine with superoxide radicals to generate peroxynitrite. On the other hand, the concentrations of endogenous antioxidants, including superoxide dismutase, catalase, and glutathione peroxidase (which antagonizes the actions of ROS), are decreased in I/R hearts. It should also be mentioned that, under in vivo conditions, the levels of transcription factors such as Nrf2, which regulate the status of several antioxidants, are also depressed upon reperfusion. Thus, an imbalance occurs between the excessive formation of ROS and the reduced levels of antioxidants due to reperfusion; these lead to the generation of oxidative stress. Although various defects occur in the I/R hearts, such as inflammation, subcellular alterations, intracellular Ca^{2+} overload, activation of proteases, and changes in cardiac gene expression, these abnormalities seem to be the consequence of oxidative stress generation during the development of I/R injury.

Impaired recovery of cardiac function due to I/R injury has been shown to be associated with depression in SL Na^{+}-K^{+} ATPase, Na^{+}-Ca^{2+} exchange, and ATP-dependent Ca^{2+} pump activities. Furthermore, I/R injury has been demonstrated to induce changes in the SR Ca^{2+} pump activity and promote the leakage of Ca^{2+} to further raise the intracellular concentration of Ca^{2+} and cause the development of MT Ca^{2+} overload, depression in the oxidative phosphorylation, and energy production, opening MT pores for the leakage of cytotoxic material and the development of programmed cellular death. The occurrence of Ca^{2+}-handling abnormalities in the SL and SR organelles in I/R hearts as a consequence of oxidative stress is also associated with the development of intracellular Ca^{2+} overload, the activation of proteases such as MMP and calpain, depression in the cardiac gene expression, and the loss of MF Ca^{2+} sensitivity. Furthermore, treatment of the heart with different antioxidants has been shown to attenuate I/R-induced Ca^{2+}-handling defects in subcellular organelles, activation of proteases, loss of MF Ca^{2+} sensitivity, and development of cardiac dysfunction. It is thus evident that both oxidative stress and subcellular Ca^{2+}-handling defects play important roles in impairing the recovery of cardiac function due to I/R injury. Accordingly, it is suggested that efforts should be made to develop safe and effective interventions for the upregulation of endogenous antioxidants for improving cardiovascular abnormalities associated with I/R injury.

Author Contributions: P.S.T. researched the literature and analyzed the data; both P.O. and P.S.T. wrote the manuscript; N.S.D. conceived, designed, and prepared the final draft of this article. All authors have read and agreed to the published version of the manuscript.

Funding: This research received no external funding.

Data Availability Statement: The original contributions presented in this study are included in the article.

Acknowledgments: The infrastructural support of this article was provided by the St. Boniface Hospital Albrechtsen Research Centre.

Conflicts of Interest: The authors declare no conflicts of interest.

References

1. Sharma, G.P.; Varley, K.G.; Kim, S.W.; Barwinsky, J.; Cohen, M.; Dhalla, N.S. Alterations in energy metabolism and ultrastructure upon reperfusion of the ischemic myocardium after coronary occlusion. *Am. J. Cardiol.* **1975**, *36*, 234–243. [CrossRef]
2. Nayler, W.G.; Panagiotopoulos, S.; Elz, J.S.; Daly, M.J. Calcium-mediated damage during post-ischemic reperfusion. *J. Mol. Cell. Cardiol.* **1988**, *20* (Suppl. S2), 41–54. [CrossRef] [PubMed]
3. Murphy, J.G.; Smith, T.W.; Marsh, J.D. Mechanisms of reoxygenation-induced calcium overload in cultured chick embryo heart cells. *Am. J. Physiol.* **1988**, *254*, H1133–H1141. [CrossRef] [PubMed]
4. Jennings, R.B.; Reimer, K.A. The cell biology of acute myocardial ischemia. *Annu. Rev. Med.* **1991**, *42*, 225–246. [CrossRef]
5. Bolli, R.; Marban, E. Molecular and cellular mechanisms of myocardial stunning. *Physiol. Rev.* **1999**, *79*, 609–634. [CrossRef]
6. Piper, M.H.; Meuter, K.; Schafer, C. Cellular mechanisms of ischemia-reperfusion injury. *Ann. Thorac. Surg.* **2003**, *75*, S644–S648. [CrossRef]
7. Hoffman, J.W.; Gilbert, T.B.; Poston, R.S.; Silldorff, E.P. Myocardial reperfusion injury: Etiology, mechanisms, and therapies. *J. ExtraCorporeal Technol.* **2004**, *36*, 391–411. [CrossRef]
8. Dhalla, N.S.; Elmoselhi, A.B.; Hata, T.; Makino, N. Status of myocardial antioxidants in ischemia-reperfusion injury. *Cardiovasc. Res.* **2000**, *47*, 446–456. [CrossRef]
9. Neuzil, J.; Rayner, B.S.; Lowe, H.C.; Witting, P.K. Oxidative stress in myocardial ischemia reperfusion injury: A renewed focus on a long-standing area of heart research. *Redox Rep.* **2005**, *10*, 187–197. [CrossRef]
10. Milei, J.; Grana, D.R.; Forcada, P.; Ambrosio, G. Mitochondrial oxidative and structural damage in ischemia-reperfusion in human myocardium. Current knowledge and future directions. *Front. Biosci.* **2007**, *12*, 1124–1130. [CrossRef]
11. Dhalla, N.S.; Saini, H.K.; Tappia, P.S.; Sethi, R.; Mengi, S.A.; Gupta, S.K. Potential role and mechanisms of subcellular remodeling in cardiac dysfunction due to ischemic heart disease. *J. Cardiovasc. Med.* **2007**, *8*, 238–250. [CrossRef] [PubMed]
12. Rodrigo, R.; Libuy, M.; Feliu, F.; Hasson, D. Oxidative stress-related biomarkers in essential hypertension and ischemia-reperfusion myocardial damage. *Dis. Markers* **2013**, *35*, 773–790. [CrossRef] [PubMed]
13. Neri, M.; Riezzo, I.; Pascale, N.; Pomara, C.; Turillazzi, E. Ischemia/reperfusion injury following acute myocardial infarction: A critical issue for clinicians and forensic pathologists. *Mediat. Inflamm.* **2017**, *2017*, 7018393. [CrossRef]
14. Zhou, T.; Chuang, C.C.; Zuo, L. Molecular characterization of reactive oxygen species in myocardial ischemia-reperfusion injury. *BioMed Res. Int.* **2015**, *2015*, 864946. [CrossRef] [PubMed]
15. Kurian, G.A.; Rajagopal, R.; Vedantham, S.; Rajesh, M. The role of oxidative stress in myocardial ischemia and reperfusion injury and remodeling: Revisited. *Oxidative Med. Cell. Longev.* **2016**, *2016*, 165450. [CrossRef]
16. Morciano, G.; Pinton, P. Modulation of mitochondrial permeability transition pores in reperfusion injury: Mechanisms and therapeutic approaches. *Eur. J. Clin. Investig.* **2025**, *55*, e14331. [CrossRef]
17. Liu, Y.; Wu, H.; Zhou, G.; Zhang, D.; Yang, Q.; Li, Y.; Yang, X.; Sun, J. Role of M6a Methylation in Myocardial Ischemia-Reperfusion Injury and Doxorubicin-Induced Cardiotoxicity. *Cardiovasc. Toxicol.* **2024**, *24*, 918–928. [CrossRef]
18. Li, J.; Zhang, Y.; Tang, R.; Liu, H.; Li, X.; Lei, W.; Chen, J.; Jin, Z.; Tang, J.; Wang, Z.; et al. Glycogen synthase kinase-3β: A multifaceted player in ischemia-reperfusion injury and its therapeutic prospects. *J. Cell Physiol.* **2024**, *239*, e31335. [CrossRef]
19. Balderas, E.; Lee, S.H.J.; Rai, N.K.; Mollinedo, D.M.; Duron, H.E.; Chaudhuri, D. Mitochondrial calcium regulation of cardiac metabolism in health and disease. *Physiology* **2024**, *39*, 247–268. [CrossRef]
20. Nakamura, E.; Aoki, T.; Endo, Y.; Kazmi, J.; Hagiwara, J.; Kuschner, C.E.; Yin, T.; Kim, J.; Becker, L.B.; Hayashida, K. Organ-specific mitochondrial alterations following ischemia-reperfusion injury in post-cardiac arrest syndrome: A comprehensive review. *Life* **2024**, *14*, 477. [CrossRef]
21. Yan, Z.; Xing, Z.; Xue, T.; Zhao, J.; Li, G.; Xu, L.; Sun, Q. Insulin-like growth factor-1 in myocardial ischemia-reperfusion injury: A review. *Medicine* **2024**, *103*, e37279. [CrossRef] [PubMed]
22. Wang, Y.; Xu, R.; Yan, Y.; He, B.; Miao, C.; Fang, Y.; Wan, H.; Zhou, G. Exosomes-mediated signaling pathway: A new direction for treatment of organ ischemia-reperfusion injury. *Biomedicines* **2024**, *12*, 353. [CrossRef]
23. Liao, W.; Wen, Y.; Yang, S.; Duan, Y.; Liu, Z. Research progress and perspectives of N-methyl-D-aspartate receptor in myocardial and cerebral ischemia-reperfusion injury: A review. *Medicine* **2023**, *102*, e35490. [CrossRef]

24. Omorou, M.; Huang, Y.; Gao, M.; Mu, C.; Xu, W.; Han, Y.; Xu, H. The forkhead box O3 (FOXO3): A key player in the regulation of ischemia and reperfusion injury. *Cell. Mol. Life Sci.* **2023**, *80*, 102. [CrossRef] [PubMed]
25. Galeone, A.; Grano, M.; Brunetti, G. Tumor necrosis factor family members and myocardial ischemia-reperfusion injury: State of the art and therapeutic implications. *Int. J. Mol. Sci.* **2023**, *24*, 4606. [CrossRef]
26. Popov, S.V.; Mukhomedzyanov, A.V.; Voronkov, N.S.; Derkachev, I.A.; Boshchenko, A.A.; Fu, F.; Sufianova, G.Z.; Khlestkina, M.S.; Maslov, L.N. Regulation of autophagy of the heart in ischemia and reperfusion. *Apoptosis* **2023**, *28*, 55–80. [CrossRef]
27. Mahdiani, S.; Omidkhoda, N.; Rezaee, R.; Heidari, S.; Karimi, G. Induction of JAK2/STAT3 pathway contributes to protective effects of different therapeutics against myocardial ischemia/reperfusion. *Biomed. Pharmacother.* **2022**, *155*, 113751. [CrossRef]
28. Bai, Y.; Wu, J.; Yang, Z.; Wang, X.; Zhang, D.; Ma, J. Mitochondrial quality control in cardiac ischemia/reperfusion injury: New insights into mechanisms and implications. *Cell Biol. Toxicol.* **2023**, *39*, 33–51. [CrossRef]
29. Liu, H.; Liu, X.; Zhou, J.; Li, T. Mitochondrial DNA is a vital driving force in ischemia-reperfusion injury in cardiovascular diseases. *Oxidative Med. Cell. Longev.* **2022**, *2022*, 6235747. [CrossRef]
30. He, J.; Liu, D.; Zhao, L.; Zhou, D.; Rong, J.; Zhang, L.; Xia, Z. Myocardial ischemia/reperfusion injury: Mechanisms of injury and implications for management. *Exp. Ther. Med.* **2022**, *23*, 430. [CrossRef]
31. Maslov, L.N.; Popov, S.V.; Mukhomedzyanov, A.V.; Naryzhnaya, N.V.; Voronkov, N.S.; Ryabov, V.V.; Boshchenko, A.A.; Khaliulin, I.; Prasad, N.R.; Fu, F.; et al. Reperfusion cardiac injury: Receptors and the signaling mechanisms. *Curr. Cardiol. Rev.* **2022**, *18*, 63–79. [CrossRef] [PubMed]
32. Zhuang, Y.; Yu, M.L.; Lu, S.F. Purinergic signaling in myocardial ischemia-reperfusion injury. *Purinergic Signal.* **2023**, *19*, 229–243. [CrossRef]
33. Casin, K.M.; Calvert, J.W. Dynamic regulation of cysteine oxidation and phosphorylation in myocardial ischemia-reperfusion injury. *Cells* **2021**, *10*, 2388. [CrossRef] [PubMed]
34. Chen, L.; Shi, D.; Guo, M. The roles of PKC-δ and PKC-ε in myocardial ischemia/reperfusion injury. *Pharmacol. Res.* **2021**, *170*, 105716. [CrossRef] [PubMed]
35. Zheng, J.; Chen, P.; Zhong, J.; Cheng, Y.; Chen, H.; He, Y.; Chen, C. HIF-1α in myocardial ischemia-reperfusion injury. *Mol. Med. Rep.* **2021**, *23*, 352. [CrossRef]
36. Jin, S.; Kang, P.M. A systematic review on advances in management of oxidative stress-associated cardiovascular diseases. *Antioxidants* **2024**, *13*, 923. [CrossRef]
37. Chen, X.; Yang, Y.; Zhou, Z.; Yu, H.; Zhang, S.; Huang, S.; Wei, Z.; Ren, K.; Jin, Y. Unraveling the complex interplay between Mitochondria-Associated Membranes (MAMs) and cardiovascular inflammation: Molecular mechanisms and therapeutic implications. *Int. Immunopharmacol.* **2024**, *141*, 112930. [CrossRef]
38. Zhang, J.; Zhao, Y.; Gong, N. Endoplasmic reticulum stress signaling modulates ischemia/reperfusion injury in the aged heart by regulating mitochondrial maintenance. *Mol. Med.* **2024**, *30*, 107. [CrossRef]
39. Zhang, H.; Dhalla, N.S. The role of pro-inflammatory cytokines in the pathogenesis of cardiovascular disease. *Int. J. Mol. Sci.* **2024**, *25*, 1082. [CrossRef]
40. Ruan, Y.; Zeng, J.; Jin, Q.; Chu, M.; Ji, K.; Wang, Z.; Li, L. Endoplasmic reticulum stress serves an important role in cardiac ischemia/reperfusion injury. *Exp. Ther. Med.* **2020**, *20*, 268. [CrossRef]
41. Shah, A.K.; Bhullar, S.K.; Elimban, V.; Dhalla, N.S. Oxidative stress as a mechanism for functional alterations in cadiac hypertrophy and heart failure. *Antioxidants* **2021**, *10*, 931. [CrossRef] [PubMed]
42. Dhalla, N.S.; Elimban, V.; Shah, A.K.; Nusier, M. Mechanisms of cardiac dysfunction in heart failure due to myocardial infarction. *J. Integr. Cardiol.* **2019**, *2*, 3–7. [CrossRef]
43. Dhalla, N.S.; Temsah, R.M.; Netticadan, T. Role of oxidative stress in cardiovascular diseases. *J. Hypertens.* **2000**, *18*, 655–673. [CrossRef] [PubMed]
44. Dhalla, N.S.; Elimban, V.; Bartekova, M.; Adameova, A. Involvement of oxidative stress in the development of subcellular defects and heart disease. *Biomedicines* **2022**, *10*, 393. [CrossRef]
45. Saini, H.K.; Xu, Y.J.; Zhang, M.; Liu, P.P.; Kirshenbaum, L.A.; Dhalla, N.S. Role of tumor necrosis factor-alpha and other cytokines in ischemia-reperfusion-induced injury in the heart. *Exp. Clin. Cardiol.* **2005**, *10*, 213–222. [PubMed]
46. Ambrosio, G.; Zweier, J.L.; Flaherty, J.T. The relationship between oxygen radical generation and impairment of myocardial energy metabolism following post-ischemic reperfusion. *J. Mol. Cell. Cardiol.* **1991**, *23*, 1359–1374. [CrossRef]
47. Sinning, C.; Westermann, D.; Clemmensen, P. Oxidative stress in ischemia and reperfusion: Current concepts, novel ideas and future perspectives. *Biomark. Med.* **2017**, *11*, 11031–11040. [CrossRef]
48. Bartekova, M.; Barancik, M.; Ferenczyova, K.; Dhalla, N.S. Beneficial effects of N-acetylcysteine and N-N-mercaptopropionylglycine on Ischemia reperfusion injury in the heart. *Curr. Med. Chem.* **2018**, *25*, 355–366. [CrossRef]
49. Ferrari, R.; Ceconi, C.; Curello, S.; Guarnieri, C.; Caldarera, C.M.; Albertini, A.; Visioli, O. Oxygen-mediated myocardial damage during ischemia and reperfusion: Role of the cellular defenses against oxygen toxicity. *J. Mol. Cell. Cardiol.* **1985**, *17*, 937–945. [CrossRef]

50. Arduini, A.; Mezzetti, A.; Porreca, E.; Lapenna, D.; DeJulia, J.; Marzio, L.; Polidoro, G.; Cuccurullo, F. Effect of ischemia and reperfusion on antioxidant enzymes and mitochondrial inner membrane proteins in perfused rat heart. *Biochim. Biophys. Acta* **1988**, *970*, 113–121. [CrossRef]
51. Dhalla, N.S.; Shah, A.K.; Adameova, A.; Bartekova, M. Role of oxidative stress in cardiac dysfunction and subcellular defects due to ischemia-reperfusion injury. *Biomedicines* **2022**, *10*, 1473. [CrossRef] [PubMed]
52. San-Martín-Martínez, D.; Serrano-Lemus, D.; Cornejo, V.; Gajardo, A.I.J.; Rodrigo, R. Pharmacological basis for abrogating myocardial reperfusion injury through a multi-target combined antioxidant therapy. *Clin. Pharmacokinet.* **2022**, *61*, 1203–1218. [CrossRef] [PubMed]
53. Matsushima, S.; Sadoshima, J. Yin and Yang of NADPH oxidases in myocardial ischemia-reperfusion. *Antioxidants* **2022**, *11*, 1069. [CrossRef]
54. Chen, C.L.; Zhang, L.; Jin, Z.; Kasumov, T.; Chen, Y.R. Mitochondrial redox regulation and myocardial ischemia-reperfusion injury. *Am. J. Physiol. Cell Physiol.* **2022**, *322*, C12–C23. [CrossRef] [PubMed]
55. Wang, M.; Liu, Y.; Liang, Y.; Naruse, K.; Takahashi, K. Systematic understanding of pathophysiological mechanisms of oxidative stress-related conditions-diabetes mellitus, cardiovascular diseases, and ischemia-reperfusion injury. *Front. Cardiovasc. Med.* **2021**, *8*, 649785. [CrossRef]
56. Hu, L.; Wang, Z.; Carmone, C.; Keijer, J.; Zhang, D. Role of oxidative DNA damage and repair in atrial fibrillation and ischemic heart disease. *Int. J. Mol. Sci.* **2021**, *22*, 3838. [CrossRef]
57. Dambrova, M.; Zuurbier, C.J.; Borutaite, V.; Liepinsh, E.; Makrecka-Kuka, M. Energy substrate metabolism and mitochondrial oxidative stress in cardiac ischemia/reperfusion injury. *Free Radic. Biol. Med.* **2021**, *165*, 24–37. [CrossRef]
58. Huang, P.; Qu, C.; Rao, Z.; Wu, D.; Zhao, J. Bidirectional regulation mechanism of TRPM2 channel: Role in oxidative stress, inflammation and ischemia-reperfusion injury. *Front. Immunol.* **2024**, *15*, 1391355. [CrossRef]
59. Liang, W.L.; Cai, M.R.; Zhang, M.Q.; Cui, S.; Zhang, T.R.; Cheng, W.H.; Wu, Y.H.; Ou, W.J.; Jia, Z.H.; Zhang, S.F. Chinese herbal medicine alleviates myocardial ischemia/reperfusion injury by regulating endoplasmic reticulum stress. *Evid. Based Complement. Altern. Med.* **2021**, *2021*, 4963346. [CrossRef]
60. Wiklund, L.; Sharma, A.; Patnaik, R.; Muresanu, D.F.; Sahib, S.; Tian, Z.R.; Castellani, R.J.; Nozari, A.; Lafuente, J.V.; Sharma, H.S. Upregulation of hemeoxygenase enzymes HO-1 and HO-2 following ischemia-reperfusion injury in connection with experimental cardiac arrest and cardiopulmonary resuscitation: Neuroprotective effects of methylene blue. *Prog. Brain Res.* **2021**, *265*, 317–375.
61. Thompson, J.; Maceyka, M.; Chen, Q. Targeting ER stress and calpain activation to reverse age-dependent mitochondrial damage in the heart. *Mech. Ageing Dev.* **2020**, *192*, 111380. [CrossRef] [PubMed]
62. Dubois-Deruy, E.; Peugnet, V.; Turkieh, A.; Pinet, F. Oxidative stress in cardiovascular diseases. *Antioxidants* **2020**, *9*, 864. [CrossRef] [PubMed]
63. Zhao, S.; Cheng, C.K.; Zhang, C.L.; Huang, Y. Interplay between oxidative stress, cyclooxygenases, and prostanoids in cardiovascular diseases. *Antioxid. Redox Signal.* **2021**, *34*, 784–799. [CrossRef]
64. Bugger, H.; Pfeil, K. Mitochondrial ROS in myocardial ischemia reperfusion and remodeling. *Biochim. Biophys. Acta Mol. Basis Dis.* **2020**, *1866*, 165768. [CrossRef]
65. Zhou, H.; Toan, S. Pathological roles of mitochondrial oxidative stress and mitochondrial dynamics in cardiac microvascular ischemia/reperfusion injury. *Biomolecules* **2020**, *10*, 85. [CrossRef]
66. Zhang, Y.; Murugesan, P.; Huang, K.; Cai, H. NADPH oxidases and oxidase crosstalk in cardiovascular diseases: Novel therapeutic targets. *Nat. Rev. Cardiol.* **2020**, *17*, 170–194. [CrossRef]
67. Fibbi, B.; Marroncini, G.; Naldi, L.; Peri, A. The Yin and Yang effect of the apelinergic system in oxidative stress. *Int. J. Mol. Sci.* **2023**, *24*, 4745. [CrossRef] [PubMed]
68. Qiu, M.; Chen, J.; Li, X.; Zhuang, J. Intersection of the ubiquitin-proteasome system with oxidative stress in cardiovascular disease. *Int. J. Mol. Sci.* **2022**, *23*, 12197. [CrossRef]
69. Szyller, J.; Jagielski, D.; Bil-Lula, I. Antioxidants in arrhythmia treatment-still a controversy? A review of selected clinical and laboratory research. *Antioxidants* **2022**, *11*, 1109. [CrossRef]
70. Adameova, A.; Shah, A.K.; Dhalla, N.S. Role of oxidative stress in the genesis of ventricular arrhythmias. *Int. J. Mol. Sci.* **2020**, *21*, 4200. [CrossRef]
71. Luan, X.; Chen, P.; Miao, L.; Yuan, X.; Yu, C.; Di, G. Ferroptosis in organ ischemia-reperfusion injuries: Recent advancements and strategies. *Mol. Cell. Biochem.* **2025**, *480*, 19–41. [CrossRef] [PubMed]
72. Wang, R.; Chen, X.; Li, X.; Wang, K. Molecular therapy of cardiac ischemia-reperfusion injury based on mitochondria and ferroptosis. *J. Mol. Med.* **2023**, *101*, 1059–1071. [CrossRef] [PubMed]
73. Fratta Pasini, A.M.; Stranieri, C.; Busti, F.; Di Leo, E.G.; Girelli, D.; Cominacini, L. New insights into the role of ferroptosis in cardiovascular diseases. *Cells* **2023**, *12*, 867. [CrossRef]
74. Yu, Y.; Yan, Y.; Niu, F.; Wang, Y.; Chen, X.; Su, G.; Liu, Y.; Zhao, X.; Qian, L.; Liu, P.; et al. Ferroptosis: A cell death connecting oxidative stress, inflammation and cardiovascular diseases. *Cell Death Discov.* **2021**, *7*, 193. [CrossRef]

75. Lillo-Moya, J.; Rojas-Solé, C.; Muñoz-Salamanca, D.; Panieri, E.; Saso, L.; Rodrigo, R. Targeting ferroptosis against ischemia/reperfusion cardiac injury. *Antioxidants* **2021**, *10*, 667. [CrossRef]
76. Tian, K.; Yang, Y.; Zhou, K.; Deng, N.; Tian, Z.; Wu, Z.; Liu, X.; Zhang, F.; Jiang, Z. The role of ROS-induced pyroptosis in CVD. *Front. Cardiovasc. Med.* **2023**, *10*, 1116509. [CrossRef] [PubMed]
77. Liu, Y.; Zhang, J.; Zhang, D.; Yu, P.; Zhang, J.; Yu, S. Research progress on the role of pyroptosis in myocardial ischemia-reperfusion injury. *Cells* **2022**, *11*, 3271. [CrossRef]
78. Adameova, A.; Horvath, C.; Abdul-Ghani, S.; Varga, Z.V.; Suleiman, M.S.; Dhalla, N.S. Interplay of oxidative stress and necrosis-like cell death in cardiac ischemia/reperfusion injury: A focus on necroptosis. *Biomedicines* **2022**, *10*, 127. [CrossRef]
79. Cinato, M.; Andersson, L.; Miljanovic, A.; Laudette, M.; Kunduzova, O.; Borén, J.; Levin, M.C. Role of perilipins in oxidative stress-implications for cardiovascular disease. *Antioxidants* **2024**, *13*, 209. [CrossRef]
80. Rongjin, H.; Feng, C.; Jun, K.; Shirong, L. Oxidative stress-induced protein of SESTRIN2 in cardioprotection effect. *Dis. Markers* **2022**, *2022*, 7439878. [CrossRef]
81. Cai, H.; Liu, Y.; Men, H.; Zheng, Y. Protective mechanism of humanin against oxidative stress in aging-related cardiovascular diseases. *Front. Endocrinol.* **2021**, *12*, 683151. [CrossRef] [PubMed]
82. Liu, Y.; Wang, M.; Liang, Y.; Wang, C.; Naruse, K.; Takahashi, K. Treatment of oxidative stress with exosomes in myocardial ischemia. *Int. J. Mol. Sci.* **2021**, *22*, 1729. [CrossRef]
83. Wang, W.; Kang, P.M. Oxidative stress and antioxidant treatments in cardiovascular diseases. *Antioxidants* **2020**, *9*, 1292. [CrossRef]
84. Wu, W.; Lai, L.; Xie, M.; Qiu, H. Insights of heat shock protein 22 in the cardiac protection against ischemic oxidative stress. *Redox Biol.* **2020**, *34*, 101555. [CrossRef]
85. Kura, B.; Szeiffova Bacova, B.; Kalocayova, B.; Sykora, M.; Slezak, J. Oxidative stress-responsive microRNAs in heart injury. *Int. J. Mol. Sci.* **2020**, *21*, 358. [CrossRef]
86. Haramaki, N.; Stewart, D.B.; Aggarwal, S.; Ikeda, H.; Reznick, A.Z.; Packer, L. Networking antioxidants in the isolated rat heart are selectively depleted by ischemia-reperfusion. *Free Radic. Biol. Med.* **1998**, *25*, 329–339. [CrossRef] [PubMed]
87. Dhalla, N.S.; Golfman, L.; Takeda, S.; Takeda, N.; Nagano, M. Evidence for the role of oxidative stress in acute ischemic heart disease: A brief review. *Can. J. Cardiol.* **1999**, *15*, 587–593. [PubMed]
88. Saini, H.K.; Machackova, J.; Dhalla, N.S. Role of reactive oxygen species in ischemic preconditioning of subcellular organelles in the heart. *Antioxid. Redox Signal.* **2004**, *6*, 393–404. [CrossRef]
89. Bhullar, S.K.; Shah, A.K.; Dhalla, N.S. Role of angiotensin II in the development of subcellular remodeling in heart failure. *Explor. Med.* **2021**, *2*, 352–371. [CrossRef]
90. Tappia, P.S.; Shah, A.K.; Ramjiawan, B.; Dhalla, N.S. Modification of ischemia/reperfusion-induced alterations in subcellular organelles by ischemic preconditioning. *Int. J. Mol. Sci.* **2022**, *23*, 3425. [CrossRef]
91. Bhosale, G.; Sharpe, J.A.; Sundier, S.; Duchen, M. Calcium signaling as mediator of cell energy demand and a trigger to cell death. *Ann. N. Y. Acad. Sci.* **2015**, *1350*, 107–116. [CrossRef]
92. Badalzadeh, R.; Mokhtari, B.; Yavari, R. Contribution of apoptosis in myocardial reperfusion injury and loss of cardioprotection in diabetes mellitus. *J. Physiol. Sci.* **2015**, *65*, 201–215. [CrossRef] [PubMed]
93. Ferrari, R.; Guardigli, G.; Mele, D.; Percoco, G.F.; Ceconi, C.; Curello, S. Oxidative stress during myocardial ischemia and heart failure. *Curr. Pharm. Des.* **2004**, *10*, 1699–1711. [CrossRef] [PubMed]
94. Neri, M.; Fineschi, V.; Di Paolo, M.; Pomara, C.; Riezzo, I.; Turillazzi, E.; Cerretani, D. Cardiac oxidative stress and inflammation cytokines response after myocardial infarction. *Curr. Vasc. Pharmacol.* **2015**, *13*, 26–36. [CrossRef]
95. Li, X.; Zhang, F.; Zhou, H.; Hu, Y.; Guo, D.; Fang, X.; Chen, Y. Interplay of TNF-α, soluble TNF receptors and oxidative stress in coronary chronic total occlusion of the oldest patients with coronary heart disease. *Cytokine* **2020**, *125*, 154836. [CrossRef] [PubMed]
96. Xiong, W.; Qu, Y.; Chen, H.; Qian, J. Insight into long noncoding RNA-miRNA-mRNA axes in myocardial ischemia-reperfusion injury: The implications for mechanism and therapy. *Epigenomics* **2019**, *11*, 1733–1748. [CrossRef] [PubMed]
97. Zhao, Z.; Sun, W.; Guo, Z.; Liu, B.; Yu, H.; Zhang, J. Long noncoding RNAs in myocardial ischemia-reperfusion inury. *Oxidative Med. Cell. Longev.* **2021**, *2021*, 8889123. [CrossRef]
98. Li, Q.; Li, Z.; Fan, Z.; Yang, Y.; Lu, C. Involvement of non-coding RNAs in the pathogenesis of myocardial ischemia/reperfusion injury. *Int. J. Mol. Med.* **2021**, *47*, 42. [CrossRef]
99. Wang, B.F.; Yoshioka, J. The emerging role of thioredoxin-interacting protein in myocardial ischemia-reperfusion injury. *J. Cardiovasc. Pharmacol. Ther.* **2017**, *22*, 219–229. [CrossRef]
100. Zhang, C.; He, M.; Ni, L.; He, K.; Su, K.; Deng, Y.; Li, Y.; Xia, H. The role of arachidonic acid metabolism in myocardial ischemia-reperfusion injury. *Cell Biochem. Biophys.* **2020**, *78*, 255–265. [CrossRef]
101. Bartekova, M.; Adameova, A.; Gorbe, A.; Ferenczyova, K.; Pechanova, O.; Lazou, A.; Dhalla, N.S.; Ferdinandy, P.; Giricz, Z. Natural and synthetic antioxidants targeting cardiac oxidative stress and redox signaling in cardiometabolic diseases. *Free Radic. Biol. Med.* **2021**, *169*, 446–477. [CrossRef] [PubMed]

102. Nagarajan, N.; Oka, S.; Sadoshima, J. Modulation of signaling mechanisms in the heart by thioredoxin 1. *Free Radic. Biol. Med.* **2017**, *109*, 125–131. [CrossRef] [PubMed]
103. Kleikers, P.W.M.; Wingler, K.; Hermans, J.J.R.; Diebold, I.; Altenhofer, S.; Radermacher, K.A.; Janssen, B.; Gorlach, A.; Schmidt, H.H.H.W. NADPH oxidases as a source of oxidative stress and molecular target in ischemia/reperfusion injury. *J. Mol. Med.* **2012**, *90*, 1391–1406. [CrossRef]
104. Yang, F.; Smith, M.J. Metal profiling in coronary ischemia-reperfusion injury: Implications for KEAP1/NRF2 regulated redox signaling. *Free Radic. Biol. Med.* **2024**, *210*, 158–171. [CrossRef]
105. Zhang, P.; Huang, C.; Liu, H.; Zhang, M.; Liu, L.; Zhai, Y.; Zhang, J.; Yang, J.; Yang, J. The mechanism of the NFAT transcription factor family involved in oxidative stress response. *J. Cardiol.* **2024**, *83*, 30–36. [CrossRef]
106. Zhang, J.; Pan, W.; Zhang, Y.; Tan, M.; Yin, Y.; Li, Y.; Zhang, L.; Han, L.; Bai, J.; Jiang, T.; et al. Comprehensive overview of Nrf2-related epigenetic regulations involved in ischemia-reperfusion injury. *Theranostics* **2022**, *12*, 6626–6645. [CrossRef]
107. Sadrkhanloo, M.; Entezari, M.; Orouei, S.; Zabolian, A.; Mirzaie, A.; Maghsoudloo, A.; Raesi, R.; Asadi, N.; Hashemi, M.; Zarrabi, A.; et al. Targeting Nrf2 in ischemia-reperfusion alleviation: From signaling networks to therapeutic targeting. *Life Sci.* **2022**, *300*, 120561. [CrossRef] [PubMed]
108. Mata, A.; Cadenas, S. The antioxidant transcription factor Nrf2 in cardiac ischemia-reperfusion injury. *Int. J. Mol. Sci.* **2021**, *22*, 11939. [CrossRef]
109. Yarmohammadi, F.; Hayes, A.W.; Karimi, G. The cardioprotective effects of hydrogen sulfide by targeting endoplasmic reticulum stress and the Nrf2 signaling pathway: A review. *Biofactors* **2021**, *47*, 701–712. [CrossRef]
110. Ucar, B.I.; Ucar, G.; Saha, S.; Buttari, B.; Profumo, E.; Saso, L. Pharmacological protection against ischemia-reperfusion injury by regulating the Nrf2-Keap1-ARE signaling pathway. *Antioxidants* **2021**, *10*, 823. [CrossRef]
111. Tavakoli, R.; Tabeshpour, J.; Asili, J.; Shakeri, A.; Sahebkar, A. Cardioprotective effects of natural products via the Nrf2 signaling pathway. *Curr. Vasc. Pharmacol.* **2021**, *19*, 525–541. [CrossRef] [PubMed]
112. Zhang, X.; Yu, Y.; Lei, H.; Cai, Y.; Shen, J.; Zhu, P.; He, Q.; Zhao, M. The Nrf-2/HO-1 signaling axis: A ray of hope in cardiovascular diseases. *Cardiol. Res. Pract.* **2020**, *2020*, 5695723. [CrossRef] [PubMed]
113. Kakavand, H.; Aghakouchakzadeh, M.; Coons, J.C.; Talasaz, A.H. Pharmacologic prevention of myocardial ischemia-reperfusion injury in patients with acute coronary syndrome undergoing percutaneous coronary intervention. *J. Cardiovasc. Pharmacol.* **2021**, *77*, 430–449. [CrossRef] [PubMed]
114. Osorio-Llanes, E.; Villamizar-Villamizar, W.; Ospino Guerra, M.C.; Díaz-Ariza, L.A.; Castiblanco-Arroyave, S.C.; Medrano, L.; Mengual, D.; Belón, R.; Castellar-López, J.; Sepúlveda, Y.; et al. Effects of metformin on ischemia/reperfusion injury: New evidence and mechanisms. *Pharmaceuticals* **2023**, *16*, 1121. [CrossRef]
115. Yang, T.; Zhang, D. Research progress on the effects of novel hypoglycemic drugs in diabetes combined with myocardial ischemia/reperfusion injury. *Ageing Res. Rev.* **2023**, *86*, 101884. [CrossRef]
116. Dragasevic, N.; Jakovljevic, V.; Zivkovic, V.; Draginic, N.; Andjic, M.; Bolevich, S.; Jovic, S. The role of aldosterone inhibitors in cardiac ischemia-reperfusion injury. *Can. J. Physiol. Pharmacol.* **2021**, *99*, 18–29. [CrossRef]
117. Ding, X.; Zhu, C.; Wang, W.; Li, M.; Ma, C.; Gao, B. SIRT1 is a regulator of autophagy: Implications for the progression and treatment of myocardial ischemia-reperfusion. *Pharmacol. Res.* **2024**, *199*, 106957. [CrossRef]
118. Lv, J.; Zhu, X.; Xing, C.; Chen, Y.; Bian, H.; Yin, H.; Gu, X.; Su, L. Stimulator of interferon genes (STING): Key therapeutic targets in ischemia/reperfusion injury. *Biomed. Pharmacother.* **2023**, *167*, 115458. [CrossRef]
119. Ding, R.; Wu, W.; Sun, Z.; Li, Z. AMP-activated protein kinase: An attractive therapeutic target for ischemia-reperfusion injury. *Eur. J. Pharmacol.* **2020**, *888*, 173484. [CrossRef]
120. Wang, J.; Liu, Y.; Liu, Y.; Huang, H.; Roy, S.; Song, Z.; Guo, B. Recent advances in nanomedicines for imaging and therapy of myocardial ischemia-reperfusion injury. *J. Control Release* **2023**, *353*, 563–590. [CrossRef]
121. Russo, I.; Barale, C.; Melchionda, E.; Penna, C.; Pagliaro, P. Platelets and cardioprotection: The role of nitric oxide and carbon oxide. *Int. J. Mol. Sci.* **2023**, *24*, 6107. [CrossRef] [PubMed]
122. Ryter, S.W. Therapeutic potential of heme oxygenase-1 and carbon monoxide in acute organ injury, Critical illness, and inflammatory disorders. *Antioxidants* **2020**, *9*, 1153. [CrossRef]
123. Li, T.; Li, Y.; Zeng, Y.; Zhou, X.; Zhang, S.; Ren, Y. Construction of preclinical evidence for propofol in the treatment of reperfusion injury after acute myocardial infarction: A systematic review and meta-analysis. *Biomed. Pharmacother.* **2024**, *174*, 116629. [CrossRef] [PubMed]
124. Yue, H.; Zhang, Q.; Chang, S.; Zhao, X.; Wang, M.; Li, W. Adiponectin protects against myocardial ischemia-reperfusion injury: A systematic review and meta-analysis of preclinical animal studies. *Lipids Health Dis.* **2024**, *23*, 51. [CrossRef]
125. Chen, K.Y.; Liu, Z.; Lu, J.H.; Yang, S.Y.; Hu, X.Y.; Liang, G.Y. The function of circular RNAs in myocardial ischemia-reperfusion injury: Underlying mechanisms and therapeutic advancement. *Cardiovasc. Drugs Ther.* **2024**, 1–12. [CrossRef]
126. Ge, T.; Ning, B.; Wu, Y.; Chen, X.; Qi, H.; Wang, H.; Zhao, M. MicroRNA-specific therapeutic targets and biomarkers of apoptosis following myocardial ischemia-reperfusion injury. *Mol. Cell. Biochem.* **2024**, *479*, 2499–2521. [CrossRef]

127. Chang, C.; Cai, R.P.; Su, Y.M.; Wu, Q.; Su, Q. Mesenchymal stem cell-derived exosomal noncoding RNAs as alternative treatments for myocardial ischemia-reperfusion injury: Current status and future perspectives. *J. Cardiovasc. Transl. Res.* **2023**, *16*, 1085–1098. [CrossRef]
128. Su, X.; Zhou, M.; Li, Y.; Zhang, J.; An, N.; Yang, F.; Zhang, G.; Yuan, C.; Chen, H.; Wu, H.; et al. Protective effects of natural products against myocardial ischemia/reperfusion: Mitochondria-targeted therapeutics. *Biomed. Pharmacother.* **2022**, *149*, 112893. [CrossRef] [PubMed]
129. Chen, C.; Yu, L.T.; Cheng, B.R.; Xu, J.L.; Cai, Y.; Jin, J.L.; Feng, R.L.; Xie, L.; Qu, X.Y.; Li, D.; et al. Promising therapeutic candidate for myocardial ischemia/reperfusion injury: What are the possible mechanisms and roles of phytochemicals? *Front. Cardiovasc. Med.* **2022**, *8*, 792592. [CrossRef]
130. Mauerhofer, C.; Grumet, L.; Schemmer, P.; Leber, B.; Stiegler, P. Combating ischemia-reperfusion injury with micronutrients and natural compounds during solid organ transplantation: Data of clinical trials and lessons of preclinical findings. *Int. J. Mol. Sci.* **2021**, *22*, 10675. [CrossRef]
131. Yoshitomi, T.; Nagasaki, Y. Self-assembling antioxidants for ischemia-reperfusion injuries. *Antioxid. Redox Signal.* **2022**, *36*, 70–80. [CrossRef] [PubMed]
132. Ertugrul, I.A.; van Suylen, V.; Damman, K.; de Koning, M.L.Y.; van Goor, H.; Erasmus, M.E. Donor heart preservation with hydrogen sulfide: A systematic review and meta-analysis. *Int. J. Mol. Sci.* **2021**, *22*, 5737. [CrossRef]
133. An, N.; Zhang, G.; Li, Y.; Yuan, C.; Yang, F.; Zhang, L.; Gao, Y.; Xing, Y. Promising antioxidative effect of berberine in cardiovascular diseases. *Front. Pharmacol.* **2022**, *13*, 865353. [CrossRef]
134. Baliou, S.; Adamaki, M.; Ioannou, P.; Pappa, A.; Panayiotidis, M.I.; Spandidos, D.A.; Christodoulou, I.; Kyriakopoulos, A.M.; Zoumpourlis, V. Protective role of taurine against oxidative stress. *Mol. Med. Rep.* **2021**, *24*, 605. [CrossRef] [PubMed]
135. Prem, P.N.; Sivakumar, B.; Boovarahan, S.R.; Kurian, G.A. Recent advances in potential of Fisetin in the management of myocardial ischemia-reperfusion injury-A systematic review. *Phytomedicine* **2022**, *101*, 154123. [CrossRef]
136. Ferenczyova, K.; Kalocayova, B.; Bartekova, M. Potential implications of quercetin and its derivatives in cardioprotection. *Int. J. Mol. Sci.* **2020**, *21*, 1585. [CrossRef] [PubMed]
137. Sun, Z.; Wang, X. Protective effects of polydatin on multiple organ ischemia-reperfusion injury. *Bioorganic Chem.* **2020**, *94*, 103485. [CrossRef]
138. Zheng, H.; Xu, Y.; Liehn, E.A.; Rusu, M. Vitamin C as scavenger of reactive oxygen species during healing after myocardial infarction. *Int. J. Mol. Sci.* **2024**, *25*, 3114. [CrossRef]
139. Shah, A.K.; Dhalla, N.S. Effectiveness of some vitamins in the prevention of cardiovascular disease: A narrative review. *Front. Physiol.* **2021**, *12*, 729255. [CrossRef]
140. Kura, B.; Slezak, J. The protective role of molecular hydrogen in ischemia/reperfusion injury. *Int. J. Mol. Sci.* **2024**, *25*, 7884. [CrossRef]
141. Saengsin, K.; Sittiwangkul, R.; Chattipakorn, S.C.; Chattipakorn, N. Hydrogen therapy as a potential therapeutic intervention in heart disease: From the past evidence to future application. *Cell. Mol. Life Sci.* **2023**, *80*, 174. [CrossRef] [PubMed]
142. Li, L.; Li, X.; Zhang, Z.; Liu, L.; Zhou, Y.; Liu, F. Protective mechanism and clinical application of hydrogen in myocardial ischemia-reperfusion injury. *Pak. J. Biol. Sci.* **2020**, *23*, 103–112. [CrossRef]
143. Sun, X.; Wu, S.; Mao, C.; Qu, Y.; Xu, Z.; Xie, Y.; Jiang, D.; Song, Y. Therapeutic potential of hydrogen sulfide in ischemia and reperfusion injury. *Biomolecules* **2024**, *14*, 740. [CrossRef]
144. Gheitasi, I.; Akbari, G.; Savari, F. Physiological and cellular mechanisms of ischemic preconditioning microRNAs-mediated in underlying of ischemia/reperfusion injury in different organs. *Mol. Cell Biochem.* **2025**, *480*, 855–868. [CrossRef] [PubMed]
145. Singh, R.B.; Hryshko, L.; Freed, D.; Dhalla, N.S. Activation of proteolytic enzymes and depression of the sarcolemma Na^+-K^+-.ATPase in ischemia-reperfused heart may be mediated through oxidative stress. *Can. J. Physiol. Pharmacol.* **2012**, *90*, 249–260. [CrossRef] [PubMed]
146. Dixon, I.M.C.; Kaneko, M.; Hata, T.; Panagia, V.; Dhalla, N.S. Alterations in cardiac membrane Ca^{2+} transport during oxidative stress. *Mol. Cell. Biochem.* **1990**, *99*, 125–133. [CrossRef]
147. Matsubara, T.; Dhalla, N.S. Effect of oxygen free radicals on cardiac contractile activity and sarcolemmal Na^+-Ca^{2+} exchange. *J. Cardiovasc. Pharmacol. Ther.* **1996**, *1*, 211–218. [CrossRef]
148. Matsubara, T.; Dhalla, N.S. Relationship between mechanical dysfunction and depression of sarcolemmal Ca^{2+}-pump activity in hearts perfused with oxygen free radicals. *Mol. Cell. Biochem.* **1996**, *160/161*, 179–185. [CrossRef]
149. Temsah, R.M.; Netticadan, T.; Chapman, D.; Takeda, S.; Mochizuki, S.; Dhalla, N.S. Alterations in sarcoplasmic reticulum function and gene expression in ischemic-reperfused rat heart. *Am. J. Physiol.* **1999**, *277*, H584–H594. [CrossRef]
150. Makazan, Z.; Saini, H.K.; Dhalla, N.S. Role of oxidative stress in alterations of mitochondrial function in ischemic-reperfused hearts. *Am. J. Physiol. Heart Circ. Physiol.* **2007**, *292*, H1986–H1994. [CrossRef]
151. Maddika, S.; Elimban, V.; Chapman, D.; Dhalla, N.S. Role of oxidative stress in ischemia-reperfusion-induced alterations in myofibrillar ATPase activities and gene expression in the heart. *Can. J. Physiol. Pharmacol.* **2009**, *87*, 120–129. [CrossRef] [PubMed]

152. Suzuki, S.; Kaneko, M.; Chapman, D.C.; Dhalla, N.S. Alterations in cardiac contractile proteins due to oxygen free radicals. *Biochim. Biophys. Acta* **1991**, *1074*, 95–100. [CrossRef] [PubMed]
153. Gajardo Cortez, A.I.J.; Lillo-Moya, J.; San-Martín-Martinez, D.; Pozo-Martinez, J.; Morales, P.; Prieto, J.C.; Aguayo, R.; Puentes, Á.; Ramos, C.; Silva, S.; et al. Safety and pharmacokinetics of a combined antioxidant therapy against myocardial reperfusion injury: A phase 1 randomized clinical trial in healthy humans. *Clin. Pharmacol. Drug Dev.* **2024**, *13*, 1051–1060. [CrossRef]
154. Lagranha, C.J.; Deschamps, A.; Aponte, A.; Steenbergen, C.; Murphy, E. Sex differences in the phosphorylation of mitochondrial proteins result in reduced production of reactive oxygen species and cardioprotection in females. *Circ. Res.* **2010**, *106*, 1681–1691. [CrossRef] [PubMed]
155. Ciocci Pardo, A.; Scuri, S.; González Arbeláez, L.F.; Caldiz, C.; Fantinelli, J.; Mosca, S.M. Survival kinase-dependent pathways contribute to gender difference in the response to myocardial ischemia-reperfusion and ischemic post-conditioning. *Cardiovasc. Pathol.* **2018**, *33*, 19–26. [CrossRef]
156. Murphy, E.; Steenbergen, C. Gender-based differences in mechanisms of protection in myocardial ischemia-reperfusion injury. *Cardiovasc. Res.* **2007**, *75*, 478–486. [CrossRef]
157. Milerová, M.; Drahota, Z.; Chytilová, A.; Tauchmannová, K.; Houštěk, J.; Ošťádal, B. Sex difference in the sensitivity of cardiac mitochondrial permeability transition pore to calcium load. *Mol. Cell. Biochem.* **2016**, *412*, 147–154. [CrossRef]
158. Ostadal, B.; Drahota, Z.; Houstek, J.; Milerova, M.; Ostadalova, I.; Hlavackova, M.; Kolar, F. Developmental and sex differences in cardiac tolerance to ischemia-reperfusion injury: The role of mitochondria 1. *Can. J. Physiol. Pharmacol.* **2019**, *97*, 808–814. [CrossRef]
159. Cross, H.R.; Murphy, E.; Steenbergen, C. Ca^{2+} loading and adrenergic stimulation reveal male/female differences in susceptibility to ischemia-reperfusion injury. *Am. J. Physiol. Heart Circ. Physiol.* **2002**, *283*, H481–H489. [CrossRef]
160. Ross, J.L.; Howlett, S.E. Age and ovariectomy abolish beneficial effects of female sex on rat ventricular myocytes exposed to simulated ischemia and reperfusion. *PLoS ONE* **2012**, *7*, e38425. [CrossRef]
161. Zhao, B.; Peng, J.; Chen, C.; Fan, Y.; Zhang, K.; Zhang, Y.; Huang, X. Innovative engineering of superoxide dismutase for enhanced cardioprotective biocatalysis in myocardial ischemia-reperfusion injury. *Int. J. Biol. Macromol.* **2025**, *286*, 137656. [CrossRef] [PubMed]
162. Tanno, S.; Yamamoto, K.; Kurata, Y.; Adachi, M.; Inoue, Y.; Otani, N.; Mishima, M.; Yamamoto, Y.; Kuwabara, M.; Ogino, K.; et al. Protective effects of topiroxostat on an ischemia-reperfusion model of rat hearts. *Circ. J.* **2018**, *82*, 1101–1111. [CrossRef]
163. Elgebaly, S.A.; Poston, R.; Todd, R.; Helmy, T.; Almaghraby, A.M.; Elbayoumi, T.; Kreutzer, D.L. Cyclocreatine protects against ischemic injury and enhances cardiac recovery during early reperfusion. *Expert Rev. Cardiovasc. Ther.* **2019**, *17*, 683–697. [CrossRef] [PubMed]
164. Curran, J.; Burkhoff, D.; Kloner, R.A. Beyond reperfusion: Acute ventricular unloading and cardioprotection during myocardial infarction. *J. Cardiovasc. Transl. Res.* **2019**, *12*, 95–106. [CrossRef]
165. Stoian, L.; Krüger, M.; Schmitt, J.; Kleinbongard, P. Is there an effect of ischemic conditioning on myocardial contractile function following acute myocardial ischemia/reperfusion injury? *Biochim. Biophys. Acta Mol. Basis Dis.* **2019**, *1865*, 822–830. [CrossRef]
166. Skrzypiec-Spring, M.; Urbaniak, J.; Sapa-Wojciechowska, A.; Pietkiewicz, J.; Orda, A.; Karolko, B.; Danielewicz, R.; Bil-Lula, I.; Woźniak, M.; Schulz, R.; et al. Matrix metalloproteinase-2 inhibition in acute ischemia-reperfusion heart injury-cardioprotective properties of carvedilol. *Pharmaceuticals* **2021**, *14*, 1276. [CrossRef]
167. Ferrari, R.; Balla, C.; Malagù, M.; Guardigli, G.; Morciano, G.; Bertini, M.; Biscaglia, S.; Campo, G. Reperfusion damage- A story of success, failure, and hope. *Circ. J.* **2017**, *81*, 131–141. [CrossRef] [PubMed]
168. Huang, J.; Li, R.; Wang, C. The role of mitochondrial quality control in cardiac ischemia/reperfusion injury. *Oxidative Med. Cell. Longev.* **2021**, *2021*, 5543452. [CrossRef]
169. Moris, D.; Spartalis, M.; Tzatzaki, E.; Spartalis, E.; Karachaliou, G.S.; Triantafyllis, A.S.; Karaolanis, G.I.; Tsilimigras, D.I.; Theocharis, S. The role of reactive oxygen species in myocardial redox signaling and regulation. *Ann. Transl. Med.* **2017**, *5*, 324. [CrossRef]
170. Buja, L.M. Myocardial ischemia and reperfusion injury. *Cardiovasc. Pathol.* **2005**, *14*, 170–175. [CrossRef]
171. Aliev, G.; Obrenovich, M.E.; Seyidova, D.; de la Torre, J.C. Exploring ischemia-induced vascular lesions and potential pharmacological intervention strategies. *Histol. Histopathol.* **2005**, *20*, 261–273. [PubMed]
172. Zhang, W.Z.; Li, R.; Liu, S.; Zhang, J.D.; Ning, X.F.; Cai, S.L. Effects of renal ischemic postconditioning on myocardial ultrastructural organization and myocardial expression of Bcl-2/Bax in rabbits. *BioMed Res. Int.* **2016**, *2016*, 9349437. [CrossRef] [PubMed]
173. Lee, K.H.; Ha, S.J.; Woo, J.S.; Lee, G.J.; Lee, S.R.; Kim, J.W.; Park, H.K.; Kim, W. Exenatide prevents morphological and structural changes of mitochondria following ischaemia-reperfusion injury. *Heart Lung Circ.* **2017**, *26*, 519–523. [CrossRef] [PubMed]
174. Shirakawa, M.; Imura, H.; Nitta, T. Propofol protects the immature rabbit heart against ischemia and reperfusion injury: Impact on functional recovery and histopathological changes. *BioMed Res. Int.* **2014**, *2014*, 601250. [CrossRef]

175. Tung, C.; Varzideh, F.; Farroni, E.; Mone, P.; Kansakar, U.; Jankauskas, S.S.; Santulli, G. Elamipretide: A review of its structure, mechanism of action, and therapeutic potential. *Int. J. Mol. Sci.* **2025**, *26*, 944. [CrossRef]
176. Guo, Z.; Tian, Y.; Gao, J.; Zhou, B.; Zhou, X.; Chang, X.; Zhou, H. Enhancement of mitochondrial homeostasis: A novel approach to attenuate hypoxic myocardial injury. *Int. J. Med. Sci.* **2024**, *21*, 2897–2911. [CrossRef]
177. Consolini, A.E.; Ragone, M.I.; Bonazzola, P.; Colareda, G.A. Mitochondrial bioenergetics during ischemia and reperfusion. *Adv. Exp. Med. Biol.* **2017**, *982*, 141–167.
178. Zhao, Z.Q. Oxidative stress-elicited myocardial apoptosis during reperfusion. *Curr. Opin. Pharmacol.* **2004**, *4*, 159–165. [CrossRef]
179. Du, B.; Fu, Q.; Yang, Q.; Yang, Y.; Li, R.; Yang, X.; Yang, Q.; Li, S.; Tian, J.; Liu, H. Different types of cell death and their interactions in myocardial ischemia-reperfusion injury. *Cell Death Discov.* **2025**, *11*, 87. [CrossRef]
180. Tsurusaki, S.; Kizana, E. Mechanisms and therapeutic potential of multiple forms of cell death in myocardial ischemia-reperfusion injury. *Int. J. Mol. Sci.* **2024**, *25*, 13492. [CrossRef]
181. Shen, Y.; Liu, X.; Shi, J.; Wu, X. Involvement of Nrf2 in myocardial ischemia and reperfusion injury. *Int. J. Biol. Macromol.* **2019**, *125*, 496–502. [CrossRef] [PubMed]
182. Boengler, K.; Eickelmann, C.; Kleinbongard, P. Mitochondrial kinase signaling for cardioprotection. *Int. J. Mol. Sci.* **2024**, *25*, 4491. [CrossRef] [PubMed]
183. Cadenas, S. ROS and redox signaling in myocardial ischemia-reperfusion injury and cardioprotection. *Free Radic. Biol. Med.* **2018**, *117*, 76–89. [CrossRef]
184. Zhong, Y.; Li, X.Y.; Liang, T.J.; Ding, B.Z.; Ma, K.X.; Ren, W.X.; Liang, W.J. Effects of NLRP3 inflammasome mediated pyroptosis on cardiovascular diseases and intervention mechanism of Chinese medicine. *Chin. J. Integr. Med.* **2024**, *30*, 468–479. [CrossRef]
185. Zhang, Y.S.; Lu, L.Q.; Jiang, Y.Q.; Li, N.S.; Luo, X.J.; Peng, J.W.; Peng, J. Allopurinol attenuates oxidative injury in rat hearts suffered ischemia/reperfusion via suppressing the xanthine oxidase/vascular peroxidase 1 pathway. *Eur. J. Pharmacol.* **2021**, *908*, 174368. [CrossRef] [PubMed]
186. Becerra, R.; Román, B.; Di Carlo, M.N.; Mariangelo, J.I.; Salas, M.; Sanchez, G.; Donoso, P.; Schinella, G.R.; Vittone, L.; Wehrens, X.H.; et al. Reversible redox modifications of ryanodine receptor ameliorate ventricular arrhythmias in the ischemic-reperfused heart. *Am. J. Physiol. Heart Circ. Physiol.* **2016**, *311*, H713–H724. [CrossRef]
187. Yang, F.; Jiang, X.; Cao, H.; Shuai, W.; Zhang, L.; Wang, G.; Quan, D.; Jiang, X. Daphnetin preconditioning decreases cardiac injury and susceptibility to ventricular arrhythmia following ischaemia-reperfusion through the TLR4/MyD88/NF-κb signalling pathway. *Pharmacology* **2021**, *106*, 369–383. [CrossRef]
188. Abdulsalam, T.M.; Hasanin, A.H.; Mohamed, R.H.; El Sayed Badawy, A. Angiotensin receptor-neprilysin inhibitior (thiorphan/irbesartan) decreased ischemia-reperfusion induced ventricular arrhythmias in rat; in vivo study. *Eur. J. Pharmacol.* **2020**, *882*, 173295. [CrossRef]
189. Das, B.; Sarkar, C. Cardiomyocyte mitochondrial K_{ATP} channels participate in the antiarrhythmic and antiinfarct effects of K_{ATP} activators during ischemia and reperfusion in an intact anesthetized rabbit model. *Pol. J. Pharmacol.* **2003**, *55*, 771–786.

antioxidants

MDPI

Review

Exploring Potential Complement Modulation Strategies for Ischemia–Reperfusion Injury in Kidney Transplantation

Dario Troise [1,2,*], Costanza Allegra [1], Luciana Antonia Cirolla [1], Silvia Mercuri [1], Barbara Infante [1], Giuseppe Castellano [3] and Giovanni Stallone [1]

1 Nephrology, Dialysis and Transplantation Unit, Advanced Research Center on Kidney Aging (A.R.K.A.), Department of Medical and Surgical Sciences, University of Foggia, 71122 Foggia, Italy
2 Division of Renal Medicine and Baxter Novum, Department of Clinical Science, Intervention and Technology, Karolinska Institutet, 141 52 Stockholm, Sweden
3 Unit of Nephrology, Dialysis and Transplantation, Fondazione IRCCS Ca' Granda Ospedale Maggiore Policlinico di Milano, 20122 Milan, Italy
* Correspondence: dario.troise@unifg.it or dario.troise@ki.se

Abstract: The complement system plays a crucial role in regulating the inflammatory responses in kidney transplantation, potentially contributing to early decline in kidney function. Ischemia–reperfusion injury (IRI) is among the factors affecting graft outcomes and a primary contributor to delayed graft function. Complement activation, particularly the alternative pathway, participates in the pathogenesis of IRI, involving all kidney compartments. In particular, tubular epithelial cells often acquire a dysfunctional phenotype that can exacerbate complement activation and kidney damage. Currently, complement-modulating drugs are under investigation for the treatment of kidney diseases. Many of these drugs have shown potential therapeutic benefits, but no effective clinical treatments for renal IRI have been identified yet. In this review, we will explore drugs that target complement factors, complement receptors, and regulatory proteins, aiming to highlight their potential value in improving the management of renal IRI.

Keywords: kidney transplantation; complement system; ischemia–reperfusion injury; Eculizumab; iptacopan; complement-targeting drugs

1. Introduction

The kidney transplantation process involves a series of events that can impact the survival of the graft, including brain or cardiac death in deceased donors, organ procurement, preservation, and reperfusion. Moreover, post-transplant immune responses and non-immune factors, including drug toxicity, hypertension, and recurrent diseases, may have a pivotal role affecting the outcomes of the kidney graft. Increasing evidence indicates that the complement system is a key regulator of both inflammatory and non-inflammatory responses throughout each stage of transplantation, potentially leading to the early decline of kidney function [1].

Due to the complex relationship between oxygen consumption, oxidative stress (OxS), renal blood flow, and glomerular filtration rate, the kidneys are considered among the organs most susceptible to hypoxic injury. Ischemia–reperfusion injury (IRI) is considered one of the main factors involved in the pathogenesis of acute kidney injury because it leads to cellular damage, which can impact outcomes, affect prognosis, and potentially limit the success of the kidney transplantation (KT) [2]. IRI occurs when a temporary loss of blood supply to the transplanted organ (ischemia) is followed by the restoration of blood flow and reoxygenation. IRI is a complex process in which hypoxic tissues are exposed to ischemic damage, marked by cellular dysfunction and death, while the subsequent reperfusion paradoxically intensifies tissue damage by amplifying the inflammatory response. The complement system participates in the pathogenesis of IRI, and its activation is considered one of the main components of renal IRI. Consequently, therapeutic strategies to prevent and treat renal IRI by targeting the complement system are being actively explored [3]. Currently, kidney damage resulting from IRI is a leading cause of delayed graft function (DGF) following KT, impacting short- and long-term graft survival [4].

This narrative review aims to emphasize the role of the complement system in renal IRI, with a focus on therapeutic strategies that target its modulation.

2. The Complement System

The complement system is considered an evolutionarily conserved component of the innate immune system characterized by an intricate network of molecules that play a crucial role in maintaining tissue homeostasis and host defense [5]. Over the years, a growing number of experimental evidence has demonstrated that the complement system has a crucial role because it carries out fundamental physiological functions, including pathogen and cell debris removal, the clearance of immune complexes, and the recruitment of components of the adaptive immune system [6]. In addition, crosstalk between the complement system and other systems and pathways has been found, including the adaptive immunity system [7], the coagulation system [8], the inflammasome [9], and toll-like receptors (TLRs) [10].

The number of identified components in the complement system is steadily increasing, with more than sixty components known to date. In addition to the nine central components of the cascade (C1 to C9), the complement system includes soluble proteins, membrane-bound receptors, and regulatory proteins [11,12]. Notably, while most complement proteins are produced in the liver and circulate largely in an inactive form, the kidney, brain, lung and intestines are among the few organs capable of locally synthesizing complement proteins [13]. In 1991, Brooimans et al. showed that human proximal epithelial tubular cells can synthesize C3 when stimulated by IL-2 [14]. Recently, the kidneys have been identified as the primary sources of complement proteins, with mesangial, endothelial, epithelial cells and podocytes being capable of synthesizing the circulating complement proteins C3, C4, and factor B and complement factor H (CFH) [15].

Complement activation is triggered by the recognition of pathogen-associated molecular patterns (PAMPs) or damage-associated molecular patterns (DAMPs), achieved via different types of pattern recognition molecules (PRMs). Based on the signaling pathway initiated, the complement cascade can be activated through one of three main pathways: the classical pathway (CP), alternative pathway (AP), or lectin pathway (LP) [16,17].

Each pathway has distinct mechanisms for the recognition of activation signals. In the CP, the recognition of immune complexes by C1q is necessary for initiation. Then, this signal leads to the subsequent activation of C1r and C1s, subsequently cleaving C4 and C2 into small fragments (C4a and C2a) and large fragments (C4b and C2b). The large fragments then combine on the cell surface to form the C3 convertase (C4bC2b). In contrast, the LP is triggered by the binding of specific pattern recognition receptors (PRRs) to PAMPs or DAMPs, leading to the activation of MBL-associated serine proteases (MASPs), the cleavage of complement components C4 and C2, and the subsequent formation of C3 convertase.

Unlike the other two pathways, the AP utilizes different C3 convertases. Priming of the AP relies on a process known as "tickover", where the circulating C3 molecule undergoes spontaneous low-rate hydrolysis in the fluid phase. Following the binding of C3 to factor B cleaved by factor D into Ba and Bb fragments, the generation of the C3 convertase of the AP (C3Bb) occurs [18]. Interestingly, the C3b generated by the classical and lectin pathways, C3 convertase, can be utilized to form the C3 convertase of the alternative pathway. Moreover, proteases not typically classified as complement components, such as neutrophil elastase and thrombin, can also cleave C3, resulting in an amplification of the alternative pathway [19].

Both the convertases cleave C3 into C3a and C3b, resulting in the formation of C5 convertase (C4b2b3b or C3bBb3b of the CP and AP, respectively), which then cleaves C5 into C5a and C5b. The latter contributes to the assembly of the membrane attack complex (MAC) alongside C6, C7, C8, and C9. Thus, all three pathways converge on the formation of the MAC and unfold sequentially. Target cells are directly lysed by the formation of the MAC, which creates 10 nm pores in the cell membrane, exerting direct cytolytic effects and leading to the release of a large number of cellular components, further activating PRMs and intensify inflammatory responses [18].

Additionally, other effector molecules, such as opsonins (C4b, C4d, C3b, iC3b, C3dg, and C3d) [20] and anaphylatoxins (C3a, C5a, and C4a), are generated as a result of complement activation. Opsonins are deposited on the cell surface and tag the cell for phagocytosis by binding to various complement receptors, a process referred to opsonization. In contrast, anaphylatoxins induce vasodilatation, histamine release, and the chemotaxis and activation of mostly macrophages and neutrophils by binding to their specific receptors, further amplifying the inflammatory response [21].

By interacting with their respective receptors—CR1, CR2, CR3, and CR4 for opsonins and C3aR, C5aR1, and C5aR2 for anaphilatoxins—these molecules can recruit other inflammatory cells to the infection site and modulate the activity of immune cells [18]. In addition, anaphylatoxin has been shown to influence endothelial cell proliferation and migration as well as cancer development [22] (Figure 1).

Moreover, under physiological condition, there are surface-bound and soluble proteins that control complement activation. These complement regulator proteins include C1esterase inhibitor (C1INH), factor H (FH), factor I (FI), decay-accelerating factor (DAF or CD55), and membrane cofactor protein (MPC or CD46); they act mainly through decay acceleration and cofactor activity. In addition, surface-bound regulators are relatively nonspecific, regulating all three complement activation pathways and inactivating both C3 and C4. In contrast, soluble regulators are more specific, targeting only the alternative, classical, or lectin pathway, and acting exclusively on either C3 or C4 [23].

An additional pathway of complement activation involving the coagulation system has also been identified. Some components of the coagulation cascade, including thrombin, activated factors XI, X, and IX, and plasmin, have been shown to mediate the proteolytic breakdown of complement components and directly activate C3 and C5, independently from the C3 convertase, leading to the introduction of the concept of a fourth complement activation pathway, known as the "extrinsic complement pathway" [24–26]. On the contrary, complement components have been shown to induce tissue factor expression and the activation of platelets or endothelial cells, which leads to the secretion of the von Willebrand factor, establishing a positive feedback loop that may serve as a powerful amplification mechanism in IRI [27–29]. Moreover, signaling crosstalk between the complement system and immunological pathways involved in the coordination of immune and inflammatory responses, such as the toll-like receptor (TLR) pathway, has been associated with increased inflammation and host tissue injury, when dysregulated. For example, common microbial molecules, including lipopolysaccharide (LPS) and bacterial CpG DNA, can act as both

TLR ligands and complement activators. In particular, LPS may induce the release of factor B of the alternative pathway in macrophages. Furthermore, epithelial and innate immune cells can be locally stimulated by TLR activators to produce key components for alternative complement activation, thereby amplifying TLR-mediated responses [30]. Among the TLRs, TLR-4 has gained attention due to its pivotal role in the pathogenesis of renal IRI. Increases in both TLR-4 expression and ligands were observed in tubular epithelial cells (TECs) and vascular endothelial cells after kidney transplantation, leading to the activation of downstream signaling pathways involved in the promotion of TEC injury and contributing to sustained inflammation and fibrosis [31]. Recently, C3 gene knockdown has been shown to downregulate the TLR-4 signaling pathway in a mouse model of renal IRI, mitigating the damage and leading to the stabilization of the podocyte cytoskeleton [32].

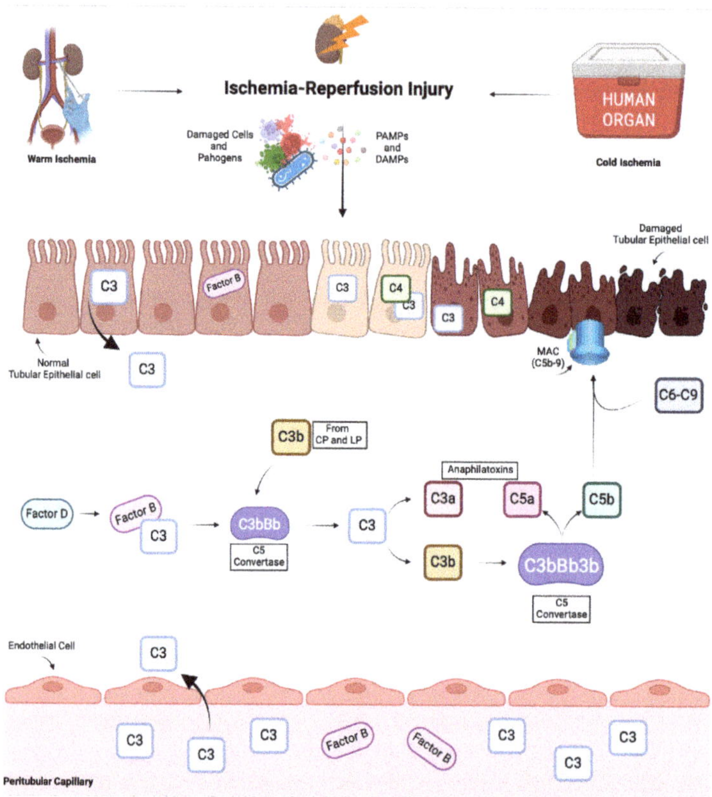

Figure 1. The kidneys are particularly susceptible to ischemia–reperfusion injury (IRI), especially in the context of transplantation, where exposure to warm and cold ischemic periods can trigger IRI. The exposition to ischemic and reperfusion phases can lead to the release of damage-associated molecular patterns (DAMPs) (and potentially pathogen-associated molecular patterns, PAMPs), which may activate the complement system. Particularly, after IRI, renal epithelial cells (RECs) undergo functional and structural changes, which leads to the amplification of the complement system and production of complement components. The alternative pathway is especially involved in the initiation of the complement cascade, leading to the formation of the membrane attack complex (MAC, C5b-9) and the release of anaphylatoxins, both contributing to cell and tissue damage. Created in BioRender.

To maintain homeostasis, the human complement system carefully balances activation and inhibition, ensuring that the intensity of the reaction is appropriately regulated. Moreover, the complement system is activated in several kidney diseases, including glomerulonephritis, vasculitis, and tubulointerstitial diseases. However, significant differences exist between the microenvironment in the glomerulus and that of the tubulointerstitial compartments. Proper complement regulation is crucial at the glomerular level to protect the kidney from the constant exposure to these proteins. In fact, all surface-bound complement regulators, including CD46, CD55, and CFH, are expressed on resident glomerular cells, as these cells are continuously exposed to high concentrations of complement proteins and immune complexes [33]. Contrarily, tubular epithelial cells are involved mainly in the activation of the complement system in response to injury. Thurman et al. demonstrated that the loss of polarity of complement receptor 1–related protein Y in the tubular epithelium after ischemic injury resulted in the activation of the alternative pathway in this compartment [34].

It is important to note that complement inhibition can be associated with serious infectious complications. Particularly, the deficiency of complement activation or terminal components has been associated with Neisseria meningitidis infection. However, the widespread use of vaccines targeting all the major invasive serotypes with vaccination prior to the initiation of complement inhibitors can significantly reduce the infection risk. Depending on the complement target, vaccination can provide different levels of protection, revealing the need for the close monitoring of vaccine efficacy over time [35]. Theoretically, the inhibition of the terminal components of the complement cascade, such as C5, preserve C3-associated effector functions, including cell opsonization and immune cell activation, leading to a lower risk of infectious complications compared to upstream C3 inhibition. Moreover, the prophylactic use of antibiotics and other antimicrobial agents active against common opportunistic pathogens, including encapsulated bacteria and fungi, can help to reduce the risk of infection [36].

Additionally, a temporary inhibition of the complement system could be a workable option, because it has been demonstrated that long-term complement inhibition may increase the risk of adverse events, while short-term inhibition is unlikely to pose significant problems [37]. Furthermore, considering the effects of complement inhibition therapies, in order to assess their efficacy as well as adverse events, it is advisable. This can be achieved by measuring circulating levels of specific complement components or activation products, or through the assessment of the functional capacity of particular pathways, in order to adjust drug dosages based on the patient's immune status, complement activity levels, and infection susceptibility, helping to identify and mitigate potential adverse events [38].

3. Oxidative Stress and Complement System

Oxygen deprivation followed by hyperoxygenation during IRI leads to the rapid generation of reactive oxygen and nitrogen species (ROS and RNS), causing rapid tissue injury and contributing to the overall inflammatory burden. During the ischemic phase of IRI, the absence of oxygen triggers anaerobic metabolic cell pathways, compromising the synthesis of ATP, which is considered the aerobic energy source of the cells. Then, during the reperfusion, the sudden influx of oxygen exceeds the cell's capacity to manage it. Both of these phases lead to the generation of OxS.

The mitochondria are considered the primary source of ROS due to the dysfunctional activity of mitochondrial complexes I and III and the subsequent ROS production that overwhelms the antioxidant defenses of the cells. Additionally, OxS can also arise from other cellular sources, including xanthine oxidase, NADPH oxidase, and endothelial nitric oxide synthase; these sources activate key pathways involved in oxidative stress responses, including the hypoxia-inducible factor (HIF) and nuclear factor erythroid2-related factor2 (NRF2) pathways [39,40]. Therefore, the excessive production of ROS impairs mitochondrial function by damaging the respiratory chain, altering mitochondrial membrane permeability, and inducing mutations in mitochondrial DNA. These effects lead to a breakdown in energy production and a progressive loss of mitochondrial efficiency [41].

The existing literature indicate that OxS can activate the complement system through all three complement pathways [42–44]. Adler et al. were among the firsts to explore the mechanisms by which MAC deposited in the glomerular mesangium could be a trigger. They stimulated rat glomerular mesangial cells with MAC derived from the purified human complement component C5b6 and measured the production of ROS, showing that MAC could induce the formation of both superoxide ion and hydrogen peroxide in mesangial cells. Interestingly, cells exposed to decayed MAC showed only mild effect or no increase in ROS production, suggesting a correlation between the deposition of MAC and OxS [45]. Moreover, Choi et al. investigated the relationship between ROS production in human umbilical vein endothelial cells (HUVECs) exposed to OxS-induced damage and complement activation. Their findings revealed, once again, that the deposition of the MAC was associated with ROS production, and treatment with the antioxidant N-acetylcysteine significantly reduced complement activation [43]. Moreover, OxS has been shown to be correlated with complement activation in studies where HUVECs were incubated with plasma from patients with thrombotic microangiopathy, demonstrating an increase in ROS production, apoptosis, and elevated C3 levels [46].

Anaphylatoxins are involved in promoting cellular responses and host defense. They have been reported to bind to their specific receptors localized on both the plasma membrane and inside the cells and correlate with OxS levels. In retinal pigment epithelial cells exposed to OxS, C3aR is internalized and can be transported to mitochondria by endosomal trafficking, where it elevates mitochondrial calcium levels and impairs respiratory function. Furthermore, the C5a/C5aR signaling axis can affect mitochondrial morphology by inducing fragmentation and an increase in the number of pyknotic nuclei. OxS also upregulates the expression of mitochondrial fusion-related proteins, mitofusin-1 and mitofusin-2. This suggests that both anaphylatoxins may play a role in sensitizing cells to ROS-induced damage [47,48]. These findings reveal the role of cellular oxidative strain in complement system-mediated injury.

Conversely, intracellular signals triggered by the complement system can stimulate ROS production and cause mitochondrial damage, resulting in the increased release of mitochondrial DAMPs. It has been shown that the intracellular activation of C5aR1 by C5a can promote the production of ROS in $CD4^+$ T cells, facilitating the assembly of a functional inflammasome system [49]. Moreover, Tsai et al. observed that C5a promotes ROS production in murine kidney endothelial cells. Elevated levels of C5a/C5aR induced cell apoptosis through cytochrome C release and caspase 3/9 activation, a process dependent on ROS generation, suggesting that C5a inhibition could directly reduce OxS and improve mitochondrial function [50].

In human proximal tubular cells, C3a has been shown to induce NOX enzymes, which are involved in the NADPH-dependent reduction of oxygen to generate superoxide, and the upregulation of alpha smooth muscle actin expression, which is a specific marker for fibrotic myofibroblasts. In an animal model of IRI, silencing NOX4 RNA resulted in decreased alpha smooth muscle actin expression, the suppression of NADPH activity, and a reduction in overall oxidative burden [51].

Collectively, these findings highlight the pivotal role of the complement system in driving OxS through a bidirectional relationship. The activation of the complement system may lead to the production of ROS, while OxS can, in turn, activate the complement system (Figure 2).

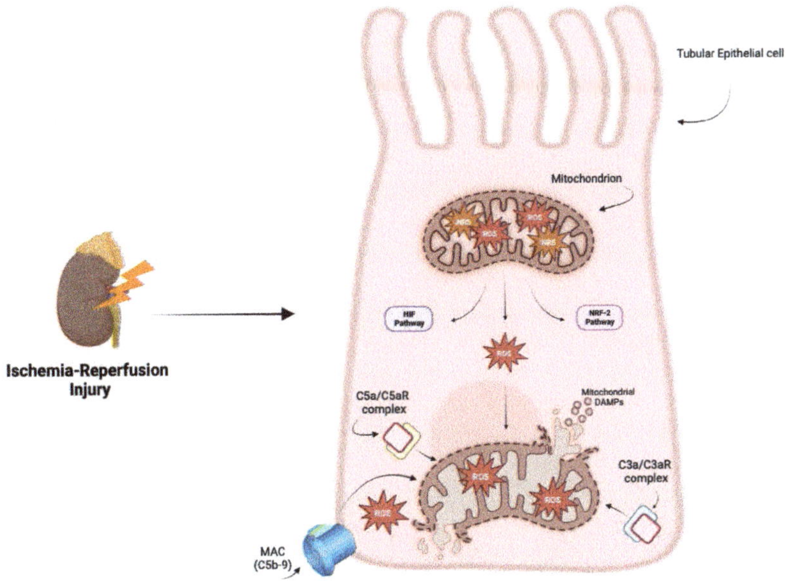

Figure 2. Ischemia–reperfusion injury triggers the production of reactive oxygen species (ROS) and reactive nitrogen species (RNS), resulting in rapid tissue damage. Mitochondria are considered the primary source of ROS; they activate pivotal pathways involved in OxS responses, including the hypoxia-inducible factor (HIF) and nuclear factor erythroid2-related factor2 (NRF2) pathways, as adaptive responses to mitigate the OxS-related damage. Moreover, OxS has been shown to activate the complement system, leading to the formation of membrane attack complex (MAC) on cells, which induces additional OxS burden. Anaphylatoxins, especially the C3a/C3aR and C5a/C5aR pathways, have also been implicated in the impairment of mitochondrial functions, sensitizing cells to ROS-induced damage. Created in BioRender.

In addition, several antioxidant agents have been proposed for the treatment of IRI, including compounds that target nuclear factor erythroid 2-related factor 2 (Nrf2), hydrogen sulfide, dexmedetomidine, edaravone, and other mitochondria-targeting antioxidants specifically designed to provide their delivery inside the mitochondria [52]. Some of them appear to be involved in the regulation of the complement system. Particularly, heme oxygenase-1, known as a key regulator of many pathophysiological processes, including apoptosis, cryoprotection, and inflammation, has recently been identified as a regulator of the complement control protein decay-accelerating factor. Natural and synthetic compounds, such as metalloporphyrins, which can modulate the expression of heme oxygenase-1, hold potential for the development of cost-effective and non-toxic strategies for the management of complement system-mediated diseases [53]. Furthermore, complement component 3 has been associated with proinflammatory effects in an animal model of IRI. Yang et al. showed that the treatment with an antioxidant compound, such as N-tert-butyl-α-phenylnitrone, reduced C3 expression, thereby reducing IRI-related damage [54]. In inflammatory and ischemia-associated diseases, complement components can cause the adhesion of leukocytes to the endothelial wall. This is considered one of the major mechanisms responsible for the production of oxygen-derived free radicals, cytotoxic oxidants, and inflammatory mediators. In this context, the oral administration of flavonoids has been demonstrated to reduce total serum complement levels and the number of adherent leukocytes, highlighting the protective effects of these compounds in mitigating proinflammatory conditions, such as IRI [55]. Therefore, strategies that modulate the complement system in conjunction with antioxidant and anti-inflammatory compounds may have a potential impact in the mitigation of complement system- and OxS-related damage during IRI.

4. The Complement System in Renal Ischemia–Reperfusion Injury

IRI is frequently an unavoidable consequence that can lead to increased morbidity and mortality in various other clinical scenarios, including myocardial infarction, stroke, vascular surgery, and trauma. The organs that may be affected by IRI include the lungs, heart, gut, brain, and, notably, the kidneys. It is important to note that, in addition to transplantation, several other factors can trigger IRI in the kidneys, such as vascular and cardiac surgeries, sepsis, trauma, and cardiocirculatory arrest followed by resuscitation [56,57] (Figure 3). Moreover, while IRI can occur in kidney grafts from living donors, it is generally more severe in organs from deceased donors. Pre-existing medical conditions, hemodynamic insults, and extended warm and cold ischemia times account for complement system activation after the release of DAMPs and inflammatory responses. Furthermore, deceased donors have increased levels of C5a and C5b-9, correlated with an increased risk of rejection compared to living donors [58,59].

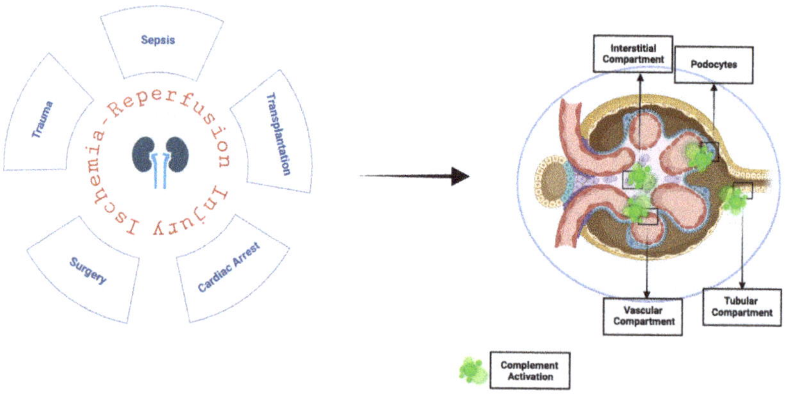

Figure 3. In the kidneys, ischemia–reperfusion injury can be triggered by several factors, such as surgical procedures, sepsis, trauma, cardiac arrest, and transplantation, leading to the activation of the complement system, which plays a key role in mediating the damage. The complement activation occurs across all kidney compartments, including the vascular, glomerular, and interstitial compartments, contributing to widespread tissue injury and dysfunction. Created in BioRender.

Metabolic changes in cells and the loss of cellular homeostasis are major players driving the pathways involved in IRI. During the transplantation process, the kidneys are exposed to phases of ischemia and reperfusions. The term "warm ischemia" refers to the time when an organ remains at body temperature after its blood supply has been interrupted but before it is cooled or reconnected to a blood supply, while "cold ischemia" is the period between cold perfusion and blood supply regeneration. Prolonged cold ischemia adversely affects the long-term survival and functional recovery of transplanted organs.

Moreover, severe oxygen deprivation leads to a shift to anaerobic metabolism across all compartments of the renal parenchyma, resulting in ATP depletion, intracellular acidosis, increased production of reactive oxygen species (ROS), and the release of DAMPs. These changes play a crucial role in activating innate immunity, particularly the complement system, as well as adaptive immunity [60].

Significant alteration in renal proximal tubular epithelial cells has been found to be associated with IRI due to its ability to drive the downregulation of complement system regulator factors and an increase in the local production of complement components from renal TECs, which are recognized as major targets of complement system activation [61], resulting in functional and structural changes, including the loss of brush borders, alterations in the cytoskeleton, and a rapid loss of surface markers that promote the activation of cell death mechanisms. Moreover, TECs acquire a dysfunctional phenotype, characterized by cell swelling, the increased expression of various cell adhesion molecules, and increased permeability, key factors contributing to prolonged kidney dysfunction. In addition, ischemia leads to interstitial inflammation and micro-vasculopathy, further exacerbating the damage [41,62].

Even if the CP has been traditionally associated with the pathogenesis of complement-mediated IRI [63], studies in animal models of renal IRI suggest that the AP and LP play a predominant role in in triggering the complement cascade during renal IRI, while the role of CP is limited. Zhou et al. evaluated renal structural and functional injury after IRI in mice, showing that C3-, C5-, and C6-deficient mice exhibited protection from the injury, while C4-deficient mice did not [4]. In addition, Thurman et al. showed that factor B-deficient mice, an essential component of the AP, developed significantly less functional and morphological injury after renal IRI than the wild-type mice, which exhibited an increased deposition of complement C3 and neutrophil infiltration, suggesting that the complement system in the kidneys is mainly activated by AP, and therapeutic strategies aiming to inhibit this pathway may offer protection against IRI [64]. Supporting this, later studies by Renner et al. in 2011 showed that the inhibition or lack of factor H, a negative regulator of the AP, worsened kidney injury [65]. Regarding the role of the LP, Møller-Kristensen et al. investigated its contribution to complement system activation in a bilateral renal IRI animal model, showing that mannan-binding lectin double-knockout mice exhibited less evident acute tubular necrosis and lower levels of C3a than wild-type mice, indicating reduced C3 deposition and overall complement activation [66]. However, recently, complement fraction C5a and membrane attack complex (MAC, C5b-9) have been found to be elevated in brain-dead donors, suggesting that downstream complement products also play a crucial role in mediating renal damage. Moreover, C5-b9 has been linked to a higher risk of kidney rejection following transplantation [67,68].

Additionally, several complement regulators and anaphylatoxins receptors have been identified as crucial in the development of IRI. Genetic deficiencies in CD55 and CD59, which are membrane-bound complement regulators, have been shown to increase renal IRI. Moreover, the modulation of their activity appears to increase the inhibition of the C3 and C5 convertases, thereby reducing IRI damage, as demonstrated by Bongoni et al., who showed that mice expressing both CD55 and CD59 exhibited improved renal parameters after experiencing moderate IRI [3]. In addition, further studies demonstrated that anaphylatoxin receptor inhibition, such as that of C3aR and C5aR1, expressed in both infiltrating immune cells and kidney parenchymal cells, with their expression levels increasing in response to IRI, prevented kidney IRI by reducing chemokine and cytokine expression and decreasing inflammatory cell infiltration [69–71].

Given the critical role of the complement system in renal IRI, identifying biomarkers or clinical indicators to select patients who might gain the most from therapies that modulate the complement system is essential for optimizing therapy and minimizing side effects. In this context, elevated levels of anaphylatoxins (C3a and C5a) and serum C5b-9 were observed 24h after IRI was correlated to organ damage. Moreover, Budkowska et al. demonstrated a positive correlation between C3a levels and C-reactive protein, an inflammatory marker, immediately after transplantation, suggesting that this relationship could represent a prognostic signature of allograft survival or rejection in an IRI liver transplantation model [72]. Elevated expression levels of complement-related mRNA were observed in a renal IRI animal model, where locally produced C3 mRNA was upregulated within 2h of reperfusion in ischemic rat kidneys, without the significant involvement of circulating C3 [73].

Additionally, significant evidence suggests that endothelial involvement in renal IRI contributes to a reduction in renal blood flow, impairing the vascular compartment of the kidney. Endothelial dysfunction may lead to retrograde complement activation, creating a vicious cycle of amplified inflammatory responses that exacerbate tissue damage and lead to organ failure [74,75]. Recently, endothelial-derived complement factor D has been associated with increased levels of endothelial dysfunction markers, including intercellular adhesion molecule-1 (ICAM-1), vascular adhesion molecule-1 (VCAM1), von Willebrand factor (VWF), and endothelin-1, suggesting that the complement factor D can mediate endothelial dysfunction [76].

Monitoring these markers could guide therapeutic approaches in order to tailor complement-targeting therapies to individual patients and optimize clinical outcomes.

5. Potential Therapeutic Strategies

An increasing number of complement system-modulator drugs have recently gained approval or are in the final stages of clinical testing for the treatment of inflammation-based conditions. Given the close relationship between complement activation and the resulting inflammatory response in renal IRI, numerous research groups have developed various therapeutic strategies to inhibit or reduce complement activation in order to mitigate kidney damage. In detail, we can arbitrarily distinguish three primary targets for intervention: complement C5 and C3, complement receptors/regulatory proteins, and complement factors B and D. The rationale behind complement system-modulating therapies in renal IRI is that targeting complement cascade factors directly blocks specific factors to prevent their activation and subsequent damage, and targeting receptors involved in the pathway leads to the disruption of the signaling and decreased recruitment of inflammatory cells, while acting on regulatory proteins could prevent the overactivation of the complement system.

5.1. *Targeting Complement C5 and C3*

Although there is currently no effective clinical treatment for renal IRI [77], a growing body of evidence indicates that complement activation at the C3 convertase and downstream C5 convertase stages plays a central role in mediating renal IRI, highlighting that targeting complement cascade factors might be a promising therapeutic target to help prevent damage in high-risk recipients [73,78].

One of the most targeted complement factors is C5 because it serves as the endpoint for all three pathways. Inhibiting C5 may effectively provide a terminal blockade without disrupting the functionality of upstream proteins, thereby minimizing the impact on basic functions of the complement, including opsonization and chemotaxis.

The first anticomplement drug approved by the US Food and Drug Administration (FDA) and the European Medicines Agency in 2007 for the treatment of paroxysmal nocturnal hemoglobinuria (PNH) [79] and later for Atypical Hemolytic Uremic Syndrome (aHUS), Generalized Myasthenia Gravis [80], and Neuromyelitis Optica Spectrum disorders [81] was the long-acting humanized anti-C5 monoclonal antibody (mAb) Eculizumab (Soliris®, Alexion Pharmaceuticals, Boston, MA, USA). However, in the field of transplantation, it has garnered significant attention for treating antibody-mediated rejection and for prophylactic use in preventing aHUS recurrences in kidney-transplanted recipients [82]. Moreover, studies are currently evaluating the efficacy of Eculizumab for the treatment of C3 glomerulopathy in kidney-transplanted patients, with promising results [83]. The mechanism of action of Eculizumab is based on the prevention of the cleavage of C5 into C5a and C5b fragments, thereby inhibiting the activation of the terminal complement pathway, including the formation of complement effectors C5a and the MAC [84].

Currently, the efficacy of Eculizumab is being investigated for several other conditions, including renal IRI in transplanted patients. Researchers are exploring whether the inhibition of terminal complement system activation could help reduce tissue damage, improve graft survival, and prevent complications in transplant patients. In 2013, Kaabak et al. described a case of renal IRI after a kidney transplantation from a deceased donor who met the standard donor criteria, where the renal IRI was completely reversed after a single infusion of Eculizumab [85]. This laid the foundation for a randomized controlled trial involving 57 pediatric kidney transplant recipients, in which half of the patients received a single dose of Eculizumab before transplantation. The results showed that the patients who received Eculizumab exhibited better early graft function, reduced arteriolar hyalinosis, and chronic glomerulopathy in early and late biopsy samples, compared to the control group [86]. However, Schröppel et al. reported data from two randomized studies regarding the use of Eculizumab in reducing DGF rate after kidney transplantation. They did not find differences between the group treated with Eculizumab and the control groups in terms of DGF rate and graft function. These results were in line with the larger phase II/III PROTECT (Prevention of Delayed Graft Function Using Eculizumab Therapy) study, which did not show significant differences in DGF rates or graft survival between the treatment and control groups [87]. The lack of efficacy of Eculizumab may be related to the specific inhibition of the downstream part of the complement pathway, without blocking the activity of upstream molecules which could be key mediators of DGF despite C5 inhibition. Future clinical studies will be needed to explore the combination of Eculizumab with other agents that regulate upstream complement system activation in order to combine their mechanism of actions.

Many pharmaceutical companies are developing alternative anti-C5 therapies inspired by the success of Eculizumab in treating various complement system-involved diseases. However, additional research is needed to confirm their effectiveness in managing renal IRI. For example, Ravulizumab (Ultomiris™, Alexion Pharmaceuticals, Boston, MA, USA) is a mAb, designated by the substitution of four amino acids in the eculizumab backbone in order to extend its half-life [88]. It is under study in the ARTEMIS protocol for the management of major adverse kidney events caused by ischemic injury, including IRI, in patients undergoing cardiac surgery [89]. Crovalimab (Roche/Genentech, South San Francisco, CA, USA), another mAb that targets an epitope on the C5 β chain (whereas Eculizumab and Ravulizumab bind to the C5 α chain [90]), is currently under investigation in a randomized phase Ib study for the management of acute uncomplicated vaso-occlusive episodes in sickle cell disease, a condition characterized by microvascular dysfunction associated with IRI [91].

Currently, one of the most important challenges in managing atypical hemolytic syndrome, which shares the common denominator of AP activation with IRI, is determining the appropriate timing for discontinuation of the therapy. A scientific consensus conference suggested that, once kidney function has improved and stabilized, discontinuation should be considered in patients without pathogenic variants in complement genes, and that close monitoring with blood tests and weekly urinary dispticks is essential to detect early relapses and restart the treatment [92]. Since renal IRI can exacerbate complement system activation and potentially increase the risk of hemolytic uremic syndrome relapses in kidney transplant patients, the prevention of IRI should be considered essential [93].

Another compelling target in the management of renal IRI is complement factor C3, because it plays a crucial role in all three activation pathways and is responsible for proximal complement activation. Currently, efforts are focused on developing drugs designed to inhibit C3. Among them, Pegcetacoplan (Apellis, Waltham, MA, USA), a pegylated anti-C3 cyclic peptide, has already been approved by regulatory agencies for the treatment of PNH in patients who do not respond adequately to Eculizumab. Pegcetacoplan is a compostatin derivative, a group of peptides that specifically bind to C3, preventing access to C3 convertases and thereby inhibiting C3 cleavage across all three complement activation pathways [94]. Moreover, there is significant interest among researchers in the field of kidney transplantation regarding the use of Pegcetacopan in the treatment of post-transplant recurrent C3 glomerulopathy or immune complex membranoproliferative glomerulonephritis [95]. Due to its small size (43.5 kDa), it may effectively reach the corticomedullary junction, a hypoxia-sensitive region of the kidney, and therefore potentially reduce the activation of the complement system during IRI [6]. In the future, clinical trials could be designed to assess the effectiveness of combining C3 and C5 inhibition in IRI to evaluate whether this combination might enhance efficacy compared to targeting C3 or C5 alone. Recently, evidence has emerged to suggest that for certain diseases, such as paroxysmal nocturnal hemoglobinuria (PNH), the simultaneous blockade of both the proximal and terminal complement pathways may be useful. In a review article by Notaro and al., the authors suggested a dual-inhibition approach to prevent C3 binding to red blood cells, thereby reducing extravascular hemolysis and preventing massive breakthrough hemolysis in PNH patients [96].

Currently, the first monoclonal antibody targeting both C5 and the C3 convertase is KP104 (Kira Pharmaceuticals, Cambridge, MA, USA); it provides both terminal and proximal complement pathway inhibition [97] and is currently under investigation in a phase II study to evaluate its efficacy and safety in patients with IgA nephropathy and C3 glomerulopathy [98]. Moreover, the potential application of KP104 in the context of renal IRI should not be ignored. The dual inhibition of the both proximal and terminal complement pathways may result in an oversuppressed fontline defense for the immune system; therefore, close monitoring of complement activation markers, prophylactic vaccinations, regular infection screenings, and regular assessment of the patient's immune status may help to maintain immune balance in this patient population.

5.2. Targeting Complement Receptors and Regulatory Proteins

The risk of recurrent infections can be increased by the use of compounds that broadly inhibit complement system activation. Therefore, a more targeted approach in order to better modulate complement system activity may offer benefits, potentially leading to similar positive outcomes for patients. In this context, the inhibition of the C5a-C5aR1 axis does not interfere with MAC formation, but it could be particularly advantageous due to the powerful chemotactic and pro-inflammatory properties of this anaphylatoxin [99].

In animal models of renal disease, blocking C5aR1 resulted in reduced small vessel inflammation and neutrophils activation in ANCA-associated glomerulonephritis [100]. Furthermore, recent studies have demonstrated that interactions between C5a and C5aR1 play a critical role in the development of renal IRI and contribute to kidney rejection. Zang et al. demonstrated that the use of recombinant C5a led to a reduction in progranulin levels, a grow factor with anti-inflammatory properties relevant in renal IRI. However, C5aR deficiency resulted in reduced NF-kB expression after IRI, which reversed the C5a-induced suppression of progranulin, supporting that the complement C5a/C5aR pathway exacerbates renal IRI by downregulating protective factors and promoting inflammation [101]. According to this, Peng et al. demonstrated that C5a caused the upregulation of inflammatory-related genes, such as interleukin-1α (IL1α), IL-6, and transforming growth factor-α in RECs. The inhibition of the C5a-C5aR1 axis significantly reduced renal injury and tubulointerstitial fibrosis, suggesting a pathogenic role for C5aR1 in the progression of fibrosis after renal IRI [102].

A powerful antagonist of C5aR1, Avacopan, has been approved by the FDA for the additional treatment of severe active cytoplasmic antibody antineutrophil (ANCA)-associated vasculitis (AAV) in combination with standard therapy in adults; it significantly improves patient kidney function by reducing proteinuria and increasing the estimated glomerular filtration rate [103]. Furthermore, C5aR expression from RECs has been reported in several kidney diseases, including diabetes, IgA nephropathy, sepsis, and IRI, suggesting its relevance in renal pathology [104].

An alternative strategy to prevent C5a signaling involves its inhibition within circulation, Vilobelimab (IFX-1), is a monoclonal IgG4 kappa antibody that selectively binds to C5a, blocking its biological activity. Authorized by the FDA for emergency use in treating COVID-19 in hospitalized adults, it is also under investigation for use in other conditions, including granulomatosis with polyangiitis, hidradenitis suppurativa, and pyoderma gangrenosum [105]. Interestingly, recent findings indicate that COVID-19 infection is related to a decreased oxygen levels and the development of IRI not only in the lungs, but also in heart, liver, and kidneys, suggesting that targeting C5a might be beneficial in attenuating renal IRI [106].

Human complement receptor 1 (CR1) is an integral membrane protein expressed on the surface of several types of cells, including podocytes, that inhibits complement activation by preventing the formation of the convertases that activate C3 and C5. Additionally, a soluble form of CR1 is also present in the circulation. Both membrane-bound and soluble CR1 help regulate complement system activity by promoting the decay of the C3 and C5 convertases and serving as a cofactor for the serine protease factor I, which degrades C3b and C4b [107]. Kassimatis et al. explored the use of Mirococept, a recombinant complement inhibitor derived from human CR1, in the EMPIRIKAL trial to evaluate its effects on reducing DGF in kidney transplantation. Initial findings showed that the ex vivo delivery of Mirococept is both feasible and safe; however, a dose calibration is necessary [108]. Based on this, the EMPIRIKAL-2 trial is now revising its human study protocol based on the optimal higher dose achieved in pigs [109].

Although the AP is considered the main pathway responsible for renal IRI, recombinant human C1 esterase inhibitor (C1INH), a powerful inhibitor of proteases of the CP and LP, has been studied in the context of renal IRI to prevent the amplification of the inflammatory responses. Castellano et al. demonstrated that the infusion of C1INH into a swine model of renal IRI was associated with a significant C4d and C5b-9 deposit reduction in the peritubular capillaries and glomerular compartments, as well as decreased infiltration of inflammatory cells [110]. Later, Danobeitia et al. investigated the use of C1INH in a mouse model of IRI, showing that the use of C1INH before transplantation significantly improved survival rates and provided protection against subsequent kidney fibrosis [111]. However, in humans, a phase I/II trial investigated the efficacy of C1INH in reducing the need for hemodialysis during the first week post deceased-donor kidney transplantation (definition of DGF [112]). While no differences in DGF were observed between the groups, those who received C1INH required significantly fewer dialysis sessions 2 to 4 weeks post transplant, suggesting that C1INH may be useful to prevent IRI and DGF in kidney allografts, but larger studies will be needed [113].

Complement factor H is a glycoprotein primarily produced by the liver which circulates in a soluble form, reaching high plasma concentrations with a complement system-inhibitory function. The interaction of factor H with certain ligands, including glycosaminoglycans, sialic acid, and C3b fragments, can anchor it to the surface of cells and membranes, thereby providing alternative pathway regulation locally. Notably, mutations in factor H can make specific cell surfaces vulnerable to alternative pathway activation, potentially disrupting normal complement regulation in those sites [114]. Goetz et al. demonstrated that in mice with a heterozygous deletion of the factor H gene there was the development of more severe kidney damage after IRI than in wild-type controls. However, complement activation was restricted to the tubulointerstitial compartment and did not occur in the glomeruli, suggesting that full factor H expression may be not necessary for controlling glomerular complement activation after IRI and that its modulation could be useful for the management of IRI-associated damage [115]. Currently, clinical trials are testing the adeno-associated virus-mediated delivery of a fusion protein that combines a complement receptor 2 fragment with the inhibitory domain of factor H for the treatment of age-related macular degeneration [116]. However, future and further studies will be essential to evaluate its efficacy for the treatment of kidney diseases, including IRI.

In addition to complement receptors and regulatory proteins that control AP, MASP-2 is an enzyme that has pivotal role in the LP. Dudler et al. developed Narsoplimab, a fully human monoclonal antibody designed to inhibit LP by binding to MASP-2. Narsoplimab is currently in phases II and III of development. Experimental models have demonstrated that the deficiency or inhibition of MASP-2 has beneficial effects in IRI and in the transplantation field, suggesting a potential application in the management of these conditions [117].

5.3. *Targeting Complement Factors B and D*

The selective inhibition of factor B or factor D offers a more targeted approach to block the AP without affecting the innate immunity of the CP and LP. As serine proteases acting upstream of C3, they reduce the activity in the proximal complement amplification loop and the terminal complement pathway. Moreover, their use is expected to lower the risk of infection and other immune-related complications compared to direct C3 inhibition. Currently, oral small-molecule inhibitors targeting complement factors B and D are being developed for use as monotherapy or in combination with a C5 inhibitor [118]. Furthermore, regarding healthcare costs, a cost-effectiveness analysis of a factor B inhibitor demonstrated that it contributes to a higher quality of life for PNH patients at a lower overall cost burden, compared to C5 inhibitors [119].

As shown, the activation of the complement system has been demonstrated in kidneys from deceased-after-brain-death (DBD) donors. Interestingly, C3 deposition was observed on glomerular endothelial cells in kidney biopsies from DBD donors, while no C3 deposition appeared in biopsies from living donors, suggesting that complement deposition is a direct consequence of brain death. In this context, the inhibition of the complement system could be a valuable approach to attenuate renal injury before the transplantation, as shown by Jager et al. They pretreated brain-dead mice with anti-factor B, showing less systemic and local complement system activation, preserved renal function, and attenuated histological injury, suggesting that this might be a promising strategy to minimize complement system-related damage from brain death [120]. Moreover, Amura et al. investigated whether blocking TLRs and the factor B pathway in an animal model of renal IRI could protect against tissue damage. Their findings showed that mice with a targeted deletion of complement factor B alone were protected from injury, while mice with deletion of both factor B and TLR-2 developed more severe damage. This suggests that, although complement and TLR-2 pathways promote pro-inflammatory signals, the selective inhibition of complement factor B may have protective effects against IRI-related damage [121]. Furthermore, Casiraghi et al. demonstrated that factor B-deficient mice underwent reduced IRI, as well as lower T cell-mediated rejection rates and impaired dendritic cell alloreactive functions. These results suggest that factor B inhibitions may have implications for prolonging graft survival, highlighting its potential utility in kidney transplantation [61]. The role of factor D has been explored in a model of gastrointestinal IRI. Stahl et al. showed that factor D-deficient mice exhibited decreased neutrophil accumulation and reduced gastrointestinal injury and suggested that the inhibition of factor D may also represent an effective therapeutic strategy for IRI [122].

Iptacopan is the first drug developed to specifically target complement factor B currently in phase II and III of development for several kidney-involved diseases, including C3 glomerulopathy, IgA nephropaty, lupus nephropathy, and aHUS [123]. Its mechanism of action is based on the inhibition of the enzymatic activity of factor B, which leads to the suppression of both convertases, resulting in an upstream and downstream regulation of the AP [97].

In addition, Danicopan is a first-in-class factor D inhibitor that has been shown to block the initiation of the AP and inhibit up to 80% of downstream events initiated by the classical or lectin pathways through amplification-loop inhibition [124]. A newer oral factor D inhibitor, Vemircopan, is currently under investigation in phase I and II trials for lupus nephritis and IgA nephropathy. While both factor D inhibitors share the same mechanism of action, Vemircopan exhibited greater potency and binding affinity for factor D [125].

6. Conclusions and Limitations

This narrative review is intended to highlight that, while many complement-modulating drugs are currently under investigation, only a few of them have been evaluated specifically for their effects on renal IRI, pointing to a significant need for targeted research in this field. One of the potential limitations of starting clinical trials for complement system inhibitors in IRI for kidney transplantation patients is that designing trials involving this specific patient population is complex due to several factors, such as the timing of intervention (pre-, during, or post-IRI), types of donors, and baseline characteristics of recipients, including the underlying cause of kidney disease. Moreover, the interpretation of the data in kidney transplant patients often leads to mixed results. For example, in the context of antibody-mediated rejection, the potential efficacy of complement system-targeting drugs is still not very clear because of the heterogeneous study findings, different drug regimens, and limited sample sizes [126]. The increased susceptibility to infection can be considered another limitation factor for the design of clinical trials in kidney transplant patients, especially given the immunosuppressive therapy required for induction during kidney transplantation. This also raises important ethical concerns about testing these drugs on human subjects. Nonetheless, animal studies can overcome some of the limitations for the use of complement system inhibition strategies in renal transplantation models of IRI, allowing for precise control over experimental conditions, and producing larger sample sizes in order to obtain extensive preclinical data.

The modulation of the complement system has shown promising results in reducing the inflammatory burden, oxidative stress, and tissue damage in many kidney diseases, with a good safety and efficacy profiles. However, studies are still needed to establish their efficacy in renal IRI, and could pave the way for novel therapeutic options in managing kidney injury and improving transplant success. By temporarily "switching off" complement system activation during the acute injury phases, these drugs may enhance renal protection, especially since the kidney itself is capable of synthetizing complement proteins [96]. Moreover, the penetrance of these molecules in the renal interstitium makes them attractive therapeutic approaches in the field of transplantation.

Author Contributions: Conceptualization, D.T.; writing—original draft preparation, D.T., C.A. and L.A.C., writing—review and editing, B.I. and S.M.; supervision, G.C. and G.S. All authors have read and agreed to the published version of the manuscript.

Funding: This work was supported by the Italian Ministry of University and Research under the Research Projects of National Relevant Interest (PRIN) project. Title of the project: "TiME-Line of Intragraft mOleculaR trAjectories: Role in Kidney Transplant ouTcomE (MELIORATE)"; Project Code P2022S9XZS (Granted to G.S.).

Conflicts of Interest: The authors declare no conflicts of interest.

References

1. Biglarnia, A.-R.; Huber-Lang, M.; Mohlin, C.; Ekdahl, K.N.; Nilsson, B. The multifaceted role of complement in kidney transplantation. *Nat. Rev. Nephrol.* **2018**, *14*, 767–781. [CrossRef]
2. Troise, D.; Infante, B.; Mercuri, S.; Piccoli, C.; Lindholm, B.; Stallone, G. Hypoxic Inducible Factor Stabilization in Pericytes beyond Erythropoietin Production: The Good and the Bad. *Antioxidants* **2024**, *13*, 537. [CrossRef]
3. Bongoni, A.K.; Lu, B.; Salvaris, E.J.; Roberts, V.; Fang, D.; McRae, J.L.; Fisicaro, N.; Dwyer, K.M.; Cowan, P.J. Overexpression of Human CD55 and CD59 or Treatment with Human CD55 Protects against Renal Ischemia-Reperfusion Injury in Mice. *J. Immunol.* **2017**, *198*, 4837–4845. [CrossRef]
4. Zhou, W.; Farrar, C.A.; Abe, K.; Pratt, J.R.; Marsh, J.E.; Wang, Y.; Stahl, G.L.; Sacks, S.H. Predominant role for C5b-9 in renal ischemia/reperfusion injury. *J. Clin. Investig.* **2000**, *105*, 1363–1371. [CrossRef]
5. Stea, E.D.; D'Ettorre, G.; Mitrotti, A.; Gesualdo, L. The complement system in the pathogenesis and progression of kidney diseases: What doesn't kill you makes you older. *Eur. J. Intern. Med.* **2024**, *124*, 22–31. [CrossRef]
6. Howard, M.C.; Nauser, C.L.; Farrar, C.A.; Sacks, S.H. Correction to: Complement in ischaemia–reperfusion injury and transplantation. *Semin. Immunopathol.* **2022**, *44*, 391. [CrossRef]
7. Lo, M.W.; Woodruff, T.M. Complement: Bridging the innate and adaptive immune systems in sterile inflammation. *J. Leucoc. Biol.* **2020**, *108*, 339–351. [CrossRef]
8. Kenawy, H.I.; Boral, I.; Bevington, A. Complement-Coagulation Cross-Talk: A Potential Mediator of the Physiological Activation of Complement by Low pH. *Front. Immunol.* **2015**, *6*, 215. [CrossRef]
9. Triantafilou, M.; Hughes, T.R.; Morgan, B.P.; Triantafilou, K. Complementing the inflammasome. *Immunology* **2016**, *147*, 152–164. [CrossRef]
10. Hajishengallis, G.; Lambris, J.D. Crosstalk pathways between Toll-like receptors and the complement system. *Trends Immunol.* **2010**, *31*, 154–163. [CrossRef]
11. Zipfel, P.F.; Skerka, C. Complement regulators and inhibitory proteins. *Nat. Rev. Immunol.* **2009**, *9*, 729–740. [CrossRef] [PubMed]
12. Nauser, C.L.; Farrar, C.A.; Sacks, S.H. Complement Recognition Pathways in Renal Transplantation. *J. Am. Soc. Nephrol.* **2017**, *28*, 2571–2578. [CrossRef]
13. Welch, T.R.; Beischel, L.S.; Frenzke, M.; Witte, D. Regulated expression of complement factor B in the human kidney. *Kidney Int.* **1996**, *50*, 521–525. [CrossRef]
14. Brooimans, R.A.; Stegmann, A.P.; van Dorp, W.T.; van der Ark, A.A.; van der Woude, F.J.; van Es, L.; Daha, M.R.A. Interleukin 2 mediates stimulation of complement C3 biosynthesis in human proximal tubular epithelial cells. *J. Clin. Investig.* **1991**, *88*, 379–384. [CrossRef]

15. Mühlig, A.K.; Keir, L.S.; Abt, J.C.; Heidelbach, H.S.; Horton, R.; Welsh, G.I.; Meyer-Schwesinger, C.; Licht, C.; Coward, R.J.; Fester, L.; et al. Podocytes Produce and Secrete Functional Complement C3 and Complement Factor H. *Front. Immunol.* **2020**, *11*, 1833. [CrossRef]
16. Franzin, R.; Stasi, A.; Fiorentino, M.; Stallone, G.; Cantaluppi, V.; Gesualdo, L.; Castellano, G. Inflammaging and Complement System: A Link Between Acute Kidney Injury and Chronic Graft Damage. *Front. Immunol.* **2020**, *11*, 734. [CrossRef]
17. Netti, G.S.; Franzin, R.; Stasi, A.; Spadaccino, F.; Strologo, A.D.; Infante, B.; Gesualdo, L.; Castellano, G.; Ranieri, E.; Stallone, G. Role of complement in regulating inflammation processes in renal and prostate cancers. *Cells* **2021**, *10*, 2426. [CrossRef]
18. Qi, R.; Qin, W. Role of Complement System in Kidney Transplantation: Stepping From Animal Models to Clinical Application. *Front. Immunol.* **2022**, *13*, 811696. [CrossRef]
19. Petr, V.; Thurman, J.M. The role of complement in kidney disease. *Nat. Rev. Nephrol.* **2023**, *19*, 771–787. [CrossRef]
20. West, E.E.; Kunz, N.; Kemper, C. Complement and human T cell metabolism: Location, location, location. *Immunol. Rev.* **2020**, *295*, 68–81. [CrossRef]
21. Cui, J.; Wu, X.; Song, Y.; Chen, Y.; Wan, J. Complement C3 exacerbates renal interstitial fibrosis by facilitating the M1 macrophage phenotype in a mouse model of unilateral ureteral obstruction. *Am. J. Physiol.-Ren. Physiol.* **2019**, *317*, F1171–F1182. [CrossRef] [PubMed]
22. Stallone, G.; Netti, G.S.; Cormio, L.; Castellano, G.; Infante, B.; Pontrelli, P.; Divella, C.; Selvaggio, O.; Spadaccino, F.; Ranieri, E.; et al. Modulation of complement activation by pentraxin-3 in prostate cancer. *Sci. Rep.* **2020**, *10*, 18400. [CrossRef]
23. Cho, H. Complement regulation: Physiology and disease relevance. *Korean J. Pediatr.* **2015**, *58*, 239. [CrossRef]
24. Keragala, C.B.; Draxler, D.F.; McQuilten, Z.K.; Medcalf, R.L. Haemostasis and innate immunity—A complementary relationship. *Br. J. Haematol.* **2018**, *180*, 782–798. [CrossRef]
25. Amara, U.; Flierl, M.A.; Rittirsch, D.; Klos, A.; Chen, H.; Acker, B.; Brückner, U.B.; Nilsson, B.; Gebhard, F.; Lambris, J.D.; et al. Molecular Intercommunication between the Complement and Coagulation Systems. *J. Immunol.* **2010**, *185*, 5628–5636. [CrossRef]
26. Heurich, M.; McCluskey, G. Complement and coagulation crosstalk—Factor H in the spotlight. *Immunobiology* **2023**, *228*, 152707. [CrossRef]
27. Foley, J.H.; Walton, B.L.; Aleman, M.M.; O'Byrne, A.M.; Lei, V.; Harrasser, M.; Foley, K.A.; Wolberg, A.S.; Conway, E.M. Complement Activation in Arterial and Venous Thrombosis is Mediated by Plasmin. *EBioMedicine* **2016**, *5*, 175–182. [CrossRef]
28. Engelmann, B.; Massberg, S. Thrombosis as an intravascular effector of innate immunity. *Nat. Rev. Immunol.* **2013**, *13*, 34–45. [CrossRef]
29. Stallone, G.; Pontrelli, P.; Rascio, F.; Castellano, G.; Gesualdo, L.; Grandaliano, G. Coagulation and Fibrinolysis in Kidney Graft Rejection. *Front. Immunol.* **2020**, *11*, 1807. [CrossRef]
30. Hajishengallis, G.; Lambris, J.D. More than complementing Tolls: Complement–Toll-like receptor synergy and crosstalk in innate immunity and inflammation. *Immunol. Rev.* **2016**, *274*, 233–244. [CrossRef]
31. Pope, M.R.; Hoffman, S.M.; Tomlinson, S.; Fleming, S.D. Complement regulates TLR4-mediated inflammatory responses during intestinal ischemia reperfusion. *Mol. Immunol.* **2010**, *48*, 356–364. [CrossRef]
32. Chen, Y.; Lin, L.; Rao, S.; Tao, X.; Cui, J.; Wan, J. Complement C3 mediates podocyte injury through TLR4/NFKB-P65 signaling during ischemia–reperfusion acute kidney injury and post-injury fibrosis. *Eur. J. Med. Res.* **2023**, *28*, 135. [CrossRef]
33. Ichida, S.; Yuzawa, Y.; Okada, H.; Yoshioka, K.; Matsuo, S. Localization of the complement regulatory proteins in the normal human kidney. *Kidney Int.* **1994**, *46*, 89–96. [CrossRef]
34. Thurman, J.M. Altered renal tubular expression of the complement inhibitor Crry permits complement activation after ischemia/reperfusion. *J. Clin. Investig.* **2006**, *116*, 357–368. [CrossRef]
35. Barnum, S.R. Therapeutic Inhibition of Complement: Well Worth the Risk. *Trends Pharmacol. Sci.* **2017**, *38*, 503–505. [CrossRef]
36. Watanabe-Kusunoki, K.; Anders, H.-J. Balancing efficacy and safety of complement inhibitors. *J. Autoimmun.* **2024**, *145*, 103216. [CrossRef]
37. Karp, D.R.; Holers, V.M. Complement in Health and Disease. In *Goldman's Cecil Medicine*; Elsevier: Amsterdam, The Netherlands, 2012; pp. 239–244. [CrossRef]
38. Mohebnasab, M.; Eriksson, O.; Persson, B.; Sandholm, K.; Mohlin, C.; Huber-Lang, M.; Keating, B.J.; Ekdahl, K.N.; Nilsson, B. Current and Future Approaches for Monitoring Responses to Anti-complement Therapeutics. *Front. Immunol.* **2019**, *10*, 2539. [CrossRef]
39. Troise, D.; Infante, B.; Mercuri, S.; Netti, G.S.; Ranieri, E.; Gesualdo, L.; Stallone, G.; Pontrelli, P. Hypoxic State of Cells and Immunosenescence: A Focus on the Role of the HIF Signaling Pathway. *Biomedicines* **2023**, *11*, 2163. [CrossRef]
40. Carcy, R.; Cougnon, M.; Poet, M.; Durandy, M.; Sicard, A.; Counillon, L.; Blondeau, N.; Hauet, T.; Tauc, M.; Pisani, D.F. Targeting oxidative stress, a crucial challenge in renal transplantation outcome. *Free Radic. Biol. Med.* **2021**, *169*, 258–270. [CrossRef]

41. Franzin, R.; Stasi, A.; Fiorentino, M.; Simone, S.; Oberbauer, R.; Castellano, G.; Gesualdo, L. Renal Delivery of Pharmacologic Agents During Machine Perfusion to Prevent Ischaemia-Reperfusion Injury: From Murine Model to Clinical Trials. *Front. Immunol.* **2021**, *12*, 673562. [CrossRef]
42. Collard, C.D.; Lekowski, R.; Jordan, J.E.; Agah, A.; Stahl, G.L. Complement activation following oxidative stress. *Mol. Immunol.* **1999**, *36*, 941–948. [CrossRef]
43. Choi, M.S.; Jeon, H.; Yoo, S.-M.; Lee, M.-S. Activation of the Complement System on Human Endothelial Cells by Urban Particulate Matter Triggers Inflammation-Related Protein Production. *Int. J. Mol. Sci.* **2021**, *22*, 3336. [CrossRef]
44. Collard, C.D.; Väkevä, A.; Büküsoglu, C.; Zünd, G.; Sperati, C.J.; Colgan, S.P.; Stahl, G.L. Reoxygenation of Hypoxic Human Umbilical Vein Endothelial Cells Activates the Classic Complement Pathway. *Circulation* **1997**, *96*, 326–333. [CrossRef]
45. Adler, S.; Baker, P.J.; Johnson, R.J.; Ochi, R.F.; Pritzl, P.; Couser, W.G. Complement membrane attack complex stimulates production of reactive oxygen metabolites by cultured rat mesangial cells. *J. Clin. Investig.* **1986**, *77*, 762–767. [CrossRef]
46. Zhang, R.; Qi, J.; Zhou, M.; Pan, T.; Zhang, Z.; Yao, Y.; Han, H.; Han, Y. Upregulation of Nrf2 Attenuates Oxidative Stress–Induced, Complement Activation–Associated Endothelial Injury and Apoptosis in Transplant-Associated Thrombotic Microangiopathy. *Transpl. Cell Ther.* **2021**, *27*, 758.e1–758.e8. [CrossRef]
47. Ishii, M.; Rohrer, B. Anaphylatoxin C5a receptor signaling induces mitochondrial fusion and sensitizes retinal pigment epithelial cells to oxidative stress. *Biochim. Biophys. Acta BBA Gen. Subj.* **2023**, *1867*, 130374. [CrossRef]
48. Ishii, M.; Beeson, G.; Beeson, C.; Rohrer, B. Mitochondrial C3a Receptor Activation in Oxidatively Stressed Epithelial Cells Reduces Mitochondrial Respiration and Metabolism. *Front. Immunol.* **2021**, *12*, 628062. [CrossRef]
49. Arbore, G.; West, E.E.; Spolski, R.; Robertson, A.A.B.; Klos, A.; Rheinheimer, C.; Dutow, P.; Woodruff, T.M.; Yu, Z.X.; O'neill, L.A.; et al. T helper 1 immunity requires complement-driven NLRP3 inflammasome activity in CD4+ T cells. *Science* **2016**, *352*, aad1210. [CrossRef]
50. Tsai, I.-J.; Lin, W.-C.; Yang, Y.-H.; Tseng, Y.-L.; Lin, Y.-H.; Chou, C.-H.; Tsau, Y.-K. High Concentration of C5a-Induced Mitochondria-Dependent Apoptosis in Murine Kidney Endothelial Cells. *Int. J. Mol. Sci.* **2019**, *20*, 4465. [CrossRef]
51. Simone, S.; Lin, W.-C.; Yang, Y.-H.; Tseng, Y.-L.; Lin, Y.-H.; Chou, C.-H.; Tsau, Y.-K. Complement-dependent NADPH oxidase enzyme activation in renal ischemia/reperfusion injury. *Free Radic. Biol. Med.* **2014**, *74*, 263–273. [CrossRef]
52. Granata, S.; Rascio, F.; Castellano, G.; Divella, C.; Chieti, A.; Ditonno, P.; Battaglia, M.; Crovace, A.; Staffieri, F.; Oortwijn, B.; et al. Oxidative Stress and Ischemia/Reperfusion Injury in Kidney Transplantation: Focus on Ferroptosis, Mitophagy and New Antioxidants. *Antioxidants* **2022**, *11*, 769. [CrossRef]
53. Detsika, M.G.; Lianos, E.A. Regulation of Complement Activation by Heme Oxygenase-1 (HO-1) in Kidney Injury. *Antioxidants* **2021**, *10*, 60. [CrossRef]
54. Yang, J.; Ahn, H.; Chang, M.; Narasimhan, P.; Chan, P.H.; Song, Y.S. Complement component 3 inhibition by an antioxidant is neuroprotective after cerebral ischemia and reperfusion in mice. *J. Neurochem.* **2013**, *124*, 523–535. [CrossRef]
55. Nijveldt, R.J.; van Nood, E.; van Hoorn, D.E.; Boelens, P.G.; van Norren, K.; van Leeuwen, P.A. Flavonoids: A review of probable mechanisms of action and potential applications. *Am. J. Clin. Nutr.* **2001**, *74*, 418–425. [CrossRef] [PubMed]
56. Soares, R.O.S.; Losada, D.M.; Jordani, M.C.; Évora, P.; Castro-e-Silva, O. Ischemia/Reperfusion Injury Revisited: An Overview of the Latest Pharmacological Strategies. *Int. J. Mol. Sci.* **2019**, *20*, 5034. [CrossRef]
57. Delaura, I.F.; Gao, Q.; Anwar, I.J.; Abraham, N.; Kahan, R.; Hartwig, M.G.; Barbas, A.S. Complement-targeting therapeutics for ischemia-reperfusion injury in transplantation and the potential for ex vivo delivery. *Front. Immunol.* **2022**, *13*, 1000172. [CrossRef]
58. Poppelaars, F.; Seelen, M.A. Complement-mediated inflammation and injury in brain dead organ donors. *Mol. Immunol.* **2017**, *84*, 77–83. [CrossRef]
59. Bartoszek, D.; Mazanowska, O.; Kościelska-Kasprzak, K.; Kamińska, D.; Lepiesza, A.; Chudoba, P.; Myszka, M.; Żabińska, M.; Klinger, M. Functional Activity of the Complement System in Deceased Donors in Relation to Kidney Allograft Outcome. *Transpl. Proc.* **2018**, *50*, 1697–1700. [CrossRef]
60. Gibson, B.; Connelly, C.; Moldakhmetova, S.; Sheerin, N.S. Complement activation and kidney transplantation; a complex relationship. *Immunobiology* **2023**, *228*, 152396. [CrossRef]
61. Casiraghi, F.; Azzollini, N.; Todeschini, M.; Fiori, S.; Cavinato, R.A.; Cassis, P.; Solini, S.; Pezzuto, F.; Mister, M.; Thurman, J.M.; et al. Complement Alternative Pathway Deficiency in Recipients Protects Kidney Allograft From Ischemia/Reperfusion Injury and Alloreactive T Cell Response. *Am. J. Transplant.* **2017**, *17*, 2312–2325. [CrossRef]
62. Arias-Cabrales, C.; Rodriguez-Garcia, E.; Gimeno, J.; Benito, D.; Pérez-Sáez, M.J.; Redondo-Pachón, D.; Buxeda, A.; Burballa, C.; Crespo, M.; Riera, M.; et al. Role of C5aR1 and C5L2 Receptors in Ischemia-Reperfusion Injury. *J. Clin. Med.* **2021**, *10*, 974. [CrossRef]

63. Weiser, M.R.; Rodriguez-Garcia, E.; Gimeno, J.; Benito, D.; Pérez-Sáez, M.J.; Redondo-Pachón, D.; Buxeda, A.; Burballa, C.; Crespo, M.; Riera, M.; et al. Reperfusion injury of ischemic skeletal muscle is mediated by natural antibody and complement. *J. Exp. Med.* **1996**, *183*, 2343–2348. [CrossRef]
64. Thurman, J.M.; Ljubanovic, D.; Edelstein, C.L.; Gilkeson, G.S.; Holers, V.M. Lack of a Functional Alternative Complement Pathway Ameliorates Ischemic Acute Renal Failure in Mice. *J. Immunol.* **2003**, *170*, 1517–1523. [CrossRef] [PubMed]
65. Renner, B.; Ferreira, V.P.; Cortes, C.; Goldberg, R.; Ljubanovic, D.; Pangburn, M.K.; Pickering, M.C.; Tomlinson, S.; Holland-Neidermyer, A.; Strassheim, D.; et al. Binding of factor H to tubular epithelial cells limits interstitial complement activation in ischemic injury. *Kidney Int.* **2011**, *80*, 165–173. [CrossRef]
66. Møller-Kristensen, M.; Wang, W.; Ruseva, M.; Thiel, S.; Nielsen, S.; Takahashi, K.; Shi, L.; Ezekowitz, A.; Jensenius, J.C.; Gadjeva, M. Mannan-Binding Lectin Recognizes Structures on Ischaemic Reperfused Mouse Kidneys and is Implicated in Tissue Injury. *Scand. J. Immunol.* **2005**, *61*, 426–434. [CrossRef]
67. van Werkhoven, M.B.; Damman, J.; van Dijk, M.C.R.F.; Daha, M.R.; de Jong, I.J.; Leliveld, A.; Krikke, C.; Leuvenink, H.G.; van Goor, H.; van Son, W.J.; et al. Complement Mediated Renal Inflammation Induced by Donor Brain Death: Role of Renal C5a-C5aR Interaction. *Am. J. Transplant.* **2013**, *13*, 875–882. [CrossRef]
68. Damman, J.; Seelen, M.A.; Moers, C.; Daha, M.R.; Rahmel, A.; Leuvenink, H.G.; Paul, A.; Pirenne, J.; Ploeg, R.J. Systemic Complement Activation I n Deceased Donors Is Associated With Acute Rejection After Renal Transplantation in the Recipient. *Transplantation* **2011**, *92*, 163–169. [CrossRef]
69. de Vries, B.; Köhl, J.; Leclercq, W.K.G.; Wolfs, T.G.A.M.; van Bijnen, A.A.J.H.M.; Heeringa, P.; Buurman, W.A. Complement Factor C5a Mediates Renal Ischemia-Reperfusion Injury Independent from Neutrophils. *J. Immunol.* **2003**, *170*, 3883–3889. [CrossRef]
70. Arumugam, T.V.; Shiels, I.A.; Strachan, A.J.; Abbenante, G.; Fairlie, D.P.; Taylor, S.M. A small molecule C5a receptor antagonist protects kidneys from ischemia/reperfusion injury in rats. *Kidney Int.* **2003**, *63*, 134–142. [CrossRef]
71. Thurman, J.M.; Lenderink, A.M.; Royer, P.A.; Coleman, K.E.; Zhou, J.; Lambris, J.D.; Nemenoff, R.A.; Quigg, R.J.; Holers, V.M. C3a Is Required for the Production of CXC Chemokines by Tubular Epithelial Cells after Renal Ishemia/Reperfusion. *J. Immunol.* **2007**, *178*, 1819–1828. [CrossRef]
72. Budkowska, M.; Ostrycharz, E.; Serwin, N.M.; Nazarewski, Ł.; Cecerska-Heryć, E.; Poręcka, M.; Rykowski, P.; Pietrzak, R.; Zieniewicz, K.; Siennicka, A.; et al. Biomarkers of the Complement System Activation (C3a, C5a, sC5b-9) in Serum of Patients before and after Liver Transplantation. *Biomedicines* **2023**, *11*, 2070. [CrossRef]
73. Farrar, C.A.; Asgari, E.; Schwaeble, W.J.; Sacks, S.H. Which pathways trigger the role of complement in ischaemia/reperfusion injury? *Front. Immunol.* **2012**, *3*, 341. [CrossRef]
74. Chaban, V.; Nakstad, E.R.; Stær-Jensen, H.; Schjalm, C.; Seljeflot, I.; Vaage, J.; Lundqvist, C.; Benth, J.; Sunde, K.; Mollnes, T.E.; et al. Complement activation is associated with poor outcome after out-of-hospital cardiac arrest. *Resuscitation* **2021**, *166*, 129–136. [CrossRef]
75. Basile, D.; Yoder, M. Renal Endothelial Dysfunction in Acute Kidney Ischemia Reperfusion Injury. *Cardiovasc. Hematol. Disord. Drug Targets* **2014**, *14*, 3–14. [CrossRef]
76. Wang, Z.; Zhang, Z.; Li, Y.; Zhang, Y.; Wei, M.; Li, H.; Yang, S.; Zhou, Y.; Zhou, X.; Xing, G. Endothelial-derived complement factor D contributes to endothelial dysfunction in malignant nephrosclerosis via local complement activation. *Hypertens. Res.* **2023**, *46*, 1759–1770. [CrossRef]
77. Bongoni, A.; McRae, J.; Salvaris, E.; Fisicaro, N.; Kiss, B.; Pál, G.; Gál, P.; Cowan, P. 228.4: Treatment with a specific inhibitor of the complement lectin pathway is protective against renal ischemia-reperfusion injury in mice. *Transplantation* **2024**, *108*, 63. [CrossRef]
78. Nieuwenhuijs-Moeke, G.J.; Pischke, S.E.; Berger, S.P.; Sanders, J.S.F.; Pol, R.A.; Struys, M.M.R.F.; Ploeg, R.J.; Leuvenink, H.G.D. Ischemia and Reperfusion Injury in Kidney Transplantation: Relevant Mechanisms in Injury and Repair. *J. Clin. Med.* **2020**, *9*, 253. [CrossRef]
79. Rother, R.P.; Rollins, S.A.; Mojcik, C.F.; Brodsky, R.A.; Bell, L. Discovery and development of the complement inhibitor eculizumab for the treatment of paroxysmal nocturnal hemoglobinuria. *Nat. Biotechnol.* **2007**, *25*, 1256–1264. [CrossRef]
80. Brandsema, J.F.; Ginsberg, M.; Hoshino, H.; Mimaki, M.; Nagata, S.; Rao, V.K.; Ruzhansky, K.; Suresh, N.; Tiongson, E.; Yamanouchi, H.; et al. Eculizumab in Adolescent Patients With Refractory Generalized Myasthenia Gravis: A Phase 3, Open-Label, Multicenter Study. *Pediatr. Neurol.* **2024**, *156*, 198–207. [CrossRef]
81. Ringelstein, M.; Asseyer, S.; Lindenblatt, G.; Fischer, K.; Pul, R.; Skuljec, J.; Revie, L.; Giglhuber, K.; Häußler, V.; Karenfort, M.; et al. Eculizumab Use in Neuromyelitis Optica Spectrum Disorders. *Neurology* **2024**, *103*, e209888. [CrossRef]
82. Barnett, A.N.R.; Asgari, E.; Chowdhury, P.; Sacks, S.H.; Dorling, A.; Mamode, N. The use of eculizumab in renal transplantation. *Clin. Transpl.* **2013**, *27*, E216–E229. [CrossRef]

83. Bartoli, G.; Strologo, A.D.; Grandaliano, G.; Pesce, F. Updates on C3 Glomerulopathy in Kidney Transplantation: Pathogenesis and Treatment Options. *Int. J. Mol. Sci.* **2024**, *25*, 6508. [CrossRef]
84. Dubois, E.A.; Cohen, A.F. Eculizumab. *Br. J. Clin. Pharmacol.* **2009**, *68*, 318–319. [CrossRef] [PubMed]
85. Kaabak, M.; Babenko, N.; Kuznetsov, O.; Matveev, A.; Minina, M.; Platova, E.; Morozova, M.; Novozhilova, T. Eculizumab reverses the potentially fatal effects of kidney graft reperfusion injury. *Pediatr. Transpl.* **2014**, *18*, E44–E47. [CrossRef]
86. Kaabak, M.; Babenko, N.; Shapiro, R.; Zokoyev, A.; Dymova, O.; Kim, E. A prospective randomized, controlled trial of eculizumab to prevent ischemia-reperfusion injury in pediatric kidney transplantation. *Pediatr. Transpl.* **2018**, *22*, e13129. [CrossRef]
87. Schröppel, B.; Akalin, E.; Baweja, M.; Bloom, R.D.; Florman, S.; Goldstein, M.; Haydel, B.; Hricik, D.E.; Kulkarni, S.; Levine, M.; et al. Peritransplant eculizumab does not prevent delayed graft function in deceased donor kidney transplant recipients: Results of two randomized controlled pilot trials. *Am. J. Transplant.* **2020**, *20*, 564–572. [CrossRef]
88. Lee, J.W.; de Fontbrune, F.S.; Lee, L.W.L.; Pessoa, V.; Gualandro, S.; Füreder, W.; Ptushkin, V.; Rottinghaus, S.T.; Volles, L.; Shafner, L.; et al. Ravulizumab (ALXN1210) vs eculizumab in adult patients with PNH naive to complement inhibitors: The 301 study. *Blood* **2019**, *133*, 530–539. [CrossRef]
89. Winterberg, P.; Solinsky, C.; LI, G.; Smith, W. #3259 Artemis: A Phase 3 Study Of Ravulizumab To Protect Patients With Ckd Undergoing Cardiac Surgery From Aki And Subsequent Major Adverse Kidney Events. *Nephrol. Dial. Transplant.* **2023**, *38*, i1110. [CrossRef]
90. Fukuzawa, T.; Sampei, Z.; Haraya, K.; Ruike, Y.; Shida-Kawazoe, M.; Shimizu, Y.; Gan, S.W.; Irie, M.; Tsuboi, Y.; Tai, H.; et al. Long lasting neutralization of C5 by SKY59, a novel recycling antibody, is a potential therapy for complement-mediated diseases. *Sci. Rep.* **2017**, *7*, 1080. [CrossRef]
91. Bartolucci, P.; Ataga, K.I.; Callaghan, M.U.; De Franceschi, L.; Minniti, C.; Alexandrou, A.; Imbs, D.-C.; Fox, R.; Patel, H.; Sostelly, A.; et al. Trial in Progress: The Randomized, Double-Blind, Placebo-Controlled Phase Ib CROSSWALK-a Trial Evaluating the Safety of Crovalimab for the Management of Acute Uncomplicated Vaso-Occlusive Episodes (VOEs) in Patients with Sickle Cell Disease (SCD). *Blood* **2021**, *138*, 3108. [CrossRef]
92. Vivarelli, M.; Barratt, J.; Beck, L.H.; Fakhouri, F.; Gale, D.P.; de Jorge, E.G.; Mosca, M.; Noris, M.; Pickering, M.C.; Susztak, K.; et al. The role of complement in kidney disease: Conclusions from a Kidney Disease: Improving Global Outcomes (KDIGO) Controversies Conference. *Kidney Int.* **2024**, *106*, 369–391. [CrossRef]
93. Frémeaux-Bacchi, V.; Legendre, C.M. The emerging role of complement inhibitors in transplantation. *Kidney Int.* **2015**, *88*, 967–973. [CrossRef]
94. Estebanez, B.T.; Bomback, A.S. C3 Glomerulopathy: Novel Treatment Paradigms. *Kidney Int. Rep.* **2024**, *9*, 569–579. [CrossRef]
95. Fakhouri, F.; Bomback, A.; Kavanagh, D.; Remuzzi, G.; Sunder-Plassmann, G.; Kanellis, J.; Daina, E.; Walker, P.; Wang, Z.; Ahmad, Z. #1467 Pegcetacoplan for post-transplant recurrent C3 glomerulopathy or immune complex membranoproliferative glomerulonephritis in NOBLE: 12-week evolution. *Nephrol. Dial. Transplant.* **2024**, *39*, i727–i728. [CrossRef]
96. Notaro, R.; Luzzatto, L. Breakthrough Hemolysis in PNH with Proximal or Terminal Complement Inhibition. *N. Engl. J. Med.* **2022**, *387*, 160–166. [CrossRef]
97. Wooden, B.; Tarragon, B.; Navarro-Torres, M.; Bomback, A.S. Complement inhibitors for kidney disease. *Nephrol. Dial. Transplant.* **2023**, *38*, ii29–ii39. [CrossRef]
98. Lv, J.; Zhang, H.; Pedagogos, E.; Ma, J.; Zhou, H.; Rabe, M.; Hart, A.; Yue, C.; Yan, A.; Tsui, P.; et al. WCN23-1154 TRIAL IN PROGRESS: AN OPEN-LABEL, PHASE 2 STUDY TO EVALUATE EFFICACY, SAFETY, PK, PD OF KP104, A BIFUNCTIONAL COMPLEMENT INHIBITOR, IN IGAN AND C3G SUBJECTS. *Kidney Int. Rep.* **2023**, *8*, S230–S231. [CrossRef]
99. Ricklin, D.; Mastellos, D.C.; Reis, E.S.; Lambris, J.D. The renaissance of complement therapeutics. *Nat. Rev. Nephrol.* **2018**, *14*, 26–47. [CrossRef]
100. Xiao, H.; Dairaghi, D.J.; Powers, J.P.; Ertl, L.S.; Baumgart, T.; Wang, Y.; Seitz, L.C.; Penfold, M.E.; Gan, L.; Hu, P.; et al. C5a Receptor (CD88) Blockade Protects against MPO-ANCA GN. *J. Am. Soc. Nephrol.* **2014**, *25*, 225–231. [CrossRef] [PubMed]
101. Zhang, K.; Li, G.-Q.; He, Q.-H.; Li, Y.; Tang, M.; Zheng, Q.-Y.; Xu, G.-L.; Zhang, K.-Q. C5a/C5aR pathway accelerates renal ischemia-reperfusion injury by downregulating PGRN expression. *Int. Immunopharmacol.* **2017**, *53*, 17–23. [CrossRef]
102. Peng, Q.; Li, G.-Q.; He, Q.-H.; Li, Y.; Tang, M.; Zheng, Q.-Y.; Xu, G.-L.; Zhang, K.-Q. The C5a/C5aR1 axis promotes progression of renal tubulointerstitial fibrosis in a mouse model of renal ischemia/reperfusion injury. *Kidney Int.* **2019**, *96*, 117–128. [CrossRef]
103. Levien, T.L.; Baker, D.E. Avacopan. *Hosp. Pharm.* **2023**, *58*, 134–142. [CrossRef]
104. Dunlap, C.; Zhao, N.; Ertl, L.S.; Schall, T.J.; Sullivan, K.M.C. C5aR expression in kidney tubules, macrophages and fibrosis. *J. Histotechnol.* **2024**, *11*, 1–19. [CrossRef]
105. Buelli, S.; Imberti, B.; Morigi, M. The Complement C3a and C5a Signaling in Renal Diseases: A Bridge between Acute and Chronic Inflammation. *Nephron* **2024**, *148*, 712–723. [CrossRef] [PubMed]

106. Ashraf, A.; Liaquat, A.; Shabbir, S.; Bokhari, S.A.; Tariq, Z.; Furrukh, Z.; Raja, A.A.; Khan, M.J. High level of lactate dehydrogenase and ischaemia–reperfusion injury regulate the multiple organ dysfunction in patients with COVID-19. *Postgrad. Med. J.* **2023**, *99*, 576–581. [CrossRef]
107. Bongoni, A.K.; Vikstrom, I.B.; McRae, J.L.; Salvaris, E.J.; Fisicaro, N.; Pearse, M.J.; Wymann, S.; Rowe, T.; Morelli, A.B.; Hardy, M.P.; et al. A potent truncated form of human soluble CR1 is protective in a mouse model of renal ischemia–reperfusion injury. *Sci. Rep.* **2021**, *11*, 21873. [CrossRef]
108. Kassimatis, T.; Greenlaw, R.; Hunter, J.P.; Douiri, A.; Flach, C.; Rebollo-Mesa, I.; Nichols, L.L.; Qasem, A.; Danzi, G.; Olsburgh, J.; et al. Ex vivo delivery of Mirocecept: A dose-finding study in pig kidney after showing a low dose is insufficient to reduce delayed graft function in human kidney. *Am. J. Transplant.* **2021**, *21*, 1012–1026. [CrossRef] [PubMed]
109. Praska, C.E.; Tamburrini, R.; Danobeitia, J.S. Innate immune modulation in transplantation: Mechanisms, challenges, and opportunities. *Front. Transplant.* **2023**, *2*, 1277669. [CrossRef]
110. Castellano, G.; Melchiorre, R.; Loverre, A.; Ditonno, P.; Montinaro, V.; Rossini, M.; Divella, C.; Battaglia, M.; Lucarelli, G.; Annunziata, G.; et al. Therapeutic Targeting of Classical and Lectin Pathways of Complement Protects from Ischemia-Reperfusion-Induced Renal Damage. *Am. J. Pathol.* **2010**, *176*, 1648–1659. [CrossRef]
111. Danobeitia, J.S.; Ziemelis, M.; Ma, X.; Zitur, L.J.; Zens, T.; Chlebeck, P.J.; Van Amersfoort, E.S.; Fernandez, L.A. Complement inhibition attenuates acute kidney injury after ischemia-reperfusion and limits progression to renal fibrosis in mice. *PLoS ONE* **2017**, *12*, e0183701. [CrossRef]
112. Ponticelli, C.; Reggiani, F.; Moroni, G. Delayed Graft Function in Kidney Transplant: Risk Factors, Consequences and Prevention Strategies. *J. Pers. Med.* **2022**, *12*, 1557. [CrossRef]
113. Jordan, S.C.; Choi, J.; Aubert, O.; Haas, M.; Loupy, A.; Huang, E.; Peng, A.; Kim, I.; Louie, S.; Ammerman, N.; et al. A phase I/II, double-blind, placebo-controlled study assessing safety and efficacy of C1 esterase inhibitor for prevention of delayed graft function in deceased donor kidney transplant recipients. *Am. J. Transplant.* **2018**, *18*, 2955–2964. [CrossRef]
114. Renner, B.; Laskowski, J.; Poppelaars, F.; Ferreira, V.P.; Blaine, J.; Antonioli, A.H.; Hannan, J.P.; Kovacs, J.M.; van Kooten, C.; You, Z.; et al. Factor H related proteins modulate complement activation on kidney cells. *Kidney Int.* **2022**, *102*, 1331–1344. [CrossRef]
115. Goetz, L.; Laskowski, J.; Renner, B.; Pickering, M.C.; Kulik, L.; Klawitter, J.; Stites, E.; Christians, U.; van der Vlag, J.; Ravichandran, K.; et al. Complement factor H protects mice from ischemic acute kidney injury but is not critical for controlling complement activation by glomerular IgM. *Eur. J. Immunol.* **2018**, *48*, 791–802. [CrossRef]
116. Schnabolk, G.; Parsons, N.; Obert, E.; Annamalai, B.; Nasarre, C.; Tomlinson, S.; Lewin, A.S.; Rohrer, B. Delivery of CR2-fH Using AAV Vector Therapy as Treatment Strategy in the Mouse Model of Choroidal Neovascularization. *Mol. Ther. Methods Clin. Dev.* **2018**, *9*, 1–11. [CrossRef]
117. Dudler, T.; Yaseen, S.; Cummings, W.J. Development and characterization of narsoplimab, a selective MASP-2 inhibitor, for the treatment of lectin-pathway–mediated disorders. *Front. Immunol.* **2023**, *14*, 1297352. [CrossRef]
118. Lee, J.W.; Brodsky, R.A.; Nishimura, J.-I.; Kulasekararaj, A.G. The role of the alternative pathway in paroxysmal nocturnal hemoglobinuria and emerging treatments. *Expert. Rev. Clin. Pharmacol.* **2022**, *15*, 851–861. [CrossRef]
119. Ito, S.; Chetlapalli, K.; Wang, D.; Potnis, K.C.; Richmond, R.; Krumholz, H.; Lee, A.I.; Cuker, A.; Goshua, G. Cost-effectiveness of iptacopan for paroxysmal nocturnal hemoglobinuria. *Blood J.* **2024**, *145*, 127–140. [CrossRef]
120. Jager, N.M.; van Zanden, J.E.; Subías, M.; Leuvenink, H.G.D.; Daha, M.R.; de Córdoba, S.R.; Poppelaars, F.; Seelen, M.A. Blocking Complement Factor B Activation Reduces Renal Injury and Inflammation in a Rat Brain Death Model. *Front. Immunol.* **2019**, *10*, 2528. [CrossRef]
121. Amura, C.R.; Renner, B.; Lyubchenko, T.; Faubel, S.; Simonian, P.L.; Thurman, J.M. Complement activation and toll-like receptor-2 signaling contribute to cytokine production after renal ischemia/reperfusion. *Mol. Immunol.* **2012**, *52*, 249–257. [CrossRef] [PubMed]
122. Stahl, G.L.; Xu, Y.; Hao, L.; Miller, M.; Buras, J.A.; Fung, M.; Zhao, H. Role for the Alternative Complement Pathway in Ischemia/Reperfusion Injury. *Am. J. Pathol.* **2003**, *162*, 449–455. [CrossRef] [PubMed]
123. Miwa, T.; Sato, S.; Golla, M.; Song, W.-C. Expansion of Anticomplement Therapy Indications from Rare Genetic Disorders to Common Kidney Diseases. *Annu. Rev. Med.* **2024**, *75*, 189–204. [CrossRef]
124. Risitano, A.M.; Kulasekararaj, A.G.; Lee, J.W.; Maciejewski, J.P.; Notaro, R.; Brodsky, R.; Huang, M.; Geffner, M.; Browett, P. Danicopan: An oral complement factor D inhibitor for paroxysmal nocturnal hemoglobinuria. *Haematologica* **2020**, *106*, 3188–3197. [CrossRef]

125. Browett, P.J.; Kulasekararaj, A.; Notaro, R.; Ogawa, M.; Risitano, A.; Yu, J.; Lee, J.W. Vemircopan (ALXN2050) Monotherapy in Paroxysmal Nocturnal Hemoglobinuria: Interim Data from a Phase 2 Open-Label Proof-of-Concept Study. *Blood* **2022**, *140*, 717–719. [CrossRef]
126. Anwar, I.J.; DeLaura, I.; Ladowski, J.; Gao, Q.; Knechtle, S.J.; Kwun, J. Complement-targeted therapies in kidney transplantation—Insights from preclinical studies. *Front. Immunol.* **2022**, *13*, 984090. [CrossRef]

MDPI AG
Grosspeteranlage 5
4052 Basel
Switzerland
Tel.: +41 61 683 77 34

Antioxidants Editorial Office
E-mail: antioxidants@mdpi.com
www.mdpi.com/journal/antioxidants

www.ingramcontent.com/pod-product-compliance
Lightning Source LLC
Chambersburg PA
CBHW061509210926
51850CB00008B/1865